Welfare rights and social policy

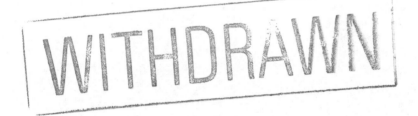

Welfare rights and social policy

Hartley Dean
University of Luton

An imprint of **Pearson Education**

Harlow, England · London · New York · Reading, Massachusetts · San Francisco · Toronto · Don Mills, Ontario · Sydney
Tokyo · Singapore · Hong Kong · Seoul · Taipei · Cape Town · Madrid · Mexico City · Amsterdam · Munich · Paris · Milan

Pearson Education Limited
Edinburgh Gate
Harlow
Essex CM20 2JE

and Associated Companies throughout the world

Visit us on the World Wide Web at:
www.pearsoneduc.com

First published 2002

© Pearson Education Limited 2002

ISBN 0130 404624

British Library Cataloguing-in-Publication Data
A catalogue record for this book is available from the British Library

10 9 8 7 6 5 4 3 2 1
08 07 06 05 04 03 02

Typeset in 11/12pt Adobe Garamond by 35
Printed in Great Britain by Henry Ling Ltd., at the Dorset Press, Dorchester, Dorset

To my mother and father

Contents

PART II *Welfare rights in practice*

PART III *Rethinking welfare rights*

List of illustrations

Acknowledgements

A number of people have contributed to the writing of this book. In so far that the book is substantially constructed on the template provided by *Welfare, Law and Citizenship*, I remain indebted to Vic George, who initially suggested the idea to me. Mike Adler's critical comments on *Welfare, Law and Citizenship* helped to inform certain of the changes I have made and his advice has been helpful. Additionally, several of my present or erstwhile colleagues – Caron Caldwell, Shane Doheny, Tony Fitzpatrick, Kathryn Ellis, Virginia MacNeill, Margaret Melrose and Ruth Rogers – similarly read and offered either encouragement or constructive comments on various draft chapters. In her capacity as a practising welfare lawyer, my daughter, Nicola Dean, provided some valuable commentary on the draft of one of the chapters. And in her capacity as my life-partner and collaborator, Pam Dean provided invaluable assistance with manuscript proof-reading and the checking of references. I am extremely grateful to them all, but responsibility for the deficiencies that remain in the pages that follow and for the interpretation that I bring to the subject matter is mine and mine alone.

We are grateful to the following for permission to reproduce copyright material:

Table 3.1 from *The Human Development Report 2000*, published by Oxford University Press (United Nations Development Project, 2000); Table 3.2 adapted from *Social Foundations of Postindustrial Economics* by Gøsta Esping-Anderson (1999) by permission of Oxford University Press, © G. Esping-Anderson, 1999.

Whilst every effort has been made to trace the owners of copyright material, in a few cases this has proved impossible and we would be grateful to hear from anyone with information which would enable us to do so.

Introduction

Rationale

This book is intended to provide an introduction to social policy through a critical discussion of welfare rights. Its purpose is to explore welfare rights and the social legislation that gives rise to them in an historical, comparative and critical context and to engage the reader, through the contested concept of 'rights', with the central questions of principle that underpin the basis of social citizenship and the welfare state.

It is a book that sets out to make connections between theory and practice, and between debate and reality. Although a single volume could not hope satisfactorily to bridge the gap, this book may at least partially heal the rift that exists between conventional academic social policy texts on the one hand, and the kind of rights guides and handbooks that are used by welfare rights practitioners on the other. The former characteristically engage with theoretical debates concerning principles of welfare citizenship without articulating this with the substantive realities of social legislation: as a result students and academics seldom have any real grasp of the practical limitations of welfare rights. The latter engage with the technical detail of prevailing social legislation without articulating this with underlying principles and theoretical debates: as a result, practitioners often function with a limited perspective upon the issues with which they contend.

The book is not so much a second edition as a successor to the author's earlier book, *Welfare Law and Citizenship* (published in 1996 by Prentice Hall/Harvester Wheatsheaf). Some of the material from that book has been retained and either developed or updated, but this volume covers a wider range of issues; it addresses new political discourses and emerging theoretical debates concerning the relationship between rights and responsibility; and it discusses the relevance of welfare rights in processes of reform and resistance.

Structure

The book is in three parts.

Part I focuses on conceptual debates concerning the relationship between welfare rights and social citizenship (Chapter 1), the significance of debates about poverty and need for differing conceptions of welfare rights (Chapter

2), the global context for the development of welfare rights (Chapter 3), and critiques of welfare rights and their consequences (Chapter 4).

Part II addresses the practical realities of welfare rights. It focuses on rights to subsistence (Chapter 5), work (Chapter 6), shelter (Chapter 7) and, more briefly, on rights to education, health and social care (Chapter 8). Chapter 9 discusses rights of redress in relation to welfare. This by no means exhausts the arena of welfare rights. Rights to welfare – or, more literally, to well-being – may be held to extend to the right to such basic infrastructural needs as a clean water supply and sanitation, or the right to physical security and freedom from fear. There are special rights to welfare that apply, for example, to children as opposed to adults and to migrants or refugees. Consumer protection rights, though they are not usually thought of as social rights, can be necessary to protect human welfare. Even if this author were competent to address such a wide range of issues, time and the limited space available within this book do not permit him satisfactorily to encompass a discussion of all the rights that might legitimately be defined as welfare rights. Although it may seem relatively arbitrary, I shall confine my attention primarily to adult rights and to those rights that flow from social legislation or that are defined through the institutions that constitute the welfare state.

Additionally, Part II focuses by and large on the situation in England and Wales and it cannot necessarily be assumed that the provisions described will affect other parts of the UK in exactly the same way. Scotland in particular has its own distinctive legal system and the powers devolved to the Scottish Parliament are significantly greater than those presently conferred on the Welsh Assembly, resulting in distinctively different legislation in certain 'non-reserved' areas of social policy. For a variety of reasons, current arrangements in Northern Ireland can also differ in certain quite significant ways from those in England and Wales. Once again, the competence of the author and the size of the book have significantly limited what can be presented here. Given that the process of devolution will probably go yet further, it will in time become necessary to bear in mind the policy nuances and differences of detail that characterise Wales and possibly even the different English regions. The greater diversity that is only beginning to emerge is undoubtedly to be welcomed, although it presents a challenge to the writers of texts such as this. To an important extent the material in Part II is intended to be illustrative: narrowing the focus has reduced the complexity and, I hope, made it easier for the reader – including readers from other countries within the UK and indeed from around the world – to establish connections between a specific account of a particular welfare rights regime and the more general arguments that I develop in Parts I and III.

The final thing to be said in advance about Part II is that, such is the ferocious pace of change (or 'reform') in social policy at present, parts of it may well be out of date before this book even appears in print. I have attempted none the less to focus on the basic underlying frameworks and principles that inform current policy and, wherever possible, to anticipate forthcoming developments. I deliberately do not explain current welfare entitlements in highly specific detail: such detail can after all be obtained from the kind of handbooks I refer to above. The account I give should, I believe, remain essentially relevant for some time to come.

Part III returns to more theoretical concerns and, specifically, a discussion of contemporary discourses of citizenship, rights and responsibility (Chapter 10) and of alternative strategies of reform and resistance (Chapter 11). Readers who are familiar with this author's more recent work may be aware that I have lately been exploring conceptual taxonomies or models around the notions of rights and citizenship. My hope is that in Part III I have brought that project to some kind of fruition. I am conscious that the models I present in Part III differ in some respects from previous offerings and it may be worth my briefly mentioning two reasons for this. First, in my previous work I fear I had become overly preoccupied with distinctions between what might loosely be called progressive discourses (rational, reflexive, egalitarian, etc.) as opposed to conservative discourses (traditional, mythologising, elitist, etc.), whereas here I shall supersede those distinctions with a more overarching distinction between systemic and agential discourses. It is a distinction that owes more than a little to Habermas's distinction between 'system' and 'life-world'. One consequence of this is that I think it becomes easier, for example, to locate internally contradictory doctrines like Benthamite utilitarianism and Fabian welfarism in relation not to liberal individualism or reformist socialism, but to their moral authoritarian implications in the sphere in which they function. Second, I am aware that my earlier attempts to engage with the systemic–agential distinction have been in some respects deficient, not least because it is not until now that I have articulated the distinction with an analysis of reformist and resistance strategies. Part III in fact draws together a number of ideas that I have already disseminated elsewhere, but I trust that I may this time have presented them in a more coherent and convincing way. Writing textbooks provides an opportunity not only to anthologise, but to reframe, correct and refine one's recent work.

The central argument

The cause of human rights is high on the global political agenda. But the status of welfare rights as an element of human rights remains curiously ambiguous. Welfare rights are a characteristic feature of welfare capitalist society and, in spite of recent cutbacks, an elaborate framework of welfare rights remains in place in countries such as Britain. Rights to social security, employment, housing, education, health and social care are critical to human well-being, but the nature of such rights can be problematic: they are invariably subordinate to the civil and political rights of citizenship, they are often fragile and difficult to enforce, and because of their conditional nature they are usually implicated in processes for the social control of individual behaviour.

The book develops a theoretical framework for understanding the different ways in which welfare rights are ideologically constructed and the different ways in which the bearers of such rights are socially constituted. Rights can be founded in doctrines that are imposed from above or upon claims that are demanded from below. Rights may flow from quite different conceptions of citizenship: from a conception that regards the relationship between the individual and the state as a form of contract, or from a conception that regards the state as the guarantor of social solidarity. Different welfare state regimes reflect different understandings of rights and different understandings of the responsibilities associated with rights. Britain's New Labour government, while it insists that rights and responsibilities go together, is seeking to enforce forms of duty, obligation and obedience while failing to engage with a reflexively ethical notion of responsibility.

Welfare rights may provide a necessary tool for social reform or a valuable weapon for social resistance. Once again, however, the nature of the rights that might be developed depend on the kind of welfare state to which we aspire. The book concludes by tentatively exploring the basis for an ethical state that properly recognises the nature of human interdependency; that regulates society so as to respond to human needs; that makes welfare rights the basis for social policy.

Part I

Welfare rights in theory

Chapter 1

The social rights of citizenship

The term 'welfare rights' is subject to a variety of interpretations. Sometimes it is used rather specifically to refer to specialised individual entitlements created by domestic social legislation, particularly those relating to social security or cash benefits. Sometimes it is used to refer to the arena of professional practice in which welfare rights specialists, advice workers and welfare lawyers engage. Sometimes it is used more generally to refer to the level of social protection that is, or that perhaps ought to be, guaranteed to the citizens of a 'welfare state'. This book is concerned with all senses of the term, including its practical and conceptual connotations.

In this chapter I am starting at the conceptual level with a discussion of what are generally defined as the social rights of citizenship. In the British context the terms welfare rights and social rights may for most purposes be coterminous, but social rights is a less parochial term than welfare rights. It is a term that I shall use here to apply as much to people's right to social participation as their right to receive socially provided services. It is concerned with a species of right that is not necessarily specific to the welfare states of the developed world and it is a term that helps us to conceptualise our own welfare rights in relation both to other kinds of rights and to the broader concept of citizenship (to which I shall return in Chapter 10).

Rights are central to social policy not only because they relate to the substantive entitlements to which the policy making process gives rise, but because they provide the basis of the rhetorical claims which drive debates and struggles over welfare. Lawyers characteristically define the first kind of rights as 'positive' or 'black-letter' rights and the latter as 'moral' rights. In social policy we usually recognise that both kinds of rights are in fact socially or ideologically constituted and later in this chapter I shall say something about the complex ways in which these two kinds of right relate to and feed off each other. I shall also say something about the extent to which provision for welfare is a matter of social rights, as opposed to private consumption.

First, however, I plan to discuss the way in which the concept of social rights has emerged as a defining feature of welfare capitalism.

The amelioration of class

Social rights, according to the sociologist T.H. Marshall (1950), were the unique achievement of the twentieth century. In Britain the struggle to achieve civil rights (i.e. civil liberties, property and legal rights) had by and large succeeded by the eighteenth century and the struggle to achieve political rights (i.e. voting and democratic rights) took major strides in the nineteenth century. The establishment of social rights – that is entitlement to basic standards of education, health and social care, housing and income maintenance – was completed with the formation of the 'modern' welfare state after the end of the Second World War. Marshall may be accused of over-generalisation, particularly in his broad-brush characterisation of different historical periods, but this ought not to obscure the importance of his argument. His contentions were, first, that social inequalities based on class divisions have been ameliorated through the development of citizenship and, second, that full citizenship requires three components – not just civil and political rights, but social rights as well.

Towards a classless society?

The first of these points finds favour in the writings of many commentators and supporters of the welfare state, especially those on the Fabian left (see George and Wilding 1985). However, T.H. Marshall's use of the term 'amelioration' had in fact been directly drawn from the works of the nineteenth-century economist Alfred Marshall. It was in a series of lectures in memory of Alfred Marshall that T.H. Marshall advanced the proposition that the welfare state as founded by the post-war Labour government represented the 'latest phase in an evolution of citizenship which has been in continuous progress for some 250 years' (1950: 7). In so doing, he claimed he was addressing a question raised by his erstwhile namesake some 70 years before, namely 'whether . . . the amelioration of the working classes has limits beyond which it cannot pass . . . [or] whether progress may not go on steadily, if slowly, till by occupation at least, every man is a gentleman' (Marshall 1873, cited in Marshall 1950: 4–5).

Marshall the nineteenth-century economist was no egalitarian (least of all so far as women were concerned). The equality he foresaw was an equality of opportunities and lifestyle rather than a material equality of incomes or wealth. Technological advances, he believed, would ameliorate the arduous nature of manual labour, while compulsory elementary education would civilise the manners of the working classes. Marshall the twentieth-century sociologist similarly believed that 'equality of status is more important than equality of income' (1950: 33). The development of a range of social services and cash benefits financed through taxation clearly did involve an equalisation of incomes, but this was not its only or even its primary achievement:

> What matters is that there is a general enrichment of the concrete substance of civilised life, a general reduction of risk and insecurity, an equalisation between the more and the less fortunate at all levels – between the healthy and the sick, the

employed and the unemployed, the old and the active, the bachelor and the father of a large family. Equalisation is not so much between classes as between individuals within a population which is now treated for this purpose as though it were one class. (*ibid.*)

The argument then is that social rights abolish class differences (gender differences were not considered). Academic commentators in the Fabian tradition, such as Titmuss (1958; 1968), argued that the development and maintenance of state welfare provision constituted a moral imperative in so far that it represented the peaceful means of mitigating the unacceptable consequences of class inequality; social rights were a civilising force which compensated for the diswelfares of the capitalist system. Other Fabians, such as the Labour politician Tony Crosland (1956), went so far as to argue that the development of social legislation and the rise of labour and trade union power had together shifted the balance so far against the capitalist class system as to promise the imminent realisation of a democratic form of socialism.

It is important, however, to grasp the extent to which T.H. Marshall's concept of citizenship was not necessarily consistent with socialist pretensions. Marshall saw citizenship, particularly through the effects of a truly meritocratic state education system, as an alternative instrument of social stratification (1950: 39). Certainly, he believed the emergence of social rights signalled the extent to which *laissez faire* capitalism had been superseded. But the result would be a society based on status and desert, rather than contract and mere good fortune: 'Social rights in their modern form imply an invasion of contract by status, the subordination of market price to social justice, the replacement of the free bargain by the declaration of rights' (*ibid.*: 40). Ironically, shorn of any commitment to economic equality, this view of social rights can be rendered consistent with a form of one-nation Toryism and the kind of call for a 'classless society' which the Conservative British Prime Minister John Major made following his 1992 General Election victory (*The Guardian*, 10.4.92).

We do not of course live in a classless society. None the less, the class structure of Britain has changed since the creation of the 'modern' welfare state, although this has been driven by changes in the nature of capitalism, rather than by any influence of the welfare state (see Bottomore 1992; Marshall 1997). The fault line in Britain's occupational structure now lies, not so much between a manual working class and a non-manual middle class, as between secure, highly trained, well-paid 'core' workers and vulnerable, low skilled, poorly paid 'peripheral' workers. What is more, since the late 1970s the growth of the welfare state has been curtailed and the extent of social and economic inequality in Britain has worsened (see Glennerster and Hills 1998; Gordon *et al.* 2000). One economic commentator has recently argued that Britain now constitutes a '30:30:40 society' in which, though 40 per cent of the population are relatively privileged in material terms, 30 per cent are chronically insecure and 30 per cent are systematically disadvantaged (Hutton 1996). I shall examine the implications of such issues – not least for social stability – in Chapter 2.

The 'hyphenated' society

For the moment, however, I shall return to the second limb of T.H. Marshall's argument, which was that civil, political and social rights are all necessary to full citizenship. Marshall recognised the sense in which citizenship based on a broad equality of rights was potentially in conflict with the workings of a capitalist market economy. In later writings, however, he stressed that full citizenship need not inhibit a market economy, provided a state of equilibrium can be sustained between political, social and civil rights in what he characterised as the 'hyphenated' society, *democratic-welfare-capitalism*. The hyphens in this formulation symbolise the interconnectedness of a democratic polity, a welfare state and a mixed economy, all functioning in harmony (1981). The maintenance of a flourishing 'hyphenated' society is therefore a matter of achieving the right balance between the three constituent components of citizenship. These components are like the legs of a three-legged stool: just as the stability of the stool depends upon the strength of each of the legs on which it stands, so the stability of society depends upon the strength of each of the three dimensions to citizenship.

Upon this premise, if too much emphasis is being placed in Britain, for example, on our rights as producers and consumers and not enough upon our rights to guaranteed living standards and social provision, this creates an imbalance between the civil and social aspects of citizenship, which in turn poses a potential threat to social stability. Similarly, the social upheavals that followed the collapse of communism in the former Soviet Union and Eastern Europe might be regarded as a consequence of violent shifts in the equilibrium of citizenship. Under former Stalinist regimes, social rights had been guaranteed, while civil and political rights were either suppressed or neglected, but now political rights have been promoted at the expense of social rights and without an adequate framework of civil rights (see, for example, Bottomore 1992).

Marshall's sociological model of citizenship clearly has its applications and attractions. It may be criticised, however, first for 'state-market essentialism' and, second, for its inherent functionalism.

The charge of state-market essentialism is levelled by Barry Hindess (1987) who complains that Marshall's model in fact assumes an overly simplistic conception of the antagonism between the state and the market. Hindess points out that there are aspects of capitalist market relations that are in tune with equal citizenship and aspects of state welfare systems that are not. As we shall see later, not all the changes to welfare systems that have been occurring since the 1970s in countries such as Britain have diminished the social rights of citizenship. Though there are obvious limitations, it is possible for the market as well as the state to contribute to the realisation of social rights. And as we shall see in Chapter 10, citizenship is a far more multi-faceted concept than that employed by Marshall and is as capable of accommodating itself as much to individualism and the needs of the market as to collectivism and the ambitions of the state.

Marshall's functionalism is evident in his treatment of social class. Although he examines the effects of social citizenship on social class, as Bottomore (1992) points out, Marshall fails to account for the impact that social classes have had on the development of citizenship. The development of civil rights and the beginnings of political rights resulted from the struggles of an emerging capitalist class to wrest power from the feudal aristocracy. The more recent development of political rights and aspects of the beginnings of social rights owed much to the struggles of working-class organisations – the Chartists, the trade unions, socialist and social democratic parties. Marshall expresses the conflicts from which citizenship has emerged in terms of clashes between opposing principles rather than between opposing classes. The development and maintenance of welfare states has been analysed by other commentators (e.g. Korpi 1983; Offe 1984; Esping-Andersen 1990) with reference to the influence of corporatism (the effect of which is more relevant in some European countries than in others). Corporatism, in this context, is a process of tri-partite negotiation between the representatives of business, workers and the government. What is often involved in the development of social rights is not an impersonally established equilibrium between formal principles, but a directly negotiated compromise between substantive class interests.

There are, as we shall see, two very different ways of looking at rights: they may be regarded as being founded on abstract or constitutional doctrines (as things that human beings are born with) or as arising from claims or demands established in the process of daily life and political struggle (as things that human society fashions for itself).

The origins of rights

The distinction I have just drawn between what might be called 'claims-based' and 'doctrinal' rights is an attempt to answer the question – where, then, do rights come from? However, it is not a straightforward distinction, because it is intended to capture two sets of overlapping conceptual distinctions: one legal and one historical. It is also bound up with competing notions of property rights on the one hand and human rights on the other.

Jurisprudential debates

I mentioned earlier the distinction that lawyers make between moral rights and 'black-letter' rights (rights that are written down and legally enforceable). The utilitarian philosopher Jeremy Bentham (1789) brutally dismissed as 'nonsense on stilts' the very idea that there can be basic moral or 'natural' rights that somehow inhere in the individual subject: what matters, he asserted, are the laws by which we might ensure the greatest good of the greatest number. However, more recent philosophers of law have sought to distinguish two underlying theories of rights: the *will* or *choice* theory and the *interest* or *benefit* theory (see, for example, Jones 1994; Campbell 1988: ch. 2; Spicker 1988: ch. V). The former is based on the idea that every human individual with free will must necessarily have some power to exercise choice and therefore to control or in certain ways limit the behaviour of other individuals. The latter is based on the idea that rights are created by rules that benefit the human individual by imposing obligations upon other individuals to protect or further her interests. The problem is that neither theory can quite account both for the material substance of our rights (the things they actually achieve) *and* for their procedural form (the way they have been set up).

A celebrated attempt to do this has been made by Ronald Dworkin (1977), who attempts to make a different kind of distinction, between concrete *institutional* rights – that are policy or goal directed and may impose certain kinds of duties on people or on government – and abstract *background* rights that embody the fundamental principles that justify political and judicial decision making. The morality that underpins Dworkin's background rights is not the supposedly 'natural' morality dismissed by Bentham, but a constructed morality based on reflexive notions of social justice (cf. Rawls 1972). None the less, how exactly do we get to the principles that inform Dworkin's background rights? The answer, MacCormick (1982: 137) suggests, is that 'to some extent we find them, and to some extent we make them'. In other words, we are forced back to the same basic distinction between the kind of rights that people might debate or assert for themselves and the kind of rights that in the name of some doctrine – whether it be secular or religious, radical or conservative in nature – are prescribed for them.

Historical evolution

The distinction must also, however, be placed in an historical context. What might once have been devised and asserted as claims-based rights, can assume the character of doctrinal rights that are defended not as rational constitutional measures or public policies, but as eternal moral verities. Conversely, morally informed demands for claims-based rights may call upon the language of constitutional or policy doctrines in order to establish themselves. The two kinds of rights exist in a fluid or 'dialectical' relationship to each other. The form of rights in 'hyphenated' democratic-welfare-capitalist societies is inescapably bound up with attempts dating from the seventeenth and eighteenth centuries to establish, first, the inalienability (or 'freedom') of property and, second, the formal separation of civil society (and in particular the economy) from the state (the political process). The modern concept of rights dates from this period when the moral claims of the Enlightenment finally displaced the doctrinal orthodoxies of the mediaeval era.

In feudal society there were no rights other than the divine right to govern which was supposedly bestowed upon the sovereign and, by delegation from the Crown, to the nobility. To the extent that there were paternalistic duties of *noblesse oblige* attaching to such rights, then privileges or customary gratuities might be conferred upon the common people (Kamenka and Tay 1975), but they enjoyed no rights in the modern sense. Though hailed for having prefigured a modern universalistic concept of rights, England's *Magna Carta* of 1215 amounted to no more than an exclusive concession of restricted liberties by the Crown to the nobility and it was not until the Petition of Right of 1628 that the process that would lead to the modern concept began to unfold (Perry 1964). The doctrines of 'natural' law on which feudal beliefs were founded were fundamentally conservative. They provided for a society that was organic, customary and hierarchical and were fundamentally inimical to the development of the forms of property ownership and market relations upon which the emergence of modern capitalism were to depend. Belief in natural law had therefore to be replaced over time by liberal beliefs in 'man-made' laws and the 'Rights of Man'. (Women, it should be noted, had little or no legal status at that time and, as we shall see in Chapter 4, can still be systematically disadvantaged before the law.)

In, for example, the philosophical writings of Locke (1690) and the political writings of Paine (1791) we see reflected a moral discourse by which 'natural' rights were first re-cast as inalienable individual rights to 'life, liberty and estate (property)' and then exchanged, as it were, to become civil rights under doctrines of liberal governance (see, for example, Goodwin 1987: ch. 11; Raphael 1989). This in essence was the discourse of rights that had informed the English Bill of Rights (1689) and a century later the American Declaration of Independence (1776), the USA Constitution (1787) and the French Declaration of Rights (1789), albeit that the impact and substantive historical relevance of these various documents were to differ rather significantly. In spite of those differences, it was not so much the claims of ordinary people that were ascendant over governments, as the interests of emerging middle classes over those of the old aristocracies. In the British case the middle classes succeeded by the nineteenth century in achieving a political ascendancy to match the advantages they had secured through the development of civil liberties and property rights.

Property rights and working-class interests

As Bob Fine has argued, the doctrines of classical jurisprudence that laid the foundations for the new 'man-made' constitutional settlement were inseparable from the doctrines of political economy. The ultimate objective was 'that of creating a synthesis between individual freedom and collective authority' (Fine 1984: 65). More particularly, liberal governance provided the right to private property and public order. The political economist Adam Smith, best known for his notion that human affairs may be governed through the 'invisible hand' of free market forces and his insistence that government should not encroach on the liberties of the property owning subject, was none the less quite clear about government's role in relation to the four 'great objects' of law, namely police, justice, revenue and arms. Smith was using the word 'police' in its archaic sense, referring not to a body of officers responsible for the maintenance of law and order (a comparatively recent invention), but to the general regulation of good order and mannerly or 'polite' conduct; to the liberal 'science' of population management (e.g. Osborne 1996). He urged that 'some attention of government is necessary in order to prevent the almost entire corruption and degeneracy of the great body of the people' (1776: 613).

To this end Smith advocated elementary state education not as a right of the poor, but as protection for the property owning classes.

Hegel's jurisprudential theory went further in advocating that 'police' within a liberal state required the provision of welfare for the poor and public health care, as well as education and public works (see Fine 1984: 59). Hegel's contribution to classical jurisprudence is significant, not only because it provided the starting point for Marxist critiques (to which I shall return in Chapter 4) but because it provided the starkest expression of the form of law and of 'rights' under liberal governance: 'Right is . . . the immediate embodiment which freedom gives itself as an immediate way, i.e. possession which is property ownership' (Hegel 1821, cited in Fine 1984: 57). In other words, the origin of rights is ownership. Rights and equality before the law are universal only in the formal and abstract sense that in an ordered (capitalist) society everybody has to relate to and respect everybody else as *proprietors*. Even people without land or goods at their disposal may 'own' (and therefore sell) their labour power.

More recent theorists have suggested that welfare rights are, or ought to be, directly analogous to property rights, and that 'government largesse' (such as welfare benefits, subsidies, grants, education, etc.) constitute a kind of property that may be subject to the same legal rules and categories as other property forms (Reich 1964). This is one way of looking at welfare rights: as an expression in legal form of the logic of individual ownership. In the case of many recipients of state welfare, this logically driven formulation may seem bizarre. Many 'clients' of the welfare state are ostensibly propertyless and their 'rights', for example to means-tested social security benefits, are governed specifically by legislation (see Chapter 5). None the less, such benefits – provided all the conditions of eligibility are met – are available as an entitlement rather than as a gift, and the principles that give rise to that entitlement are supposed to operate with indifference to the personality and status of the recipient. They are rights within the liberal definition of the rule of law, but this makes them appear as products of a doctrinal fiction, rather than a politically determined reality.

In contrast, working-class agitation for the development of social rights has generally appealed to morally or ontologically founded convictions (albeit with rhetoric that often acknowledges the hegemony of property and market relations). For example, the opposition of the Owenites and Chartists to the Poor Law Amendment Act of 1834 was founded on the romantically conceived 'birth rights' of free Englishmen, that is to say

> the right to have a living out of the land of our birth in exchange for labour duly and honestly performed; the right in case we fell into distress, to have our wants sufficiently relieved out of the produce of the land, whether that distress arose from sickness, from decrepitude, from old age, or from inability to find employment.
> (William Cobbett, cited in Thompson 1968: 836)

The contemporary equivalents of such demands are the right to work, the right to a living wage, the right to an adequate income in the event of incapacity, unemployment or retirement and the right to education, health care and affordable housing: claims demanded out of moral conviction, but which can only become substantive rights through processes of negotiation and concession. This is an issue to which I shall return in Chapters 9 and 11, when we consider the role of the contemporary welfare rights movement.

Human rights and human welfare

However, there is a forum in which such rights have achieved doctrinal status of a sort, namely in human rights discourse and in particular the symbolically important United Nations' Universal Declaration of Human Rights (UNDHR) of 1948. Though human rights are often regarded as a class of natural or pre-legal rights, Clarke (1996: 119) points out that 'human' is no less a social and political construct than 'citizen' and, historically speaking, it is a term of more recent provenance. Citizen rights, Clarke contends, provide the model for human rights and not the other way round. Any charter or declaration of rights assumes that its signatory states – whether local, national, supranational – are, or will at least *potentially* be, capable of guaranteeing such rights. Declarations of human rights characteristically contain a mixture of rights that actually exist, in so far that they are universally enforceable, and rights that should exist, but that are not yet universally enforceable (e.g. Bobbio 1996); what Feinberg has called 'manifesto rights' (cited in Campbell 1983: 19). The important feature of the UNDHR for our purposes is that it incorporates not only civil and political rights (to life, liberty, property, equality before the law, privacy, fair trial, religious freedom, free speech and assembly, to participate in government, to political asylum and an absolute right not to be tortured), but also what it refers to as 'economic, social and cultural' rights. What are here referred to as economic and cultural rights might legitimately be encompassed within an expanded concept of 'social' rights and include rights to education, work and even leisure. Most particularly, Article 24 states:

> Everyone has the right to a standard of living adequate for the health and well being of himself and his family, including food, clothing, housing and medical care and necessary social services, and the right to security in the event of unemployment, sickness, disability, widowhood, old age or other lack of livelihood in circumstances beyond his control.

It is commonly supposed that, during the negotiations that led up to the promulgation of the UNDHR, provision for social rights was included only at the insistence of the Soviet bloc and reflected a very different view of what freedom required (Goodwin 1987: 240). In the event, it has to be noted not only that the Soviet bloc nations all abstained when the Declaration was eventually adopted, but also that there were other ideological forces at work. US President Roosevelt (whose widow, Eleanor, went on to be the US delegate to the United Nations General Assembly and was one of the principal architects of the UNDHR) had clearly signalled in an address in 1941 that 'freedom from want' was one of the freedoms to be achieved in any post-war international order and, famously, that 'necessitous men are not free men' (see Eide 1997). Arguably, it is to the doctrine of social liberalism rather than that of socialism that we owe the social rights provisions of the UNDHR. I shall address

critiques of the UNDHR at various points later in the book, but suffice it here
to say that its influence in advancing social rights has been limited. In 1950 the
Council of Europe, drawing upon the UNDHR, adopted its own European
Declaration of Human Rights (though this relates only to civil and political
rights) and in 1961 a separate sister document, the Social Charter (that relates
to economic and social rights). Only the former provided a means of enforcing the rights it created through the European Court of Human Rights and it
is only the former that has recently been directly incorporated into English
law by the Human Rights Act 1998 (and by parallel legislation into the law
of the other nations of the UK (see Wadham and Mountfield 1999)). The
constitutional status of social rights remains at best weak.

Does this in practice matter? Is it possible to advance the cause of social
rights without recourse to constitutional declarations or doctrinal principles?
Such an approach is implied, for example, by Paul Hirst's critique of liberal-
democratic rights (1980). Like Bentham, Hirst rejects the notion that rights
can have any natural or ontological attributes, and argues that rights serve
socially determined policy objectives. The rights that social legislation bestow
do no more than assign or regulate the responsibilities and conduct of persons
appointed to fulfil particular tasks. Rights are no more and no less than specific
capacities, conferred by law. The rights created, for example, by social security
legislation do not relate to any inherent or unconditional claim by the citizen,
but to the precise duties of state departments and officials. These rights merely
define the more or less limited circumstances in which social policy will permit
assistance to be given. Unlike Bentham, Hirst does not seek to establish a
utilitarian regime of social control, but to envisage the basis on which a socialist
society might promote human welfare through self-regulation. His concept of
a right as a specific capacity, rather than as something possessed by a unitary subject or individual, is important since it represents a clear if counterfactual example
of what a more strictly claims-based approach to social rights might entail.

Social rights and 'privatisation'

The final set of preliminary debates that this chapter must address relates to
the distinctive nature of social rights as 'positive' demands for resources, the
implications of providing such resources collectively through public spending,
and recent trends by which the fundamental character of social rights is being
transformed by processes of 'privatisation'.

Social rights as 'positive' rights

The language or 'discourse' of rights, as we have already seen, is shot through
with ambiguities and dichotomies. In addition to the array of overlapping
distinctions discussed above, there is a distinction that is sometimes made
between 'negative' rights, which protect the individual from external interference,
and 'positive' rights, which guarantee state intervention. The distinction between
negative and positive 'liberties' was drawn by Berlin to mark the difference

between a 'right' to forbearance by others, as opposed to 'the freedom which consists in being one's own master' (1967: 149). Here the term 'positive' is being used in a quite different sense to that applied by 'legal positivists', that is the sense we have already discussed in which 'positive' has been used to refer to prescribed or 'black-letter' rights, as opposed to abstract or 'moral' rights. Hohfeld (cited in Weale 1983) identified four kinds of rights: liberties, claims, immunities and powers. Liberties and immunities are what might be called negative rights because they signal a *freedom from* something, whereas claims and powers are positive rights because they signal an *entitlement to* something.

Crudely speaking, negative rights ('freedoms from') have been supported from the political Right, while positive rights ('entitlements to') have more usually been championed on the political Left. This, however, is a generalisation. The entitlements created by positive rights are often subject to conditions. As will be seen in Chapter 4, welfare rights in particular may also be the means of enforcing certain duties of citizenship. Authoritarians and utilitarians of the right may therefore be supportive of positive welfare rights where these are closely tied to the performance of obligations, particularly such private obligations as the duty to work and/or to support dependants (see Roche 1992). Conversely, there are those on the libertarian left who are mistrustful of the conditional nature of positive welfare rights and seek also to emphasise the negative rights of citizens against the welfare state such as the right to 'privacy, dignity and confidentiality' (Esam *et al.* 1985: 38).

The development of the modern welfare state has been achieved through a body of social legislation, which has extended 'positive' rights of citizenship by expanding public services. Whereas civil and political rights primarily entail 'negative' rights (e.g. freedoms of movement and opinion), social rights entail 'positive' rights (i.e. entitlements to welfare provision). Social rights are positive in the sense that they entail the provision of the goods and services required for human welfare. Social rights came on to the agenda when the state began to make provision for the goods and services required for human welfare rather than leaving their provision to the mechanisms of the market: in other words, when certain goods and services were 'de-commodified'. We have seen that, according to T.H. Marshall, social rights developed after the development of the negative rights that secured the legal and economic infrastructure required for a free market economy, in which goods and services, and even land and labour power, can be traded as commodities. However, Marshall has been challenged by the neo-Marxist theorist Claus Offe, who has argued that the development of positive social rights were necessary to the development of capitalism; that 'a supportive network of non-commodified institutions is necessary for an economic system that utilises labour power as if it were a commodity' (1984: 263).

Public welfare and de-commodification

The development of social rights has undoubtedly been messier and more complex than T.H. Marshall suggested and, in order to account for the various ways in which welfare states have emerged, Esping-Andersen has developed the concept of 'de-commodification' not directly to describe the ways in which non-commodified forms of welfare provision have developed, but 'the degree to which individuals, or families, can uphold a socially acceptable standard of living independently of market participation' (1990: 37). I shall return to Esping-Andersen's work in Chapter 3, where I discuss how welfare rights can differ between countries. For now, however, I am concerned to draw out three different ways in which, according to Esping-Andersen, social rights may be understood as a means of de-commodification, or as a response to the process of commodification that characterised the advent of capitalism (cf. Marx 1887; Polanyi 1944). He defines these responses in terms of the classical paradigms of conservatism, liberalism and socialism.

The conservative approach resists commodification because it undermines traditional authority. Characteristically therefore this approach favours 'rights' in a paternalistic sense: the kind of rights which come from imposing obligations on employers to look after their workers; from encouraging corporatist guilds and mutual self-help societies; or from state intervention in a paternal-authoritarian mode (e.g. compulsory national insurance schemes). The liberal approach does not resist commodification and seeks to intervene only to the extent that intervention will assist the commodification process or correct 'market failures'. Characteristically, this approach favours 'rights' of a highly conditional nature (such as strictly means-tested social assistance schemes). The socialist/social democratic approach resists commodification because it is the basis of social alienation and class exploitation. Characteristically, this approach favours 'rights' which are emancipatory; which minimise stigmatising conditions and maximise equality. What Esping-Andersen's analysis seeks to demonstrate is that all welfare state regimes are in fact compromises between these competing notions of what social rights should achieve.

Those critics of the welfare state whom George and Wilding (1985) have aptly characterised as 'anti-collectivists' complain that the degree of state intervention involved and the scale of public services have been at the expense of the 'negative' rights that we discussed above. The freedoms that citizens must enjoy if a market economy is to prosper have been eroded by an interfering state, which stifles initiative (Hayek 1960), and public spending, which crowds out productive investment (Bacon and Eltis 1978). In the late twentieth century this kind of thinking informed the political project of the New Right, whose manifestation in the UK was 'Thatcherism' (Gamble 1988). Like the middle-class utilitarians of the nineteenth century, the Thatcher governments of the 1980s were concerned to promote both a free market *and* a strong state; a project based not on classic liberalism, but a combination of economic liberalism and moral authoritarianism. This involved strengthening the 'negative' rights of businesses (through tax cuts and deregulation), while using the power of the state to control the rights of trade unions, unemployed people and welfare dependants. In practice, the degree of retrenchment suffered by the welfare state was relatively modest (Glennerster and Hills 1998). Of far greater significance was a restructuring of welfare spending and a transition to what is widely termed the 'mixed economy of welfare' or 'welfare pluralism' (see, for example,

Johnson 1987). It is a process that has been furthered in Britain since the election in 1997 of a New Labour government committed to a 'Third Way' (Blair 1998; Giddens 1998). New Labour's approach to social rights belonged, it claimed, neither to the New Right nor to the socialist/social democratic traditions of the past and has embraced the compromise that welfare pluralism represents, entailing as it does elements of a tendency that Offe had predicted and termed 'administrative recommodification' (1984: 124).

Welfare pluralism

In the process of the shift to welfare pluralism, welfare rights have also been restructured, or at least a different dimension has been introduced to the social rights of citizenship. There is a sense in which many rights have been 'privatised' or 'recommodified', although both terms run the risk of obscuring the complexity of the processes involved.

The concept of welfare pluralism rests on the idea that, instead of the public sector (the state) being the principal provider of welfare goods and services, a significant level of provision should also come from the 'informal' sector (families and communities), the 'voluntary' sector (independent self-help or non-profit making organisations) and the 'commercial' sector (private enterprise). The suggestion is not that the state should no longer guarantee the welfare rights of the citizen, but that that guarantee should not necessarily be honoured through the direct provision of services by public sector organisations. The state might instead fund the provision of services by other agencies, or it might do no more than regulate the standards of provision made by such agencies.

The promotion of the *informal* sector lies at the heart of the development of policies of community care. In practice the greater part of everyday health and social care takes place within households (Rose 1988) and, for everyday needs, most people do tend in the first instance to look for help from members of their family (Beresford and Croft 1986). At the same time, there has for nearly half a century been widespread agreement throughout the Western world that the institutional forms of care – for physically disabled people, people with severe learning difficulties, people with mental health problems and frail elderly people – should be replaced by alternative forms of community-based care. In seeking to give expression to this objective in the 1980s, the British Conservative government emphasised that care *in* the community should increasingly mean care *by* the community and that the contribution to care by family, relatives, friends and neighbours should be maximised (see, for example, Walker 1990). The government justified this in terms of giving people the right to choose where and how they should be looked after (DHSS 1989). In practice, as we shall see in Chapter 8, choices may be limited. The intention was that, as far as possible, care in public institutions should be avoided and that people should be 'enabled' to live independently in their own homes. The character of the citizen's right has been altered to the extent that the provision of a direct service may in some circumstances become contingent upon the imposition of an obligation upon a close relative to act as an informal carer.

The promotion of the *voluntary* sector has been accompanied by attempts to advance the concept of 'active citizenship'. Towards the end of the 1980s ministers of the Conservative government sought to ameliorate the ostensibly amoral premises of Thatcherism by encouraging voluntary action, especially on the part of successful citizens. Active citizenship was described as 'a necessary complement to that of the enterprise culture' (Hurd 1989) and entailed charitable giving and voluntary service. As a concept of citizenship it was one which emphasised, not the rights of disadvantaged citizens, but the duties of those with time and money to spare. Lister (1990) has suggested that this amounted to an attempt to 'privatise' citizenship and negate welfare rights. The implication of a shift of social obligations from the sphere of tax financed benefits to the sphere of charitable and voluntary service is a return to the feudal notion of *noblesse oblige* (that the divine rights bestowed upon the nobility obliged them to be charitable to their subjects). Appeals to the ideal of active citizenship were renewed under the New Labour government which sought, once again, to counter the socially corrosive consequences of liberal individualism by promoting communitarian ideas (Driver and Martell 1997), including initiatives to promote volunteering, to foster partnership between local government and voluntary groups and to introduce the teaching of active citizenship into the school curriculum. From the 1980s onwards, continued support has been given by government to the use of voluntary organisations and volunteers in the provision of social services and, for example, voluntary sector housing associations have become the favoured providers of social rented housing (Kemp 1999; DETR 2000).

The promotion of the *commercial* welfare sector (see Papadakis and Taylor-Gooby 1987) has affected citizenship rights in a number of ways. The encouragement given during the 1980s to insurance-based private health care and pensions was given on the basis that such arrangements would afford citizens independence from the state: the intention was that people should substitute civil rights (based on a contract of insurance) for social rights (based on citizenship status). The New Labour government's pensions policy maintains a trend by which private funding arrangements are to be promoted at the expense of public funding (Ward 2000). The promotion of home ownership through the Right to Buy scheme for public sector tenants similarly sought directly to substitute property rights for social rights. In other areas of social policy, however, the partial privatisation of public welfare was intended to create competition between public and private sector providers and so alter the ethos of public service provision. Where citizens had a right to a service, they should have a choice between providers: even if no payment was required at the point of service delivery, the rights of a service user should be more akin to the civil rights of a paying customer than the social rights of a citizen.

The 'marketisation' of welfare

What is more, this could be achieved without transferring services to the private sector, through a process that is sometimes referred to as 'marketisation'. In the 1980s and 1990s three methods were employed towards this general goal.

The first of these devices found expression in the doctrine of New Public Management (NPM) (Hood 1991; Gray and Jenkins 1993; Clarke and Newman 1997). The idea was that, if public services were not to be relocated in the commercial sector, the business practices of the commercial sector could none the less be imported into public services. To this end, for example, the principles of general management were introduced into the National Health Service (Butler 1993); the administration of social security benefits was hived off to an 'arm's length' executive agency governed by performance targets (Dean 1993). The essence of the NPM doctrine is a change in the culture of public service delivery and a deliberate attempt at the level of discourse to reconstitute the client, the patient or the claimant as a 'customer'. Under subsequent New Labour government, though the overtly managerialist language of NPM became less prominent, many of its essential objectives have been subsumed within the government's 'modernisation' agenda (Cabinet Office 1999). This included the introduction of Best Value reviews for all local government services and a technocratic emphasis on 'evidence-based' policy and practice.

Second, in a number of social policy areas the emphasis in the late 1980s and early 1990s shifted in favour of the introduction of 'quasi-markets' (LeGrand 1990). This found its most explicit expression in the National Health Service 'internal market', in which District Health Authorities and fund-holding General Practitioners became the 'purchasers' of health care on behalf of their patients, while hospitals and community health care trusts became 'providers' competing for the custom of the purchasers. The community care reforms described above have had a similar effect for local authority Social Services Departments which must now operate separate commissioning and provider operations with contracts for residential care, daycare and domiciliary services being placed both internally and externally (Lawson 1993). In education the introduction of open enrolment and formula funding has effectively put state schools in competition with each other for pupils and funding (Taylor-Gooby 1993). Though New Labour claims, for example, to have abolished the internal market in the NHS in favour of partnership and long-term planning agreements, the division between purchasers (or commissioners) and providers (including new species of primary care groups and trusts) remains, as do the essential elements of the Conservative's approach to funding for education and the social services (Powell 1999).

Third, in 1991 Prime Minister John Major introduced the Citizen's Charter (Prime Minister's Office 1991). At first sight the Citizen's Charter, aimed at improving the standards of public services, represented a retreat from Thatcherism and a return to a more social democratic concern with the positive rights of the citizen (Miller and Peroni 1992). The stated aim of the Charter was to make services more open and accountable, but as Miller and Peroni put it: 'it creates few new rights. The drafting skilfully blurs the distinction between what is new and what merely confirms past practices and promises' (1992: 256).

The Charter claimed to provide a 'tool kit' of initiatives and ideas, among which were:

more privatisation; wider competition; further contracting out; more performance related pay; published performance targets – local and national; comprehensive publication of information on standards achieved; more effective complaints procedures; tougher and more independent inspectorates; better redress for the citizen when things go badly wrong. (Prime Minister's Office 1991: 5)

As we shall see in Chapter 9, stemming from the Citizen's Charter there has been a proliferation of more specific charters for the users of different welfare services, a process that was enthusiastically continued under New Labour. Central to the idea of the Citizen's Charter is the link between payment for services (whether directly or through taxes) and the quality of those services. The competent citizen is therefore the successful consumer, able to get the best out of services. The users and providers of services are cast as opponents of each other's interests. What is more, the 'business' of service provision is uncoupled from the 'politics' of welfare: policy makers may evade responsibility for policy failures (because customers are encouraged to blame the providers of services) and the collectivist ethos of the welfare state is diluted (because service provision is driven by individualised incentives rather than policy, or vocational or professional commitment). In T.H. Marshall's terms, the Citizen's Charter strengthened civil rights (the kind of rights 'customers' enjoy in the market place) *at the expense* of both political rights and social rights.

To say that social rights are being privatised or re-commodified is not to suggest that rights to welfare are necessarily being extinguished, rather that they are being made more akin to the property rights of classical jurisprudence. Social rights are now less about enabling people to exist independently of the market, and rather more about requiring them to participate in markets (including 'quasi-markets' for welfare services). The shift is occurring on a global scale since the World Trade Organisation has made clear that health and social services provided under governmental authority should not be exempt from free trade and competition requirements under the General Agreement on Trade and Services (see Deacon 2000). In Britain the New Labour government has made clear that 'where it makes sense to use private or voluntary sectors better to deliver public services, we will' (Blair 2001). Paradoxically, however, welfare rights are no less administrative in nature, it is simply that administrative power has been made more technical than political in character.

Summary/conclusion

All our rights are ideological constructions. When we speak of welfare rights we are dealing with abstract ideas rather than concrete realities. None the less, it is welfare rights that give expression to the effects (if not always the intentions) of social legislation and the substantive exercise of state power. This chapter has examined a range of theoretical explanations concerning the basis of welfare rights.

We have been concerned first with the extent to which welfare rights are founded in a form of mature citizenship, which has displaced class as a basis for social organisation. If this view were accepted, in place of a society founded on class antagonisms and inequalities we would now have a society based on a broad equality of citizenship. It is difficult, however, to reconcile this view with the realities of contemporary welfare state societies, although there is a sense in which the idea of welfare (or social) rights represents only a part of a wider project in which property (or civil) rights and democratic (or political) rights must also play a part if capitalism is to work.

We have also considered the extent to which the concept of rights under capitalism is problematic. Essentially, the basis of individual 'rights' stems from the definition of private property. Welfare rights, however, are bestowed by the collective authority of the state. While it is possible to speak of welfare rights as if they are property rights, in practice they are defined with reference to obligations imposed both on those who administer and those who benefit from such rights. To this extent, welfare rights are also political in character, because they may represent negotiable claims made by or on behalf of groups in society and we have sought to tease out an important but elusive distinction between the kinds of rights that are prescribed by doctrine and the kinds of rights that people establish for themselves through struggle.

Clearly, therefore, welfare rights are not static attributes of citizenship. They change over time and we have considered how recent welfare reforms have resulted in sometimes subtle transformations to the nature of welfare rights and social legislation. In particular, we have examined how the privatisation of certain aspects of welfare and changes to the way in which public services are administered have been reflected in a more consumer oriented form of rights. In the process, we have discussed commodification, de-commodification and re-commodification, concepts that provide a particular perspective upon the development of welfare rights in capitalist societies, and an explanation both of the contradictory potential of welfare rights (as rights to an existence independent of the market) and their ambiguous status (when deflected into the form of consumer rights).

The next chapter will move on from broad definitions of social rights as a component of citizenship to a discussion of poverty and need and, specifically, the extent to which welfare rights address poverty and need.

Chapter 2

Poverty and need

The last chapter discussed welfare rights as a component of citizenship within a democratic-welfare-capitalist state. Just as rights to political participation and legal protection are supposedly guaranteed, so citizens are also entitled to have certain basic needs satisfied: but which needs and to what extent?

The Beveridge Report (1942), which provided the blueprint for Britain's post-war welfare state, identified five metaphorical 'giants' to be banished; Disease, Idleness, Ignorance, Squalor and Want. The social ills for which these giants stood reflected those needs that the welfare state promised to underwrite; the need for health, employment, education, housing and the means of subsistence. Of the five giants, it is Want (or what we might now call poverty) that has proved the most difficult to defeat, especially since this giant can be sustained by all or any of its companions. The right to an adequate means of subsistence is difficult to guarantee, not least because over-all adequacy of living standards can be dependent upon a complex array of life chances, including good health, employment prospects, educational opportunity and decent housing. An issue to which I shall return is that of whether Want, in the sense that Beveridge spoke of it, implies a universal conception of human need and therefore a set of rights to welfare which are both specifiable and general, or whether needs – like the rights by which we give expression to them – are socially or ideologically constructed.

First, however, this chapter will discuss the concept of poverty. Poverty – its definition and measurement, its relief or prevention – has been one of the central preoccupations of Social Policy. The classic debates to which that preoccupation gives rise provide a necessary backdrop for any discussion of the relationship between human needs and welfare rights, and for any attempt to articulate recent debates about social inequality, social exclusion and social citizenship.

Under the Poor Laws, which preceded the 'modern' British welfare state, people who received state assistance were defined as 'paupers'. Paupers were not citizens. They were disqualified, for example, from voting in elections. By finally repealing the Poor Laws the modern welfare state sought to banish not simply poverty, but pauperism. Welfare rights for all implied a formal equality of citizenship. Poverty represents 'a strategically important *limit* for the concept of social citizenship' (Roche 1993: 55). If poverty persists in capitalist welfare states this implies a failure of citizens to secure their rights and a failure by the welfare state to honour those rights. Poverty is the 'limit case', the 'litmus test' or 'yardstick' against which the effectiveness of welfare rights is to be defined and judged.

Defining poverty

The trouble with 'poverty' is that politically and technically it is a highly contested concept (for a basic introductory text see Alcock 1993/1997) and at the level of popular discourse it is an especially elusive and ambiguous term (see Dean with Melrose 1999).

Absolute or relative?

The traditional battle lines in the debate about poverty have been drawn between those who subscribe to an *absolute* definition of poverty and those who subscribe to a *relative* definition. The absolute definition, broadly speaking, has been that favoured by Victorian poverty investigators (Booth 1889; Rowntree 1901) and, more recently, by politicians of the New Right (Joseph and Sumption 1979; Moore 1989). It is a definition that restricts the term poverty so as to apply only to people with insufficient resources for physical survival. The relative definition is that favoured characteristically by Fabian academics (Townsend 1979; Donnison 1982) and the so-called 'poverty lobby' (e.g. Oppenheim and Harker 1996). It is a definition that expands the term poverty so as to apply to people with insufficient resources for normal social participation. From this classic debate stem a number of related controversies of a technical, explanatory, political and sociological nature.

First, there is no agreed way of measuring poverty. Rowntree, for example, sought in his research to apply an absolute or primary poverty line based upon the cost of providing 'the minimum necessaries for the maintenance of merely physical efficiency' for a household of any given size or composition. This is now called the 'budget standard' approach to poverty measurement. It has been extended in recent years in Britain by the Family Budget Unit, which has developed not only a 'low cost but acceptable' budget standard, but also a 'modest but adequate' budget standard – reflecting as it were a relative as well as an absolute definition (Bradshaw 1993; Parker 1998). The Family Budget Unit calculated that, at 1993 prices, families with young children in the UK needed incomes around one third higher than the prevailing levels of social assistance benefit in order to achieve even a 'low cost' budget standard and when the exercise was repeated, using a more rigorous methodology in 1998, it was found that the social assistance entitlement of a couple with two dependent children fell at least £32 per week below the low cost standard. Alternatively, it is common practice in some Western countries, officially or unofficially, to define a 'poverty line' with reference to the level of income at which people qualify for means-tested social assistance benefits or a level of income equivalent to some arbitrary proportion (often 50 per cent) of average household incomes, though neither of these indices is, strictly speaking, a measure of poverty (see Veit-Wilson 1994; 1999). Other commentators prefer statistical or 'income proxy' measures that identify the level of income below which need demonstrably replaces choice as the principal determinant of household expenditure (Orshansky 1969) or below which prevailing public opinion believes it impossible to make ends meet (van-Praag *et al.* 1982). Rather than only measure incomes, some sociologists have sought to measure 'deprivation'. This may be achieved by applying either a range of expertly determined indicators relating to diet, consumption patterns, housing, working conditions, family and community activity levels (Townsend 1979) or a consensually determined range of 'socially perceived necessities' identified through public opinion surveys (Mack and Lansley 1985; Gordon and Pantazis 1997; Gordon *et al.* 2000).

Second, there are explanatory controversies. The conflict here is between explanations of poverty based on pathology and those based on structural causes (Holman 1978). Pathological explanations blame poverty on the failures of the poor. Poverty is seen to arise because of the inadequacies of the individuals, families or communities affected. As a result of their genetic make-up, their personalities or sheer bad luck, individuals may be inept, lazy or incapacitated. Deficient parenting or a deprived family background may result in the transmission of poverty and inappropriate behaviour patterns from generation to generation (Joseph 1972). In certain localities or communities a ghetto subculture may develop which reinforces and perpetuates economic dependency and poverty (Murray 1984). The alternative structural explanations focus upon the part played by society. This blames poverty on the inevitable 'diswelfares' of the competitive market economy (Titmuss 1968), the nature of class relations (Townsend 1979), or on the consequences of patriarchy and racism (e.g. Williams 1989).

Third, there are political controversies concerning what role (if any) the state should play in relation to poverty and whether the objective of social policy is to prevent or to limit relative poverty, or merely to relieve or abate absolute poverty when, or if, it occurs. There are those on the far Right who are critical of the welfare state, not only for eroding individual freedoms (see the discussion of 'negative rights' in Chapter 1), but also for perpetuating poverty by frustrating the wealth creating propensities of a free market (Boyson 1971; Murray 1984). They suggest that the kindest thing the state can do for 'the poor' is to stand out of their way. Most right wing opinion, however, acknowledges that the state should have a minimalist role in relieving extreme poverty (Hayek 1944; Anderson 1991), as indeed the British state had done for three and a half centuries under the Poor Laws. To the centre and left of the political spectrum it is widely believed that the state should provide more than an 'ambulance' service to relieve the casualties of poverty, and that it should attempt to cure the causes of poverty and so prevent poverty and relative deprivation from occurring in the first place. The social legislation to which such an approach gives rise ranges from social insurance to the provision of universal benefits and these will be discussed in Chapter 5.

Fourth, there are sociological controversies about the meaning of poverty as a social or symbolic construct. Though social attitude data suggest that popular opinion in Britain strongly favours an absolute or 'breadline' definition of poverty, as opposed to a relative definition (Taylor-Gooby 1990 and 1995), qualitative studies reveal a more complex picture. Popular understandings of the distinction between 'poor' and 'not poor' are in one sense inherently relativist. On the one hand, people who are 'poor' in terms of the kinds of criteria outlined above are often disinclined to regard themselves as poor: poverty is generally regarded as something that happens to 'other' people (Dean 1992). On the other hand, a fear of poverty can extend to people on middle to moderately high incomes for whom the risk of falling into poverty is quite negligible (Dean with Melrose 1999). Poverty is not an objective state – in either an absolute or a relative sense – but a discursively created spectre that can impact on the personal experiences and private identities of everybody.

For the moment, I should like to go behind the old debate about absolute and relative poverty since this has been in some respects eclipsed – first, by new debates about the relationship of poverty to inequality and social exclusion and, second, by new approaches to the definition of human need. To the second of these issues this chapter will turn shortly, but first it would be useful to open up a rather different distinction, between *distributional* concepts, which equate poverty with inequality, and *relational* concepts, which equate it with social exclusion.

Inequality and social exclusion

The figure who can claim the greatest credit both for Britain's 'rediscovery' of poverty in the 1960s and for major advances in the theory and analysis of poverty in the 1970s is Peter Townsend. Townsend pioneered a structural analysis of poverty and devised an index of relative deprivation based on living patterns. From the findings of a major survey he sought to demonstrate that people with incomes of up to one and a half times the prevailing level of social assistance benefits were likely to suffer relative deprivation; that is to a greater or lesser extent to be excluded from socially acceptable living patterns. Townsend's contention was that there is an income band or threshold below which the risk of relative deprivation increases disproportionately (1979). In 1981, in the columns of the periodical *New Society*, a celebrated exchange occurred between Townsend and David Piachaud. Piachaud criticised Townsend's index of relative deprivation because it did not allow for the diversity of people's lifestyles and behaviour; it assumed uniformity and so denied individual choice and freedom. At first glance, Piachaud's attack appears 'absolutist', but the main thrust of his argument lies in his contention that 'There is a continuum from great wealth to chronic poverty and along that continuum a wide diversity of patterns of living' (1981: 118). Piachaud readily concedes that 'The term "poverty" carries with it an implication and a moral imperative that something should be done about it' (*ibid.*: 119), but it is precisely because this requires the making of political or value judgements that there can be no objective measurement of relative deprivation.

Poverty, in this sense, is quite simply 'the unacceptable face of inequality' (Alcock 1993: 255). Poverty might, as I have already indicated, be regarded as a socially or culturally unacceptable human experience or threat. On the other hand, it may also be understood in terms of, or in relation to, an unacceptable degree of structural inequality in society, or the inadequacy of the individual or household resources available to people at the bottom of the income distribution. It is because of their preoccupation with the empirical definition and measurement of what amount to standards or thresholds of *acceptability* in the context of an unequal distribution of resources that even avowed relativists like Townsend appear in practice to 'vacillate' between absolutism and relativism (Doyal and Gough 1991: 33).

For this reason, Room (1995) has argued that the intellectual tradition that has informed research and debate on 'poverty' – especially in the English speaking world – is distinctively *distributional*. Even when commentators seek to break out from the prevailing assumptions of market liberalism to question the underlying relations of power that determine the life chances of the individual, the focus has usually been on the distribution of resources. In contrast, the concept of 'social exclusion', which is informed by intellectual traditions more characteristic of socially conservative continental Europe, is *relational*. Social exclusion as a concept is not concerned with distributional inequality, but with inadequate social participation and lack of social integration. It is a term that has become increasingly prominent within social policy discourse at the European level (Room 1995) and more recently under a New Labour government in Britain (SEU 1997; Levitas 1998; Oppenheim 1998).

Poverty and social exclusion are not the same thing. While one is ultimately concerned with the (mal)distribution of incomes, goods and services, the other is concerned with the processes by which people may become marginalised within society. It is possible for people to be poor but socially included, or affluent but socially excluded. In practice, however, poverty and social exclusion are closely related and tend to occur together. The concept of social exclusion and its use have been criticised for the way in which they can actually obscure questions of material inequality (e.g. Levitas 1996). The concept assumes a consensual, functionalist model of society that ignores the potentially exploitative nature of capitalism. Often, the opposite of social exclusion that is implied, Levitas argues, is not social inclusion, but social integration. The preoccupation of the emergent discourse of social exclusion is with social cohesion as a prerequisite of effective market relations. When married to market economics, the concept focuses upon maximising economic competitiveness through the promotion of inclusion in labour market processes, and minimising social expenditure through the promotion of inclusion within supportive and self-help social networks. In much of the recent policy discourse, it would appear that the language of social exclusion is associated with a socially conservative form of communitarianism that is inherently authoritarian (Driver and Martell 1997; Jordan 1996 and 1998).

None the less, the concept of social exclusion chimes in some important respects with the concerns of relative theorists of poverty. Williams and Pillinger (1996) have suggested that, in one sense, social exclusion represents an intermediate concept that potentially mediates between macro-level concerns with structural poverty or social inequality and micro-level concerns with poverty as it is culturally constituted and individually experienced. While there is plainly some ambiguity about the way in which the term social exclusion is currently being deployed, it can facilitate a relational as well as a distributional understanding of poverty.

Defining need

Closely related to the concept of 'poverty' is that of 'human need'. Need is no less a problematic concept, albeit for rather different reasons. The controversies tend to stem more from philosophical than political concerns. At root, however, human need, like poverty, is also beset by a dichotomy between absolute and relative definitions.

Absolute or 'basic' human needs might be supposed to arise from the requirements of biological survival and protection from physical harm. Relative needs or mere 'wants' might be supposed to arise from culturally or socially determined expectations. The distinction, however, is one that melts away as soon as one tries to specify what is 'basically' necessary to human survival. What constitutes adequacy of diet or shelter, for example, is fundamentally related not only to socio-cultural considerations, but also to physiological, physical, geographical and climatic factors. Exact scientific or clinical criteria even for 'starvation' and 'hunger' are not easy to find (Townsend 1993: 132) and strict medically or biologically derived definitions are likely to be at best arbitrary and at worst meaningless unless they can be situated in a substantive human context.

Theoretical approaches to human need have tended to be polarised not simplistically between the absolute and the relative, but between notions of needs which are *inherent* to the human individual and *interpreted* needs which are creatures of policy processes and debates.

Inherent need

An early instance of the former was provided by Maslow (1943) who argued that humans' basic drives are (in descending order of potency): first, physiological; second, for physical safety; third, for love and belonging; fourth, for self-esteem; and fifth, for 'self-actualisation'. Maslow's approach cannot account for the potency of socially constituted needs and the fact that, for example, in affluent societies people on low incomes may literally go hungry in order to maintain forms of consumption by which to 'keep up appearances'.

Probably the most systematic attempt to wrestle with such questions has been provided by Doyal and Gough (1984 and 1991). They start from the premise that a conception of human need is implicit in almost every ideological stance, even those that reject the possibility of defining basic human needs:

- Market liberals who believe that the market is the ideal medium through which needs or 'preferences' may be formulated and expressed must none the less concede that – for a variety of reasons – markets will sometimes fail to meet the needs of everybody.

- Critical theorists of all kinds – including Marxists, anti-racists, feminists and ecologists – though they may reject the false needs that are defined for, and imposed upon, oppressed people – by the capitalist economic process, imperialism, patriarchy or scientism – are by implication subscribing to some notion of the rights or needs that these same forces have violated.
- Even the most radical democrats and extreme relativists are obliged to recognise that society must be able to respond to those needs that may arise from objective realities or external threats (e.g. natural, economic or military) that are capable of occasioning harm to its members.

Doyal and Gough go on to advance and defend a theory of human need as a 'universal' rather than a relative concept and to provide an absolute definition of need – with explicit distributional consequences – capable of application in a relative context across different cultures and societies. They specify the universal preconditions for human action and interaction in terms of physical health and personal autonomy. The need for physical health requires the protection of all people from harm as well as the provision of the means of subsistence, shelter and health care. The need for personal autonomy requires that all people should have knowledge, capabilities and opportunities, which would seem to imply education or training and the prospect of productive and satisfying work. Personal autonomy, however, has societal preconditions and the historical process of human liberation may be construed as the struggle to optimise the satisfaction of human need. Like Rousseau and Durkheim before them, Doyal and Gough argue that to be a social being is to be the bearer of responsibilities. However, unlike modern communitarians, they contend that the moral reciprocity that is the universal foundation for all human societies is such that the needs of all people should be satisfied not only to a minimal, but to an optimal extent:

> For if humans do possess the power to alter history, the task is to keep trying to bring about those alterations which are necessary conditions for human liberation – the satisfaction of the health and autonomy needs of as many humans as possible to the highest sustainable levels. (1991: 110)

This is a powerful defence for a positive conception of welfare rights. It is a conception very much in the Enlightenment tradition. That is to say, it is a normative conception of how progress in history is to be made and of the relationship between abstract ideals and individual conduct.

Interpreted need

The inherent needs which Doyal and Gough define are universal in an *a priori* sense. It may be argued that such 'needs' are no more than abstract formulations and that what is objective and concrete is not 'need' so much as 'dependency' (see Dean and Taylor-Gooby 1992: 174). What defines our social being is not our individual moral responsibility, but our mutual interdependency as human subjects. Rights, duties and morality flow from the manner in which people are dependent upon each other. The seminal interpretive concerns of sociology had been with the growing complexity of the social order in the Western world. The greater the social division of *labour* within a society, the greater the extent of human interdependency. It was within this tradition that theorists of the 'modern' welfare state, such as Titmuss (1958), began to analyse social divisions of *welfare* and the basis upon which to posit collective (i.e. state) responsibility for 'dependent people' (*ibid.*: 42).

Spicker (1993) has suggested that the problem of defining or conceptualising 'need' can in fact be resolved when one interprets needs as claims. Chapter 1 has already considered an argument that 'rights' are not propensities that vest naturally in every individual but represent specific demands or claims for resources and/or services. Certainly, a 'need' becomes a 'right' when it is formulated as a 'claim'; but there is a sense in which needs, rights and claims are all expressions of human dependency. They are neither absolute (capable of *a priori* prescription) nor relative (mere cultural artefacts) but relational and therefore negotiable. They are created neither by rational precept, nor chance of circumstance, but through the way people interact in time and space. Needs, rights and claims may be defined or satisfied by family members, kinspeople, lovers, friends, community members, voluntary associations, within a market or by a welfare state, but their common moral nexus is the dependency of all upon all.

The issue that this still leaves is how and by whom are our needs as interdependent beings to be interpreted for the purposes of social policy making? Bradshaw (1972) has proposed a taxonomy of need, distinguishing: the 'normative' needs defined on our behalf by professionals and experts; the 'felt' needs which we might identify when asked what we need; the 'expressed' needs articulated through political demands for the delivery of services; and the 'comparative' needs which may be said to exist when there is a shortfall or deficiency in the services received by one person or group relative to those received by another similarly placed person or group. Bradshaw's approach fails to prioritise different kinds of need or to say which needs should inform the development of social policy. Should people be allowed to determine their own needs and interests? Given that people are not always best placed to identify or to safeguard their own interests, who should be the arbiter and guarantor of their needs?

There is arguably a distinction between the universal or basic needs objectively defined by Doyal and Gough that must be met if people are to survive and autonomously function and the more subjectively defined needs that people must satisfy in order truly to flourish (cf. Ignatieff 1984: 11). One way to conceptualise the distinction is to think of the former as 'thin' and the latter as 'thick' needs (Fraser 1989: ch. 8; Drover and Kerans 1993: 11–13). Interpreting thick needs requires an understanding of the cultural context in which people name their needs. From a feminist perspective Nancy Fraser (1989: ch. 7) has made the case for a 'politics of need interpretation'. She proposes an oppositional form of politics by which to give 'publicity' to the needs of oppressed groups in society; that is to project into the sphere of public policy those demands that had hitherto been subordinated as private needs. For her part, Fraser is in no way advocating that thick needs should take precedence over thin ones, but it is important to note that a claims-making approach based on the interpretation of thick needs could be advocated as readily by populist or conservative communitarians as by radical feminists or other new social movements (Soper 1993); that is by those who seek to challenge not only the unwarranted authority, but also the redistributive power of the welfare state and to privilege the needs of included social groups at the expense of the excluded.

A quite different way to conceptualise the same distinction is provided by Amartya Sen (1984 and 1985). Sen distinguishes between the 'space of capabilities', that is the sphere of human functioning in which people's needs must be met, and the 'space of commodities', the goods that are necessary to satisfy need. His contention is that poverty is absolute in the space of capabilities, but relative in the space of commodities. What is required for physical and social functioning may vary between societies, but the fundamental capabilities that all people require are the same. In a social context in which daily journeys are unnecessary, the absence of a bicycle, a car or the inaccessibility of public transport will not be a problem, but in a context in which one must travel to obtain the means of subsistence such things are not luxuries but essentials. Doyal and Gough (1991: 155–9) equate Sen's space of capabilities with universal or basic need, and the space of commodities with 'basic needs satisfiers' or 'intermediate needs'. The important point about this argument, as I understand it, is that this does allow for the development of human capabilities, the expansion or 'thickening' of intermediate needs and a progressive enhancement of welfare rights.

Sen's account articulates with the 'relational' view of needs, rights and claims, which I outlined earlier, and with the idea that needs, rights and claims are materially grounded in social practice. It also chimes with Paul Hirst's definition of 'rights' as 'capacities' conferred by law (see Chapter 1 above). Hirst's argument is that rights 'serve socially determined policy objectives and interests' (1980: 104); that they represent codified objectives by which a democratic society must secure its own regulation, whether that be a utopian socialist society or a democratic-welfare-capitalist society. In a later work Hirst (1994) elaborates a concept of 'associative democracy' in which voluntary, self-governing associations would replace existing unaccountable forms of governance. In a broadly similar vein, Giddens (1994) has envisaged a form of 'dialogic democracy'. As with Nancy Fraser's politics of needs interpretation, these are scenarios in which rights to need satisfaction could be negotiated. They are all scenarios redolent of, or informed by, Habermas's (1987a) notion of the 'ideal speech situation' that might occur in an un-coerced and inclusive communication community. However, like a strictly claims-based notion of rights, a strictly relational interpretation of need remains a counterfactual premise. In other words, it makes for an interesting discussion, but it does not advance our understanding of the selective and partial ways in which certain needs have been, however inadequately, translated into rights.

Rights and equality

Welfare rights are rights to needs satisfaction. A fundamental question for this book is the effect that welfare rights have had in alleviating poverty. Has the formal equality of citizenship promised by the welfare state succeeded in banishing Want? During the 1970s and 1980s it was widely argued that the welfare state had failed (see, for example, Taylor-Gooby 1991). The more theoretical or ideologically based critiques of state welfare will be visited in Chapter 4, but here I should like briefly to mention debates concerning the empirical effects which state welfare has had on social equality.

A strategy of equality?

The basis of the post-war welfare consensus (see, for example, Mishra 1984: ch. 1) was a general acceptance that the state should play some role in ameliorating Want, through the provision of a 'national minimum'. Implicitly, the formal equality of citizenship was to be accompanied by a greater degree of substantive equality, albeit at such a level as to provide a modest floor below which none should fall, rather than a generous ceiling above which none might climb (Beveridge 1942). Kincaid, however, suggested that by 'extraordinary ingenuity' the welfare state managed to avoid any considerable influence in levelling post-tax incomes (1975: 219). In fact, the income share of the poorest tenth of the UK population fell from 4.2 per cent of national income in 1961 to 3.0 per cent in 1991, while that of the richest tenth rose from 2 per cent to 25 per cent (Goodman and Webb 1994: 66).

Worse still, in a highly influential book entitled *The Strategy of Equality*, Julian LeGrand (1982) found that public expenditure in such areas as health, education, housing and transport exacerbated inequality by benefiting higher and middle income groups more than lower income groups. In a later review of the welfare state in Britain between 1974 and 1987 LeGrand more reassuringly concluded that, in spite of the economic difficulties faced by Labour governments of the 1970s and the ideological hostility to welfare exhibited by Conservative governments of the 1980s, the welfare state had continued successfully to 'smooth income over the life-cycle of each individual' and progressively to reduce 'the gap between "original" (i.e. market) incomes and "gross" incomes (original incomes plus cash benefits)' (1990a: 340). He was obliged none the less to concede that the welfare state had been less successful in ameliorating a widening gap since 1979 between the richest and the poorest in terms of original incomes. A further edition of that review, extended to 1993, concluded that:

> despite the combined effects of a somewhat more pro-poor redistribution from the in-kind welfare services such as health, education, and housing and the increased targeting of cash social security benefits, the gap between rich and poor grew. The driving force was not social welfare policy but a combination of the widening rewards in the labour market and labour market inactivity combined with the decline in benefit levels relative to earnings and tax policy, roughly in that order of importance. (Glennerster 1998: 325)

It is too soon to say at the time of writing whether the policy changes of the New Labour government, first elected in 1997, will result in a significant reduction in poverty and/or social exclusion. A study by the New Policy Institute (Rahman *et al.* 2000), based mainly on official statistics, has revealed that in 1998/99 14 $^1/_4$ million people (about one quarter of the population) were living in households with less than half average income, after housing costs. Not only was this more than double the number in the early 1980s, but it was half a million greater than the previous high point in 1992/93. While the same study could point to some recent improvements in basic educational standards and housing conditions, it also indicated that significant health inequalities persist. While unemployment has lately been falling from its high level in the 1980s and 1990s, low pay and job insecurity mean that poverty and social exclusion, even if we were to achieve full employment, will not disappear (cf. Gordon *et al.* 2000). The raft of policy changes introduced by the New Labour government, which we shall discuss in Chapters 5 to 8, have been especially framed with the objective of ending child poverty by 2019 and recent projections by Piachaud and Sutherland (2001) suggest that these should succeed in lifting around 1 million children out of poverty by 2002 (applying the government's preferred measurement of poverty). This will, however, leave some 2 million children still in poverty and the task of redressing their plight will be less tractable.

In spite of the welfare state, Britain is a more unequal society than it was 50 years ago. Whether this means the welfare state has failed depends, as Taylor-Gooby puts it, 'on how redistributive you expected it to be in the first place' (1991: 40). Hindess (1987) for example has taken issue with the supposition that the welfare state ever embodied a grand 'strategy of equality' and has suggested that the development of social policy has been informed by rather more limited and pragmatic objectives.

Differential outcomes

It is difficult therefore to establish in any overall sense how effective welfare rights have been, although it is possible to establish who has benefited least from such protection as welfare rights do afford. While accepting that poverty is a contested concept, it is possible to observe the extent to which the composition of the poorest section of the population changes over time. Such changes, both in Britain and in other developed countries (see, for example, Room *et al.* 1989) have led to the emergence of what are sometimes called the 'new poor'. The 'old poor' of the Beveridge era were principally pensioners and 'large' working families, for whom the risk of financial hardship arose from the vicissitudes of the life-course. The 'new poor' of the late twentieth century tended to be unemployed people (especially young and long-term unemployed people), lone parents and both workless and low-paid working families (regardless of size) for whom the risk of financial hardship arises because of the consequences of economic restructuring and social change.

Table 2.1, based on households below average income (HBAI) figures, shows the changing proportions of different family types and economic groups

Table 2.1 The changing risk of 'poverty' in the UK: 1979–1998/99[1]

| | As a proportion of total population | | | As a proportion of poorest 10%[2] | | | | | |
	1979 %	1998/99 %	Change	1979 %	1979 under/over-representation	1998/99 %	1998/99 under/over-representation	Change	Change of risk factor[3]
By family type									
Pensioner couple	9	9	0	20	(+11)	5	(−4)	−15	−15
Single pensioner	8	7	−1	11	(+3)	5	(−2)	−6	−5
Couple with children	47	36	−11	41	(−6)	39	(+3)	−2	+9
Couple without children	18	22	+4	9	(−9)	13	(−9)	+4	0
Single with child	4	8	+4	4	(+5)	16	(+8)	+7	+3
Single without child	14	17	+3	10	(−4)	22	(+5)	+12	+9
By economic status									
Self-employed	6	9	+3	10	(+4)	14	(+5)	+4	+1
Single/couple all in FTW[4]	24	23	−1	2	(−22)	3	(−20)	+1	+2
1 FTW[4] and 1 PTW[5]	20	15	−5	2	(−18)	2	(−13)	0	+5
1 FTW[4] and 1 not working	21	12	−9	9	(−12)	8	(−4)	−1	+8
Single/couple all in PTW[5]	6	8	+2	10	(+4)	13	(+5)	+3	+1
Head/spouse aged 60+	15	17	+2	33	(+18)	13	(−4)	−20	−22
Head/spouse unemployed	3	4	+1	16	(+13)	21	(+17)	+5	+4
Other	5	11	+6	18	(+13)	26	(+15)	+8	+2

Notes:
1 Sources: Department of Social Security (1993) *Households Below Average Income: A statistical analysis 1979–1990/91*, HMSO, London (*Crown Copyright*) and Department of Social Security (2000) *Households Below Average Income: A statistical analysis 1994/95–1998/99*, CDS, London (*Crown Copyright*).
2 i.e. as a proportion of the bottom income decile group *after* housing costs.
3 i.e. overall change in under/over-representation in poorest decile.
4 FTW – full-time work (>30 hours per week).
5 PTW = part-time work (<30 hours per week).

both within the general UK population and within the bottom income decile, whose incomes fall well below the government's own accepted definition of poverty and are in one sense the poorest of the poor. To the extent that the poorest tenth of the population in the 1990s were in fact worse off than they were in the 1970s (Jenkins 1994), we are not dealing here with a consistent, still less an objective measure of poverty (see Veit-Wilson 1994). However, changes in the number of percentage points by which groups are under or over-represented within the poorest tenth may be taken as a crude index or 'change of risk' factor. It may be seen clearly that during the last 20 years of the twentieth century:

- Pensioners faced a reduced risk of extreme poverty, though single pensioners (among whom women are disproportionately represented) remained more at risk than pensioner couples. This demonstrates the considerable impact of occupational pensions, from which, however, the oldest pensioners tended not to benefit. What is more, in spite of the improvement, there were still a greater number of pensioners living on below half average household incomes than was the case even in the 1960s (see Goodman and Webb 1994).
- Couples with children were demonstrably at greater risk of extreme poverty than in the 1970s. This related partly to the extremely high risk of poverty faced by workless households, but also – as dual earner households and a low-wage economy became the norm (Dean 2002) – to the increased risk of poverty faced by the declining proportion of families with only one earner. While households containing a full-time worker were consistently under-represented in the poorest tenth, it is significant that their overall risk of poverty still increased.
- Lone parent households remained consistently over-represented in the poorest tenth. It should be borne in mind that the proportion of households with children to be headed by a lone parent increased very dramatically during the 1970s (Burghes 1993) and has proceeded since then to double. Though lone parents' risk of extreme poverty increased only slightly during the 1980s and 1990s, it remained proportionately very high and, in one sense, could not have got much worse.
- Single people without children faced an increased risk of poverty and this risk was visited disproportionately on young single people, for whom rights to social security benefits were significantly curtailed (Dean 1997) while the youth labour market collapsed (Coles 1995).

One conclusion is that rights to welfare have not been consistently secured over time or for all social groups. This was a concern expressed in Titmuss's (1958) seminal analysis of the social division of welfare. Titmuss had identified a three-fold division between the fiscal, occupational and state welfare systems and he pointed to the relative advantages and disadvantages that these systems created for different social classes. Those who are most marginal to the labour process must place greatest reliance on rights to (inferior) state welfare, rather than more highly prized fiscal or occupational alternatives. More recent theorists have additionally pointed to a sexual division of welfare (Rose 1981) and indeed a case can be made 'for identifying a racial division of welfare, an age division and other specific divisions based on the failure of welfare to cater for the needs of the various and disparate groups which constitute the poor' (Mann 1992: 26).

'Rights', as socially and politically constructed phenomena are with few exceptions unmindful of such dimensions as gender, 'race', age and disability and welfare rights may be seen in many respects to have failed women, minority ethnic groups, older people and people with disabilities. The implicit assumptions on which the 'modern' welfare state was founded have been outlined by Hermione Parker as including:

> . . . that all poverty is due either to 'interruption or loss of earnings' or to 'failure to relate income during earning to the size of family'; . . . that society consists of happily married couples (no divorce), widows (no widowers) and heterosexual celibates living either alone or with their parents; . . . that all married women are financially dependent on their husbands; . . . that it is within the power of governments to maintain full employment; . . . that full employment means regular full-time work for men, aged 15 to 65, with minimal job changes . . . (1989: 23–9)

The legacy of these assumptions, in spite of more recent piecemeal reform, is that women (see Glendinning and Millar 1992; McLaughlin 1999), minority ethnic groups (see Amin and Oppenheim 1992; Craig 1999), older people (see Townsend 1991; Evason 1999) and people with disabilities (see Oliver 1990; Barnes and Baldwin 1999) have been systematically marginalised from welfare citizenship's mainstream. In Part II we shall explore some of the ways in which the explicit rights accorded to such groups may in practice have been compromised, but here I simply underline the point that welfare rights are not equal rights.

Citizenship and welfare

The promise of universal rights to meet universal needs that had been held out in T.H. Marshall's concept of social citizenship has not been fulfilled. Referring to the disparities of power and resources that continue in practice to divide citizens, Ruth Lister has argued that:

> These inequalities – particularly class, race and gender – run like fault lines through our society and shape the contours of citizenship in the civil, political and social spheres. Poverty spells exclusion from the full rights of citizenship in each of these spheres and undermines people's ability to fulfill the private and public obligations of citizenship. For people with disabilities, this exclusion is often compounded . . . (1990: 68)

In a later work Lister goes on to argue for a form of citizenship based on 'differentiated universalism' (1997): a citizenship in which rights give expression both to equality and difference, to universal and to particular needs. I shall address controversies about the nature and potential of citizenship as a concept in Chapter 10, but demands like Lister's raise a critical issue that must be addressed while we are discussing poverty and need: how is any such vision of citizenship to be realised? What seems to be implied is the kind of approach characterised by Alan Hunt as an 'oppositional project conceived of as if it were constructed "elsewhere", fully finished and then drawn into place, like some Trojan horse of the mind, to do battle with the prevailing dominant hegemony' (1990: 313).

Constructing citizenship

One answer to this is to be found in Bryan Turner's (1990 and 1991) discussion of the different historical kinds of citizenship. One of the key distinctions he draws is between passive citizenship derived from a 'descending' view and active citizenship derived from an 'ascending' view: 'In the descending view, the king is all powerful and the subject is the recipient of privileges. In the ascending view a free man was a citizen, an active bearer of rights' (1990: 207). The first is typified by the English constitutional settlement of 1688 by which the rule of the sovereign-in-parliament was established over subjects-as-citizens. The latter is typified by the aspirations of the French revolution of 1789. The essential critique of 'bourgeois' citizenship within modern parliamentary democracies by Marxists such as Mann (1987) is that it is passive: that it represents a ruling class strategy for the regulation of citizens (an argument to which I shall return in Chapter 4). In contrast, Turner argues thus:

> active and radical forms of citizenship will be grabbed from below by struggle in societies which emphasise the moral importance of the public domain . . . Radical citizenship should produce norms which would challenge the marginalisation of the elderly, the alienation of unemployed youth or the isolation of the chronically sick. Active traditions of citizenship should produce an inclusive and extensive social policy of reform. In short, active citizenship should be the basis of an extensive social welfare programme. (1991: 36)

Clearly, this is a very different kind of 'active citizenship' to that envisaged by either the Conservative government of the 1980s (see above) or the New Labour government of the 2000s (see Chapter 10). It should be noted that, harking back to Habermas (1976), Turner expresses the fear that this form of active citizenship runs the risk of generating expectations that cannot be fulfilled, of creating a 'legitimation deficit' and therefore social instability. In practice, what is more, the kind of citizenship that is forged by the seizure of rights 'from below' can follow from processes of incremental negotiation as much as from violent struggle. What distinguishes the descending from the ascending view of citizenship has less to do with passivity and activity than with the manner in which power is exercised.

The late twentieth century witnessed a wave of postmodernist and post-Marxist thinking (e.g. Laclau and Mouffe 1985; Hall and Jacques 1990; Pakulski and Waters 1996) which argued that the politics of class, that had once generated demands for citizenship from below, had been superseded by a politics of discourse. Abandoning the possibility of class struggle and class interest as the driving force of history they embraced the relativist notion of the 'discursive position': political struggles over needs and rights in a postmodern age will be conducted, they believed, not between classes but at the level of discourse; in terms not of universal but of particular claims. Critiques of Laclau and Mouffe have been provided by Wood (1986) and Callinicos (1989), both of whom seek to hold on to a theory of structural determination, while recognising the necessity of human agency; the belief that human welfare can result from reasoned human action; 'the idea that there is no cure for the wounds of Enlightenment other than the radicalised Enlightenment itself' (Habermas 1986, cited in Callinicos 1989: 95). Doyal and Gough's theory of human need, which I have outlined above, is very much an attempt to recapture that Enlightenment tradition. They argue for a compromise or 'dual strategy' that combines a mixed economy of welfare with elements of central planning. The 'tragedy' of relativism, they say, is that 'through proclaiming the incoherence of debates about how [the optimisation of needs satisfaction] should be achieved, its supporters – whatever their intentions might be – lend support to those who wish to prevent such change' (1991: 110–11).

System and agency

As we have seen, the development of citizenship has extinguished neither social inequality (i.e. class), patriarchy, nor racism. However, as Lister emphasises (1997: 41), citizenship must be understood both as a status and as a practice: there are some rights that we enjoy by virtue of *being* a citizen and others we exercise when we *act* as a citizen. To my mind the distinction is in some ways analogous to that which Marx (1847) made between a class that exists objectively *in* itself and a class that exists self-consciously *for* itself. Albeit for a very different purpose, Giddens has drawn a not entirely unrelated distinction between hierarchical and 'generative' power (1991): the former relates to the power that groups or individuals exert over others; the latter to the capacity for autonomy or the power of 'self-actualisation'. Underpinning all these distinctions is the essential distinction between system and agency. It is possible, I would argue, to distinguish between *systemic* and *agential* notions of citizenship: the former acknowledges the conceptual and structural parameters of the social settlement and the latter the capacity for human action – both individual and collective; whether repressive or emancipatory. Citizenship co-exists with or encompasses both the systems in which power operates and the living agents of that power, and it may be regarded from either perspective. This draws on Habermas's celebrated and overarching distinction between system and life-world and the idea that we live with the consequences of the separation and continuing tensions between, on the one hand, the technical systems by which rights of citizenship are formulated and administered and, on the other, the life-world which gives meaning to social participation and in which the well-springs of behaviour and aspiration are located (Habermas 1987a).

A good way of understanding the competing notions of rights that were discussed in Chapter 1 and the competing notions of citizenship that are discussed above is through the pivotal distinction developed in this chapter

Table 2.2 Competing views of poverty and need and their correlative perspectives on rights and citizenship: a model

correlative nature of rights	approaches to poverty and need	correlative basis of citizenship
'doctrinal' or *a priori*	absolutist (in the space of capabilities)[1] or 'distributional'	'descending'[2] or systemic
'claims-based' or negotiable	relativist (in the space of commodities)[1] or 'relational'	'ascending'[2] or agential

Notes:
1 Cf. Sen (1984; 1985).
2 Cf. Turner (1990; 1991).

between distributional and relational conceptions of need (which relates in turn to Sen's account of absolute poverty as it occurs in the space of capabilities and relative poverty as it occurs in the space of commodities). The associations that I wish to draw upon are illustrated in Table 2.2. Distributional/absolutist notions of human need/poverty correlate with notions of rights that are *a priori* and with what I have defined as the doctrinal perspective on rights; with notions of citizenship that are systemic and with what Turner defines as the descending perspective on citizenship. Relational/relativist notions of human need/poverty correlate with notions of rights that are negotiable and with what I have defined as the claims-based perspective on rights; with notions of citizenship that are agential and with what Turner defines as the ascending perspective on citizenship.

The distinctions outlined in Table 2.2 may be understood as dichotomies, or we can investigate those distinctions as dialectical relationships. On the one hand, we have here a dilemma. Do we address poverty by imposing citizenship from above and regulating people's capabilities or capacities; or is such an objective to be achieved by seizing citizenship from below and democratically reconstituting the discourses through which needs are identified, formulated and legitimised as claims? On the other hand, as will become clear later in this book, we have here an explanatory model that helps to cast light on the competing forces that have together shaped and will continue to shape our welfare rights.

Summary/conclusion

The modern welfare state was ostensibly created to remedy poverty and meet needs through the creation of social rights of citizenship.

This chapter has tried first of all to tease apart some of the complex arguments about how to define poverty and human need. A central theme in both sets of arguments is the conflict between absolutism and relativism. At one level absolutism is associated with individualist explanations of poverty and restrictive approaches to state welfare, while relativism is associated with structural explanations of poverty and expansive approaches to state welfare. At another level, however, relativism can also be associated with forms and notions of citizenship which are potentially authoritarian, and with a failure to specify and therefore to guarantee that which may be fundamental to human emancipation.

Second, this chapter has sought to demonstrate that social rights of citizenship have not made Britain a more equal society. Indeed, some groups in society (women, minority ethnic groups, older people and disabled people) remain more unequal than others. This has led to a discussion about what it is that social citizenship should achieve. Remedying poverty and meeting need requires a society that is inclusive not exclusive, but this need not imply any single model of citizenship. There is a tension between an essentially relativist vision of a discursively constructed citizenship of postmodernity, and what is in one sense an absolutist vision of a regulated citizenship in the Enlightenment tradition. There is, however, a more essential distinction that may be drawn between citizenship as a systemic construct and citizenship as an arena of human agency.

It may be seen that controversies about the fundamental nature of welfare rights do not always fit neatly with the left/right political conventions with which readers may be familiar. It should also be emphasised that such issues are certainly not unique to any one country, nor will they necessarily be resolved in the same way in all parts of the world. Accordingly, the next chapter will extend the analysis to consider welfare rights in a global context.

Chapter 3

Welfare rights in global perspective

This book is primarily concerned with welfare rights in a particular democratic-welfare-capitalist state, namely Britain. There are however dangers in concentrating on the British case. First, the classic view of social citizenship expounded by T.H. Marshall (see Chapter 1), because it related so specifically to the British case, is profoundly ethnocentric and provides only a limited understanding of the scope and limits of social citizenship. Second, the future of the welfare state in Britain and elsewhere is increasingly dependent upon global influences. This chapter aims to open up the discussion and to consider the role that social rights might play in alleviating poverty in different parts of the world. It will consider the different ways in which democratic-welfare-capitalism has emerged in the Western or developed world and the extent to which, in an era of 'globalisation', social rights and social policy may extend to other parts of the world. I shall also return to the issue of human rights and the emergent discourse of global citizenship.

To begin, however, we need to address the concept of 'development'; the implicit assumption that democratic-welfare-capitalism is the irresistible or desirable outcome of a universal process; and the relationship between economic development on the one hand and social or human development on the other.

Social rights and social development

We saw in Chapter 2 that different explanations are offered for the existence of poverty in its national context. Broadly speaking, these divide between individualist explanations based on notions of pathology, and structuralist explanations based on the idea that poverty has social causes. Vic George has observed that explanations of wealth and poverty at the international level – or of what is often called 'development' and 'underdevelopment' – can be divided along similar lines. There are commentators who attribute the failure of some countries to 'modernise'; to technological, cultural or political deficiencies that are internal to those countries. Other commentators attribute the continued disadvantage of developing countries to external factors and, in particular, the historical and structural economic dependency of poor and economically weak nations upon rich and powerful ones (George 1988: ch.1); to the ways in which poor nations are more vulnerable than rich ones to the power of transnational capital and the transnational corporations; or to the systematic ways in which the participation by poor nations in the global economy is regulated by supranational bodies such as the International Monetary Fund and the World Bank (Deacon 1997).

Whether we blame the losers for their own incompetence or the winners for unfair competition, the assumption it seems is that poverty at the international level reflects the outcome of a global race for economic development. Social ecologists have argued that while it would seem on the one hand that 'Capitalism needs poverty in order to survive' (Kemp 1990: 3), on the other hand there are finite global limits to economic growth (Meadows *et al.* 1972). Certainly, the ascendancy of international capitalism and the universal quest for economic growth must at least raise questions about how feasible it is for poor nations ever to 'modernise' and to develop their economies in the manner of their richer competitors. Even if we were to accept the contention by proponents of 'ecological modernisation' that it may yet be possible to sustain economic growth in spite of environmental constraints (see, for example, Dryzek 1997), there appears to be a logical and empirically demonstrable limit to the process (cf. Hirsch 1977).

That the world is divided between rich and poor is beyond dispute. Average income in the world's richest 20 countries is 37 times that in the poorest 20 countries (World Bank 2001). Table 3.1 compares the 'richest' and the 'poorest' ten countries in the world in 1998, measured by Gross Domestic Product per head of population. It may be seen that the GDP per capita in each of the tiny, but affluent, nations of Luxembourg and Switzerland was more than 400 times higher than that in war-torn Ethiopia in the Horn of Africa. By this criterion the richest ten nations of the world include the USA (which, with its huge population, is *collectively* the richest nation on earth), some seven Northern European nations (among which Britain is *not* included), Japan (whose economic fortunes, however, have waned since 1998) and Singapore (a small but spectacularly economically successful nation that, paradoxically, because it is not one of the 30 nations subscribing to the Organisation for Economic Co-operation and Development (OECD), is still classified as a developing country). By the same criterion the poorest ten nations are all in sub-Saharan Africa.

Knowing a country's GDP per capita does not tell us how its relative affluence or poverty might be translated into the living standards of its inhabitants (cf. Wilkinson 1996) and the United Nations Development Programme (UNDP) has constructed a number of composite indices, including the Human Development Index (HDI) by which it is possible to rank countries in terms of their achievements with regard to life-expectancy, adult literacy and education participation rates, as well as GDP per capita. In 1998 the highest-ranking country was Canada (which does not feature among the ten richest nations in Table 3.1) and the lowest-ranking was Sierra Leone (which does, but isn't quite the poorest nation in terms of GDP per capita). Obviously, some measure of economic development is essential if countries are to develop health and education services, but it is not the only factor. Nor is it the only factor in the direct alleviation of poverty. So as to reflect the fact that poverty is likely to be absolute in poor countries but relative in rich ones, the UNDP applies

Welfare rights in theory

Table 3.1 'Richest' and 'poorest' countries, 1998

'Richest' 10 countries

	GDP per capita 1998 (US$[1])	Population 1998 (millions)	HDI ranking 1998	% Population living on <US$[1]14.40 per day (1989–95)[2]
Luxembourg	46591	<5	17	4.3
Switzerland	44908	<7	13	–
Japan	42081	126	9	3.7
Denmark	37449	5	15	7.6
Norway	36806	<10	2	2.6
Germany	31141	82	14	11.5
Singapore	31139	<5	24	–
Austria	30869	8	16	8.0
USA	29683	274	3	14.1
Iceland	29488	<5	5	–

'Poorest' 10 countries

	GDP per capita 1998 (US$[1])	Population 1998 (millions)	HDI ranking 1998	% Population living on <US$[1]1 per day (1989–98)[3]
Niger	215	10	173	61.4
Mozambique	188	19	168	37.9
Eritrea	175	<5	159	–
Tanzania	173	32	156	19.9
Guinea-Bissau	173	<5	169	–
Malawi	166	10	163	–
Sierra Leone	150	<5	174	57.0
Burundi	147	7	170	–
Congo	127	49	152	–
Ethiopia	110	60	171	31.3

Notes:
1 Adjusted for purchasing power parity.
2 At 1995 values.
3 At 1993 values.
Source: United Nations Development Project (2000) *Human Development Report 2000*, New York: Oxford University Press (Human Development Indicators 4, 5, 7 and 19).

different measures of poverty in the developing as opposed to the developed world. In Norway, which was second in the HDI rankings in 1998 and has one of the most extensively developed welfare states in the world, fewer than 3 per cent of the population were in poverty by the relevant UNDP standard, whereas in Ethiopia, even by an adjusted standard, over ten times that proportion were in poverty, and in Niger over 20 times that proportion.

Of the world's 6 billion people, some 2.8 billion live on the equivalent of less than US$2 per day and 1.2 billion on less than US$1 per day (World Bank 2001). Most of those people were concentrated in the poorest countries, with over two-thirds of those living on less than US$1 per day being in either South Asia or sub-Saharan Africa, but it is also estimated that even in OECD countries there were in 1998 some 8 million people who were undernourished (UNDP 2000). Economic growth does not guarantee the elimination of poverty. So what is the role of social rights in protecting against poverty and what is the relationship between social rights and economic prosperity?

The so-called 'modernisation' theorists referred to above have assumed that there is a set path with predetermined stages that all nations must traverse in order to become mature civilisations. Sometimes associated with this view is the idea that, in a free world market, wealth will eventually 'trickle down' from rich to poor nations, just as it should 'trickle down' from rich to poor people within each nation. What matters, from this perspective, is that the engine of economic growth and development should be kept running. Within the spectrum of modernisation theories, however, there is another influential view, first propounded by Wilensky (1975), that the development of social rights follows as a direct result of economic prosperity. Wilensky sought to demonstrate a positive correlation between social security spending as a proportion of GNP and economic development as measured by per capita GNP and he inferred a causal relationship between the two.

So-called 'dependency' theorists and structuralists, on the other hand, would hold that economic growth does not invariably lead to social development and the enhancement of welfare. In fact, there is some evidence that the opposite can apply. Research by Newman and Thompson suggests that provision for basic needs (measured by indices of basic literacy, perinatal mortality and life expectancy) *precede* rather than result from economic development (1989). This research involved correlations over a 20-year period (from 1960 to 1980) of data from some 46 developing countries. More recently, Wilkinson (1996) has amassed a considerable body of evidence to demonstrate that health variations within countries relate not to the extent of their economic development, but to their degree of social equality. The more egalitarian and internally cohesive a society can contrive to make itself, he suggests, the better the general health of its people is likely to be. Not only is there no automatic link between economic growth and social development (UNDP 1993) but there is a positive association between economic growth and income equality (UNDP 1996). Social integration may actually be economically functional and measures that enhance 'social quality' through social rights may enhance rather than impair economic competitiveness (e.g. Gough 1997). Regardless of whether social rights help or hinder economic development, opponents of Wilensky's thesis – that welfare rights are a spin-off from economic prosperity – have argued that it takes insufficient account of the part that political processes play in determining the level of spending on things like social security provision (e.g. Castles 1982). Welfare rights are political achievements in their own right and not an incidental outcome of the capitalist development process.

Welfare state capitalism

It is in the capitalist welfare states that welfare has become a matter of rights. This does not, however, mean that there is any one example of the way in which social rights of citizenship have typically emerged. Nor does it mean that there is any dominant form of democratic-welfare-capitalist state.

Different roads to welfare citizenship

As has already been said, T.H. Marshall's theory of citizenship was based entirely on the British case, yet it is often presented as an evolutionary schema to account for all welfare states. That this is unsatisfactory has been pointed out by many writers, including Michael Mann (1987). For Mann, the strength of Marshall's thesis was that it showed how the development of modern citizenship served to render class struggle innocuous. Its weakness was that it failed to demonstrate the full variety of the strategies by which *ancien regimes* of the West have sought to institutionalise their conflict with class movements, both of the bourgeoisie and the proletariat. Mann suggests that, prior to the main phase of industrialisation, the West was divided into three kinds of regime:

- constitutional regimes (Britain and the USA) in which civil citizenship and a limited form of political franchise had already developed;
- absolutist regimes (such as Prussia, Austria and Russia) in which the monarch's despotic power was exercised partly by selective tactical repression, but also through 'divide and rule' negotiations with powerful corporate groups in society;
- 'contested' or 'merged' regimes in which conflict between absolutism and constitutionalists was either highly turbulent (as in France) or relatively peaceful (as in the Scandinavian countries).

From the nineteenth century onwards:

i Initially, the constitutional regimes took different paths – the USA, liberalism; Britain, reformism. The early extension of a universal franchise (i.e. full political rights) in the USA meant that class struggles were diverted and fragmented into interest group politics. The consequent absence of a developed labour and trade union movement accounts for the late and relatively limited development of social rights in the USA. In comparison, the much later development of political rights in Britain permitted the emergence of a strong labour and trade union movement requiring the accommodation of reformist strategies, more extensive social rights and the Beveridgean welfare state.

ii The absolutist regimes turned to 'authoritarian monarchy'. They had no intention of granting universal citizenship rights, but found ways to incorporate both bourgeoisie and proletariat through 'modernisation'. The civil legal code required for the successful development of capitalist production, distribution and exchange was conceded and limited forms of social citizenship were offered to stem the threat of organised labour. The classic example is that of late nineteenth century Germany, where Bismarck pioneered the introduction of social insurance. However, to the extent that political citizenship was allowed to develop, prior to the First World War, this was little more than a sham. Subsequent geopolitical upheavals were to play some part in the (temporary) emergence of fascism in Germany and authoritarian socialism in Russia.

iii The 'contested' regimes, such as France and Italy, endured protracted political upheavals until broad alliances between bourgeoisie, labour and small farmers could attain a lasting corporatist compromise. The 'merged' regimes of Scandinavia in fact pursued a kind of reformism which, as Mann points out (1987: 344), is probably closer to Marshall's vision than the British case!

Different kinds of welfare state

This returns us to the point made earlier, that social rights represent the outcome of political processes. It also returns us to the work of Esping-Andersen and the idea that there are different political responses to the process of 'commodification', which characterises capitalism (see Chapter 1). Esping-Andersen (1990) has suggested that there can be liberal, conservative or social democratic responses that will modify the consequences of market relations by allowing, respectively, a relatively low, medium or high degree of 'de-commodification'. He constructed a quantitative index by which to measure the extent to which the social security systems of different OECD countries will allow aged, sick and unemployed workers to exist on a 'de-commodified' basis, that is to say outside the labour market. He complemented this analysis by the construction of 'stratification indices', which measured the extent to which the social security systems of different countries are based on selective social assistance principles (a liberal approach), class or status reinforcing social insurance principles (a conservative approach), or on egalitarian universal benefit principles (a social democratic approach). Using contemporary empirical data, rather than an historical analysis, Esping-Andersen was able to demonstrate the existence of three 'clusters' of countries, exhibiting the characteristics of three different kinds of welfare state regime.

The first cluster contains liberal regimes. These are countries with minimalist welfare states such as the USA, Canada and Australia. State welfare in these countries is founded in the poor relief tradition, with emphasis on selectivity and means-testing of benefits and only modest levels of provision through social insurance or universal transfer schemes. Entitlement rules tend to be strict and benefit levels low, with encouragement being given to occupational fringe benefits and private or market-led forms of welfare provision.

The second cluster contains conservative or 'corporatist' regimes. These are countries such as Austria, France and Germany. State welfare provision in these countries is founded in a corporatist tradition; that is to say there is an emphasis upon policy negotiation between major corporate interest groups (especially tripartite negotiation between capital, labour and the state) rather than upon democratic/parliamentary processes. It is a tradition preoccupied less with free markets than with the preservation of status differentials and, for example, a privileged and influential civil service. The emphasis is on social insurance type benefits and universal family allowances. Levels of provision are usually high and occupational and private market welfare provision is marginal. Services such as daycare are underdeveloped, since motherhood and the 'traditional' family are encouraged. Benefits for those excluded from the labour market or traditional family support may be selective and poor.

The third cluster contains socialist or, more precisely, social democratic regimes, most notably the Scandinavian countries – Sweden, Norway and Denmark. In these countries, state welfare provision is founded in a universalist tradition concerned to promote an equality of high standards. The emphasis is on universal transfers, supplemented by earnings-related social insurance. Levels of provision are or have been high (for some, even luxurious) and occupational and private market provision is or has been effectively excluded. Full employment is an integral objective of policy, as are benefits and services for children and for parents wishing to work.

It is important to emphasise that what Esping-Andersen is describing are 'ideal-types' embodying features, tendencies or propensities that may be present in any given instance only to a greater or lesser extent and the balance of which will never be static. Changes in the political complexion of national governments can bring about shifts in the relative emphasis of policy. Also, not all countries 'fit' the typology and may in fact represent 'hybrids', combining features of different regime types. So, for example, although Britain in the mid-twentieth century had a certain amount in common with the social democratic welfare state model, by the end of the century it appeared – in spite of having near universal health care provision – to have more in common with the liberal welfare state regime category: far from providing a model by which to understand the nature of modern welfare states, Britain is an atypical and ambiguous case. The Netherlands, similarly, has certain features in common with social democratic welfare regimes (e.g. Goodin *et al.* 1999), though Esping Andersen continues to argue (1999: 87–8) that it should probably on balance be assigned to the conservative regime category.

An attempt is made in Figure 3.1 to map Esping-Andersen's typology on to Mann's historical typology of citizenship strategies. This illustrates the development of strategies adopted or negotiated to accommodate the class conflicts and economic restructuring associated with the rise of industrial capitalism. From the old European absolutism eventually emerged corporatist welfare regimes, providing developed social rights for workers, rather than citizens. From the early constitutionalist resistance to absolutism have emerged two very different kinds of welfare state: those in the English speaking world have tended to give rise to restrictive welfare regimes providing minimalist welfare rights primarily for the poor; the Scandinavian states have given rise to extensive welfare regimes, providing universal social rights for all citizens.

Esping-Andersen's typology has been criticised on several grounds. First, Leibried (1993) has argued that the Southern European nations – Spain, Italy and Greece – have rudimentary welfare states that do not directly compare with

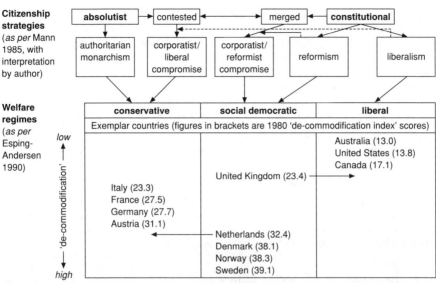

Figure 3.1 Citizenship strategies and welfare regimes

those of Northern continental Europe. Second, Castles and Mitchell (1993) have argued that the Antipodean nations – Australia and New Zealand – have what might be termed a 'wage-earner' welfare state that is more than residual in nature. Esping-Andersen has responded to both criticisms by admitting that any typology is problematic, 'because parsimony is bought at the expense of nuance' (1999: 71), while arguing none the less that Southern European states are essentially conservative and Antipodean states essentially liberal. A third criticism is that the typology does not easily accommodate Japan or any of the other East Asian capitalist states and I shall return to this issue later in the chapter. A fourth criticism, to which I shall return in Chapter 4, is that the typology fails to take account of the distinctive and different ways in which women's labour may be decommodified (e.g. Langan and Ostner 1991; Lewis 1992). To this final criticism Esping-Andersen has responded by admitting that his original formulation failed to take sufficient account of a process parallel to that of de-commodification, namely 'de-familialisation' or the process by which welfare provision may lessen individuals' reliance upon families. Esping-Andersen now argues that it may be changes in the household economy that will impact most upon the future trajectory of welfare regimes, but he insists none the less that his original model, while empirically focused on state benefit provision, was intended to take account of the differential role of family, market and state, and that the classification remains sustainable. Whether that is entirely true, the typology has been, as we shall see, hugely influential. Table 3.2 is a version of a summary of the regime characteristics posited by Esping-Andersen, adapted to demonstrate the relationship the regimes bear to the basis upon which welfare rights are constructed. Probably every capitalist welfare state can lay claim to aspects of all three regimes, and Britain is no exception. This, however, need not of itself diminish the explanatory value of the typology.

Table 3.2   Characteristics of capitalist welfare state regimes

	Conservative	Social democratic	Liberal
Role of:			
family	central	marginal	marginal
market	marginal	marginal	central
state	subsidiary	central	marginal
Degree of de-commodification	high (for bread winner)	maximum	minimal
Dominant locus of solidarity	family	state	market
Dominant form of welfare rights	compensatory rights for workers	universal rights for citizens	conditional rights for the poor

Source: adapted from Esping-Andersen 1999: Table 5.4, p. 8.

The globalisation of social policy

The concept of economic globalisation, though it is in many respects contested (e.g. Held *et al.* 1999), captures the extent to which, especially since the collapse of communism in the former Soviet Union and Eastern Europe at the end of the twentieth century, capitalism has become globally ascendant. In so far that globalisation limits the power of nation states (Horsman and Marshall 1994), Esping-Andersen (1996) himself has acknowledged that we have perhaps witnessed the end of the 'golden age' of the protective welfare state. Welfare statism, increasingly, is giving way to welfare pluralism (see Chapter 1 above). The triumph of capitalism in the 'late-modern age' has revitalised a normative interest in the role of civil society or 'community' – as a sphere that is conceptually distinct from state, market and family – in which social values may be fostered and welfare guaranteed without recourse to formal rights (Putnam 1993; Etzioni 1995).

On the other hand, there are elements of the welfare state, as will be argued later in this chapter, that are remarkably durable in spite of globalisation. What is more, despite the constraints on social policy at the level of the nation state, Deacon has argued that we are now witnessing a process that he describes as 'the globalisation of social policy and the socialisation of global policy' (1997: 4). Deacon's argument is that, with the end of the cold war, with the growing potential for economic migration from poor countries to rich countries, and with the realisation of the transnational consequences of environmental degradation, the governments of rich nations, supranational organisations (such as the World Bank and the International Monetary Fund) and transnational capital itself are all becoming increasingly conscious of the need to regulate global capitalism. The preoccupations of policy makers at the global level – at least prior to the terrorist atrocities in New York and Washington in September 2001 and the US-led military response – had been shifting from military and security concerns, through trade and economic concerns, to social and environmental concerns. As a consequence global capitalism, ostensibly, has begun to develop a more human face and has sought, for example, to co-ordinate debt relief for developing countries and to link such relief to their compliance with principles of good practice in social policy (see Deacon 2000). However, the precise nature of such principles remains contested. Deacon suspects that the model that will be imposed will entail elements characteristic of the liberal welfare regime outlined above. Whether or not this is so, the point to be grasped is that it is the dominant models represented by welfare regime theory that tend to inform the process.

There is a danger that principles with their own distinctive socio-historical provenance may be inappropriately applied (cf. Mamdani 1996). Outside the context of the political struggles that gave rise to them the principles that have informed the different kinds of capitalist welfare regime may simply be irrelevant. Wood (2001), for example, has argued that the welfare regime typology defined by Esping-Andersen relies on two key assumptions – a legitimated state and a pervasive labour market – that may not apply in some developing countries. There are parts of the 'non-Western' world where the state and the market have emerged or are emerging in ways that make it possible analytically to apply welfare regime typologies, albeit in a manner that must accommodate quite different historical and cultural conditions, but there are others where it is necessary to acknowledge that economic activity remains embedded in social relations; where the formalisation process or 'great transformation' (Polanyi 1944) that has characterised the process of economic development has not occurred in any functional sense; and where informal community based social networks and movements still in practice have primacy as determinants of human welfare over such institutions as the state, the market and even the family. There is scope within this chapter to do no more than briefly skirt over the current state of welfare rights in three broad types of country: post-communist, new capitalist and non-capitalist.

The post–communist world

Prior to 1989 the political, economic and social regimes that characterised the Soviet Union and its satellite states in Central and Eastern Europe were sufficiently distinctive to justify their classification as a sphere of influence quite separate from that of either Western-style capitalism or the less industrialised portions of the globe. The collapse of Soviet-style communism has dissolved the basis for that distinction. While some Central-Eastern European countries are now on the verge of joining the 'First World' club of capitalist nations by acceding to membership of the European Union, it is unclear whether the principal members of the Commonwealth of Independent States (broadly speaking, the nations of the former USSR) should be regarded as a part of the developed or the developing world.

Although Soviet-style communism manifestly failed to protect its citizens from poverty, it provided social rights through guaranteed employment, subsidised prices and extensive state-enterprise-based social benefits. The demands that led to the fall of that system were for the political and civil rights that it withheld. In the months preceding the Soviet Union's final collapse in 1991, President Gorbachov's attempts at *perestroika* were not only too late, they also entailed a top-down reconstruction of the system rather than reform from below. The people of the communist world continued to covet the political freedoms and economic rewards of the capitalist world and they were in practice little enamoured of the social rights at their disposal.

The welfare systems of the Soviet Union and Eastern Europe had guaranteed: a right to work; minimum wages at levels representing a high proportion of average wages; a free health service; free daycare for children, 3-year childcare grants for women and the right to return to work; highly subsidised housing; social insurance provision for retirement and sickness. Set against these benefits, however, there were drawbacks: the jobs that the state guaranteed to provide were often unproductive in nature or in reality non-existent; minimum wages fell consistently below poverty levels, while party and state bureaucrats enjoyed many valuable perks and undeserved privileges; health services were under-developed and bribes were often required to secure access to more advanced treatments; although women had the opportunity (if not an obligation) to work, they were still expected to shoulder the burden of domestic and care work; state housing was often of poor quality and strictly rationed, with the best housing often going to state or party bureaucrats; social insurance benefits were not index-linked and, because the existence of unemployment and poverty was denied, there had been no unemployment benefit and grossly inadequate social assistance (George 1993).

Under the guidance of foreign 'advisers' from the West, the precipitous transition of these command economies to market capitalism entailed a process of 'shock therapy' (Standing 1996). Price subsidies were withdrawn and state enterprises exposed to competition before any provision was made to develop alternative forms of social protection. The result was staggering increases in poverty and social inequality and a decline in health and life-expectancy indic-ators. When attempts were made to develop a social safety-net, these were strongly influenced by thinking characteristic of the liberal or residual welfare state model.

Deacon (1993) initially identified four main problems facing the transition process. First, while the old system in many respects failed, it did create popular expectations of what housing, health care and pensions should be like. To compound this, domestic politicians and Western free-market ideologues also generated expectations that free markets would be more efficient and could deliver what central planning had not. Second, the standards of public health and housing and the extent of poverty had been such that the scale of the investment and expenditure required to meet such expectations was con-siderable. Third, unemployment, which had in any event been rising, could be expected with the deregulation of the economy to reach crisis levels. Fourth, the collapse of the Soviet and Eastern European economies would mean that, pending a market-led recovery, there would be an insufficient and dwindling tax base from which to raise the revenue to address these issues. While predicting that some countries such as Hungary and the Czech Republic might take a different course, Deacon predicted that most former Soviet and Eastern European countries would end up not as liberal welfare regimes, but as 'post-communist conservative corporatist' states. His argument was that the historical legacy of countries like Russia was absolutist. In the absence of a democratic or constitutionalist tradition, and in spite of transnational influences, the powerful and adaptable *nomenklatura* that make up the emergent capitalist class, the communist 'old guard' and organised segments of the working class would broker a pragmatic social deal in which unrestrained economic growth would be traded for modest social protection.

Although elements of Deacon's analysis were prescient, it is still too early to say whether his characterisation of a post-communist conservative corporatism is right. In most of the larger countries it remains uncertain whether the influence of the World Bank and the IMF will result permanently in conditional forms of welfare rights; whether employers and workers will succeed in establishing processes of representation through which to negotiate compensatory forms of welfare rights; or whether the state can re-establish a position of legitimacy from which to develop universal forms of welfare rights (cf. Standing 1996: 249–50). In the meantime, struggles over social rights remain locked in a contest between a liberal intelligentsia that is generally hostile to social rights and a fragmented array of paternalistic non-governmental organisations (Stephenson 2000).

The new capitalist world

The term 'newly industrialised countries' has been applied to a variety of nations, some of which have been industrialised for many years and some of which are at least if not more economically successful than established capitalist nations. My concern here, however, is with two regions of the world that stand apart from both the English speaking and the continental European industrialised worlds, namely East Asia and Latin America. Most of the countries in both these regions are characterised by having relatively low social spending, but relatively high (or at least medium ranking) Human Development Index scores.

East Asia, prior to the financial crisis that beset the region in 1997, had witnessed impressive economic growth accompanied by falling levels of poverty. Catherine Jones (1993; 1999) has coined the term 'Confucian welfare states' to characterise not only Japan – which first industrialised in the late nineteenth century – but the emerging 'little tigers' of Hong Kong, Singapore, South Korea and Taiwan. More recent analyses, while expressing scepticism about Jones's terminology, have sought to include countries such as Malaysia, Indonesia and the Phillipines as examples of an East Asian regional welfare regime (Gough 2001). These nations all spend proportionately less on welfare than Western-style welfare states and they certainly do not conform to the liberal ideal; '... there is far too much social direction and too little sense of individual rights' (Jones 1993: 214). These are welfare states without social rights in the sense defined by T.H. Marshall and are run not so much democratically as by top-down consensus, '. . . in the style of a would be traditional, Confucian, extended family' (*ibid.*). The approach to social provision is pragmatic rather than doctrinaire, sometimes borrowing and sometimes avoiding Western examples to make up their 'own brand' welfare states. Characteristically, these states offer education, limited housing and health care provision, a deliberately constrained social security system and no personal social services. Where services are provided, there is heavy reliance on voluntary action. The economic 'miracles' contrived by these countries rested upon self-conscious policies of hierarchical community building. Within the tradition of popular Confucianism, government is supposed to represent a hierarchy with responsibility for national 'housekeeping'. It is not the voice or the moral conscience of the people and it is not responsible for those duties that fall to families and communities.

Esping-Andersen (1999) now insists that this is commensurate with the criteria by which he defines a conservative-corporatist welfare regime, although Japan in particular – as an OECD country – has often been presented as an 'exceptional' or 'hybrid' case. Goodman and Peng (1996) have argued against applying concepts derived from a Western framework and suggest that the East Asian region as a whole has been influenced by what might legitimately be termed a 'Japanese style welfare-system' appropriate to a meritocratic society in which class and class struggle have little salience. It is clear, none the less, that the Japanese/East Asian model has itself deliberately adopted and adapted Western welfare policies and, in the circumstances, it is not unreasonable to characterise the regimes in relation to the variety of sources upon which they have drawn. Holliday (2000) has defined them as 'productivist welfare regimes' (because social policy is subordinated to economic production) and Baldwin (1990) as 'Bonapartist' regimes (because social policy is used by social elites to maintain the status quo). Within the region, countries have been responding quite differently to the economic crisis that befell East Asia in the late 1990s (Gough 2001) and it is important not to overplay the similarities between them. It is significant none the less that both in Japan and elsewhere in East Asia there have been 'internal cultural debates' about 'the issue of "rights" – for which a whole new vocabulary has had to be constructed – and "obligations", which draws on the traditional Confucian ideas that applied essentially to the elites in the pre-modern period . . . but has been invoked consistently over the past decades in a number of different social contexts' (Goodman and Peng 1996: 215).

The Latin American region, which is usually taken to include Central and South America and the Caribbean, is at least as diverse as East Asia, but is very different in character. While certain East Asian countries were held up in the late twentieth century as examples of a capitalist economic miracle, Latin American countries have been held up as examples of a pernicious late-modern form of *laissez faire* capitalism. The terms 'Latinamericanisation' or 'Brazilianisation' were coined to describe an economic development strategy premised on unregulated inward investment and minimal welfare provision. Brazil has often been singled out as an example of a country in which extreme affluence and poverty were permitted to co-exist (e.g. George 1988) and Chile as the originator of neo-liberal private pensions policy (e.g. Midgley 1997). Barrientos (2001) has recently argued that, as a region, Latin America provides a rare example of a welfare regime shift. Several of the larger Latin American countries in fact had relatively well-developed welfare states from quite early in the twentieth century. These were characterised by highly stratified and fragmented social insurance arrangements, quite extensive employment protection measures and reasonably well-developed public health and education provision. Barrientos suggests that such arrangements represented a liberal-conservative hybrid regime with many parallels with the Mediterranean regimes with which, of course, the region enjoys historical links. As Huber (1996: 159) points out, 'these welfare states reinforced class and status distinctions and made the nexus of the labour market pivotal'. In the 1980s, however, the entire region was gripped by an economic crisis and was dependent for recovery upon assistance from international financial institutions, such as the IMF and the Inter-American Development Bank, conditional upon the implementation of neo-liberal 'structural adjustment' policies. These entailed the privatisation of social insurance arrangements, the deregulation of labour markets and the decentralisation of health and education provision, coupled with a shift from an industrialisation strategy based on import substitution to one that was strictly export-led. The result of these austerity measures, as in the post-communist countries, was a rise in poverty and inequality and a compensatory expansion in the amount of informal economic activity.

It would seem, however, that whereas East Asian countries were prepared to adapt Western social policy prescriptions on a selective and pragmatic basis, Latin America was more inclined to accept the underlying ideology, including and particularly in relation to the shrinking of the state (Huber 1996). That this was so reflects the extent to which democratic traditions in Latin America were weak (the region has experienced numerous military dictatorships and authoritarian governments) and political support for existing welfare institutions was fragmented (just as their coverage had been fragmented). Even when countries have sought to implement more universal forms of welfare provision (as has happened lately in Brazil), this is impeded by the legacy of local clientalism, especially in rural areas. In any event, Barrientos suggests, Latin America – subject to some important exceptions, such as Costa Rica – is now characterised by liberal welfare regimes. The high level of social risks faced by citizens across the region is associated, he implies, with a low level of rights (Barrientos 2001: 28).

The non-capitalist world

Finally, in this section, I shall turn very briefly to four parts of the developing world that do not have economies that may be described as capitalist or which cannot be meaningfully located as welfare regimes: the Middle East; South Asia; sub-Saharan Africa; and China. In each case, albeit for different reasons, it is difficult to equate welfare with rights.

The Middle Eastern region, which is normally so defined as to include the Arabic nations of North Africa, includes several spectacularly rich oil-producing nations, such as Saudi Arabia and Oman, as well as several much poorer countries such as Morocco, Iraq and Yemen. As nation states they are all relatively modern creations, but they encompass relations of power and patterns of social organisation that remain in some respects pre-modern. Destremau (2000) has characterised these states as 'rentier states'. They do not, by and large, have productive economies but are substantially dependent on external revenues from oil exports, financial revenues, royalties and tourism. Welfare provision consists in the distribution of such revenues. There is very little taxation and usually limited (if any) political representation. Acquired shares in a nation's 'rent' do not generally extend to groups such as migrant workers, peasants or nomadic pastoralists. None the less, prior to the 1980s, many of these states had developed extensive public service provision, generating public employment for an emerging middle class. The global economic crisis of the 1980s and its consequences exposed the Middle East to the influences of international financial institutions and 'structural adjustment', resulting in reduced social expenditures, an increase in poverty – not only for those that had always been excluded, but also among middle-class public sector workers – and the ceding of power to a fragmented range of non-governmental organisations. Though this has moderated the authoritarian power of state elites, the welfare outcomes are poor (especially for women) or inconsistent and there are no rights to welfare.

The South Asian sub-continent is mainly composed of countries with low social spending and poor human development outcomes, of which the largest is India. India is a country with an incipient welfare state owing much to its British colonial history. A substantial government bureaucracy produces impressive five-year plans, which have included rural employment creation programmes, water supply schemes, health centres, education facilities and housing. The plans also purport to give special attention to the needs of women and vulnerable minorities. In practice, the bureaucracy and local oligarchies reputedly misappropriate much of the resources and benefits of anti-poverty programmes. Western inspired egalitarianism fails to penetrate the *dharma* ethic that informs the Indian caste system. Imported Western health care and education practices are often ill suited to local needs and aspirations. At the same time India has, since independence, allowed most land and industry to remain concentrated in private hands and it has relied heavily on overseas aid and expertise for its industrialisation strategy. As a result, India produces cash crops and cheap consumer goods for the industrialised world, rather than subsistence crops and staple goods for its own population, and it remains locked into the world banking and finance system (see Townsend 1993: ch. 8). The situation in the other main countries of the region, Pakistan and Bangladesh, is similar (e.g. Davis 2001). To the extent that there is 'welfare' provision, especially in rural areas, it comes in the form of Food for Work programmes (that, despite the involvement of NGOs, can be subverted by patronage and clientalism at the local community level) and micro-credit schemes such as those operated by the widely acclaimed Grameen bank (that, none the less, often do little more than support income smoothing strategies for poor households, rather that the development of small enterprises).

However, the poorest region of the world, as we have already seen, is sub-Saharan Africa, a region in which, for most countries, colonial domination has been succeeded not so much by Western inspired models of governance as by a form of modernity without development (Bevan 2001) and in which, outside the urban centres, the populations are not citizens so much as subjects (Mamdani 1996). It is a region in which, for the most part, European social policy concepts have little purchase and a combination of pre-modern patrimonial social relations, illegal international trading networks and dysfunctional clientalist state forms hold sway. In the sub-Saharan African context, Bevan (2001) has argued for a concept of 'in/security regimes', rather than welfare regimes. While South Africa and Zimbabwe have higher levels of economic development and countries such as Botswana and Namibia enjoy diamond and mineral wealth, the majority of countries in the region are best described as insecurity regimes, ranging from the 'war lord regime' of Sierra Leone at one extreme to the 'humanitarian aid regime' of Sudan at the other. Even more than is the case in South Asia, the labour market and the state have not permeated as universal institutions. In such conditions, as Wood has argued (2001 and see above), entitlement to welfare stems largely from the 'rights of adverse incorporation'; from codes of fairness negotiated under the rule of local elites and community leaders, war lords, chieftains, mafia bosses, corrupt state bureaucrats and/or benign aid officials.

Turning lastly to China, as the world's most populous country and the last major communist nation it represents a unique case. Comparisons are often drawn between China and India and the radically different courses pursued by these very large developing nations (e.g. George 1988). In the early 1950s China nationalised most land and industry and gave it over to local collectives and co-operatives. The country accepted very little external aid and it emphasised a self-reliant path to industrialisation and endogenous styles of education and health provision. China's centrally planned approach has extended to the curtailment of population movements and other freedoms, but the result has been much higher economic growth than India has managed to achieve (George 1988: 77–8) and, lately, a dramatic reduction in income poverty – from 33 per cent in 1978 to 7 per cent in 1994 (UNDP 2000: 4). The People's Republic of China has been able substantially to honour the 'five guarantees' it makes its citizens – enough food, enough clothes, enough fuel, an honourable funeral and education for the children.

Critics of communism commonly complain that, notwithstanding the great strides China has made in realising the social rights of its citizens, it has also suppressed (with appalling brutality) the civil and especially the political rights of those citizens. This is true so far as it goes, but it misses the point that China does not provide *any* rights in the democratic-liberal sense. There are no rights vesting in the individual Chinese citizen. Pepinsky (1975), for example, has drawn a contrast between China, where there is no (or very little) formally promulgated legislation or written law, and a country like the USA, where rights and prohibitions are minutely prescribed by substantive written rules contained in public legislation. Western citizens have their freedoms guaranteed in writing and are enabled to calculate in advance whether any particular action may be liable to coercive restraint by agents of the state. By contrast, the Chinese citizen appears to the Western observer to enjoy no assurances against the prospects of social disorder and to be subject potentially to unlimited social control. Pepinsky argued, however, that very different kinds of freedom are involved. He contrasted the 'freedom of social mobility', enjoyed by citizens of Western countries, with the 'freedom of collective accomplishment'. Westerners are characteristically entitled to a high degree of spatial and occupational mobility, they are free (subject to the rules of marriage and divorce) to enter or to leave relationships with other human beings, and, increasingly, they rely on state authorities to resolve the disputes they may have with other human beings. Chinese citizens live and work where they are assigned and within a culture that emphasises reconciliation between disputants, the reintegration of the excluded, and open criticism and 're-education' of the delinquent. Yet, for all that, Chinese citizens are not subject so directly to the prescriptions of written law and substantive intrusion by the state. Official pronouncements in the People's Republic of China do not have the status of legislation: they may prescribe what collectives and communes should achieve but they do not prescribe the conduct required of individuals. Within the confines and strictures of their communities, Chinese citizens have freedoms to debate and participate, to adapt and to innovate, to work and co-operate in ways which formal written law might even inhibit. This is not to romanticise what is in many respects a semi-feudal form of society. Indeed, policies of market liberalisation in the 1980s have resulted in a weakening of the collective social protection that had been in force when Pepinsky was writing and an increase in social inequalities (see Leung 1994). The purpose here has been to underline the culturally circumscribed way in which rights to welfare are guaranteed in 'developed' Western countries. It is possible to have welfare without rights (see Rose 1993).

Global citizenship and human rights

In this final section I shall first return to consider why welfare rights remain an established feature of the developed world before enquiring whether, through the 'globalisation' of citizenship and human rights, it may yet be possible that they will in time extend in some form to all parts of the world.

The resilience of capitalist welfare states has given rise to a number of explanations or theses, which Mishra (1990) succinctly summarises as the irreversibility, maturity and pluralist theses. Irreversibility theses claim that state welfare has become essential to the survival of capitalism and cannot be dismantled. Maturity theses claim that, after a period of rapid development, most welfare states have no need for further growth and can be expected to consolidate. Pluralist theses claim that, in the process of surviving recent crises, the tendency has been for welfare states to adapt and to restructure their

commitments away from direct services in favour of the funding and regulation of welfare provision in the household, voluntary and market sectors. The
suggestion implicit in all such theses is that there is a natural level of state
welfare activity to which most developed countries will tend to approximate.
If this were true, it would leave two questions unanswered. First, given the
diversity of capitalist welfare states, is it likely that just one kind of welfare regime
will come in time to dominate in the developed world? Second, will this regime
eventually be exported, adopted by or imposed upon developing countries?

Prospects for convergence

Turning to the first of these questions, the part of the world where the
impetus for convergence between welfare regimes is greatest (but the direction
of convergence is least certain) is Western Europe. This is a consequence of
the 'widening' and 'deepening' of the European Union, as a supranational
governing body. While it is probable that the EU will continue to widen its
membership it is widely prophesied that there is a limit to this process and
that eventually the Union will shore itself up economically against the USA
and Japan on the one hand and against the interests of its poorer neighbours
to the East and the rest of the developing world upon the other (e.g. Simpson
1993). The sense in which the EU might also be 'deepened' reflects a desire
that the union between member states should extend beyond the economic
level to the monetary and political level and into the 'social dimension' (CEC
1993). It had always been envisaged that European integration should have a
social as well as an economic dimension though, in practice, this was seen to
relate largely to labour market issues and, for example, to the application of
modest levels of structural funding to help improve the economic infrastructure of disadvantaged regions. The 1989 EU Charter of Fundamental Social
Rights and subsequent instruments (discussed in Chapter 6 below) have sought
to give greater momentum to the process, but such binding directives and
policy statements as have emerged have tended to reflect a conservative/
corporatist concern for the rights of workers, rather than citizens. In so far
that the EU is concerned to address the social consequences of economic
integration, it seeks to combat not poverty and social inequality, but social
exclusion and risks to social cohesion (Townsend 1992; Gold and Mayes
1993; Room 1995; Levitas 1996).

I shall discuss the impact of this in the UK in later chapters, but here we
should note that Leibfried (1993) suggests there are two ways in which the
EU might bring about convergence in social policy. The first he defines as the
'Europeanisation' of poverty policy '. . . from the top down'. This would entail
the institutions of the EU imposing, for example, a European formula for
minimum income protection. Potentially, this might result in ascendancy for
a conservative/corporatist welfare model, but in practice there is little prospect
of a systematic pan-European harmonisation of social security policy so much
as a 'convergence of objectives' (Berghman 1991; Keithly 1991). The second
way in which European social policy might develop, Leibfried describes as

'Americanisation from the bottom up' (1993). Current EU social legislation is mainly procedural rather than substantive, leaving the implementation of welfare policy at the level of the nation state. This makes it possible for the EU to develop as a United States of Europe, in a manner that constitutionally would be similar to the USA. In the USA social rights of citizenship developed only after political citizenship had been fully established and to a much lesser extent than in Western Europe. Leibried argues that with the development of EU citizenship it will become possible and indeed necessary to develop procedural legislation that enables citizens from one European state to claim poor relief or medical treatment in any other European state. To an extent, this is already beginning to happen but, ultimately, it could progress beyond the present reciprocal funding arrangements to the provision of automatic EU-wide rights for all EU citizens and for the setting of minimum standards of provision. As happened in the USA, the assertion of individual rights to free movement might eventually draw concessions at federal government level so as to create new kinds of rights and new (generally minimal) duties for member states.

Different commentators have advanced other reasons for supposing that the liberal/residual welfare state regime characteristic of North America may represent a more dominant paradigm than that of the conservative/corporatist or social democratic regimes that characterise continental Western Europe and Scandinavia. Mishra, for example, has argued that economic globalisation, the attendant shift in power from labour to capital and greater political pluralism will have had a greater impact on Western Europe than North America, and are likely 'to bring the political economy (though *not necessarily* the social policy) of European welfare states somewhat closer to that of North America' [emphasis added] (Mishra 1993: 28). It is too early to be sure whether the welfare regimes of the developed world may converge upon a European or an American model. It is also too early to speculate about whether and in what way social rights in the rest of the world might converge.

Global citizenship

This, however, has not prevented discussion of the possibility that a form of 'global citizenship' might emerge, predicated on a global conception of human rights. Falk (1994), for example, has suggested that, quite apart from the consequences of economic globalisation, there are several other intimately interconnected grounds upon which it is possible to conceive or advocate forms of global citizenship: the longstanding aspirational demands for global peace and justice; emergent modes of transnational political mobilisation arising both from regional movements and new social movements; and the emerging ecological crisis. Although such a vision of global citizenship is far from being realised, Soysal (1994) has demonstrated how the institution and meaning of citizenship is none the less changing. She argues that two institutionalised principles of the global system – namely, national sovereignty and universal human rights – are now colliding (cf. Turner 1993). The concept of human rights is more global than traditional ideas of citizenship in so far that it encompasses notions of entitlement that transcend considerations of nationality. Soysal illustrates how one consequence of this is to be observed in the rights that are begrudgingly afforded by developed nations to foreign guestworkers. None the less, to the extent that it is the developed nation states that are accorded responsibility for maintaining human rights, paradoxically this can also fortify their authority in relation to developing countries and may justify humanitarian or even military intervention in other parts of the world. Soysal implies that as our concepts of rights become globalised they become abstracted and detached from our sense of local belonging or identity; from our capacity to regulate our own lives. Returning to the distinctions I developed in Chapter 1, human rights discourse tends to be abstract, doctrinal and 'top down', rather than concrete, claims-based and 'bottom up' in nature.

In this context, it is significant that the UNDP in the *Human Development Report 2000* should seek to concert its demands for human development with demands for human rights. Recognising that in the past 'the rhetoric of human rights was reduced to a weapon in the propaganda for geopolitical interests' (UNDP 2000: 3), the end of the cold war, UNDP argues, has created a climate in which it is possible to realise the common vision and common purpose that informs the respective concepts of human rights and human development: the former is concerned with basic human freedoms, the latter with the enhancement of human capabilities. The language of the *Human Development Report* is explicitly influenced by Amyarta Sen, whose work we discussed in Chapter 1 and who is acknowledged as the author of the report's first chapter. Sen's contribution to the report draws carefully upon Kant's distinction between perfect and imperfect duties, which he uses to underline the point that just because rights may not be fulfilled, this doesn't mean they do not exist. Sen's argument – as I read it – is that rights may be constituted through the aspirations and demands of the dispossessed even when the powerful repudiate or neglect the duties that such rights would impose upon them. This, however, is not quite the reading that the UNDP would seem to adopt in the rest of its report in which Sen's notion of human capability is subtly appropriated as a malleable concept more akin to that of human or social *capital* (cf. Coleman 1988; Putnam 1993). Development is assumed self-evidently to require economic growth; while rights require liberal democracy. Both require a pluralistic and apolitical social context in which NGOs and civil society groups can play a role as much as government (though, conspicuously, trade unions are never mentioned). The enforceability of rights, it is assumed, requires mechanisms akin to those by which global *trade* is governed. As it identifies the gaps that exist in the global order, the UNDP begins to draw upon managerialist expressions. It speaks of the need for incentive structures, for regulatory jurisdiction and for adequate participation. It speaks of the need for poor countries to avail themselves of the *opportunities* that globalisation offers (UNDP 2000: 9), but it seems not fully to recognise that while the powerful may interpret the risks of a globalised capitalist economy in terms of opportunity, the vulnerable may interpret them in terms of insecurity (cf. Vail 1999).

We can only welcome the UNDP's demand that – in the pursuit of human development – economic, social and cultural rights should be given as much attention as civil and political rights (2000: 13). None the less, the document contains many hallmarks of what has elsewhere been characterised as new managerialist doctrine (e.g. Hood 1991; Clarke and Newman 1997): its demands for better use of information is couched in the depoliticised language of evidence-based policy making; the processes by which the achievement of human rights can be managed invoke such recognisable techniques as self-assessment, benchmarking, culture change – drawn from the repertoire of new managerialism. Human rights have in a sense become colonised in the cause of a managerialist approach to human development. There is a danger perhaps that the powerful ideological ambiguity of welfare rights may be eclipsed by the market individualism that provides the unspoken ideological foundations of global managerial orthodoxy.

Summary/conclusion

Welfare rights are by no means the automatic outcome of capitalist development. This chapter has sought to illustrate this in four ways.

First, we have discussed the different ways in which capitalist welfare states have been formed. The social rights of citizenship provided in the former absolutist monarchies of Western Europe tend to differ in character from the social rights provided in constitutionalist English speaking countries. What is more, the social democratic ideal embodied in T.H. Marshall's notion of 'democratic-welfare-capitalism' has best been exemplified in Scandinavian countries.

Second, we have discussed the extent to which social rights in the post-communist world are in retreat. The efficacy of social rights under former communist regimes may have been impaired by the absence of a complementary framework of civil and political rights, but as the countries of the former Soviet Union and its Central and Eastern European neighbours struggle to adopt capitalism, the evidence is that this has been at the expense of social rights.

Third, we have discussed the extent to which social rights have or have failed to develop in the so-called 'developing' world. Particular attention has been drawn to the way in which notions of 'rights', founded in Western tradition, may be culturally inappropriate or even practically irrelevant to some parts of the developing world and to the possibilities that welfare provision may be developed without 'rights' in the sense that they are understood within the traditions of the West.

Finally, this chapter has considered the idea that social rights may in time converge towards a universal globalised form. The future of welfare rights both in Britain and throughout the world will be subject to global influences, but the outcome remains uncertain and the likelihood that a single type of welfare state will emerge as ascendant seems remote.

Having therefore underlined the point that the British form of social rights is far from being the only or an inevitable form, the next chapter will consider the extent to which social rights are necessarily an unambiguous good.

Chapter 4

Critiques of welfare rights

It should be clear from the preceding chapters that this book treats welfare rights as an ambiguous phenomenon. T.H. Marshall, whose concept of social rights was discussed at length in Chapter 1, looked upon social rights as a civilising influence, a form of 'class abatement' with consequences both for the stability of society and for the structure of social equality. Implicitly, this civilising influence would not only tame the excesses and redress the diswelfares of the capitalist system, but it would also temper or refine the conduct of the working class. The nature of this inherent ambiguity is most clearly brought out by Ian Gough, who has written of the welfare state that:

> It simultaneously embodies tendencies to enhance social welfare, to develop the powers of individuals, to exert control over the blind play of market forces; and tendencies to repress and control people, to adapt them to the requirements of the capitalist economy. (1979: 12)

In so far that modern welfare state and social security provisions have their historical origins within discretionary systems of poor relief, the extension of social rights can quite easily be portrayed as an extension of the crude controls exercised against the poor during capitalism's earlier stages (see Piven and Cloward 1974; Novak 1988). However, even allowing for the cross-national variations discussed in Chapter 3, the social rights that characterise the welfare systems of advanced capitalism differ significantly from the discretionary forms of poor relief that they have superseded, in their form and scale on the one hand and in their substance and sophistication on the other. Social rights are still associated with correlative duties and conditions of entitlement, but the nature of these is different in character. Challenges to the idea that citizens can have 'rights' to welfare and as to the nature of such rights have issued from several quarters and this chapter will explore certain of these.

Giving citizens rights is ostensibly one way of protecting their liberties; of safeguarding them from arbitrary power. This was fundamental to the strategy by which the property owning bourgeoisie, in their bid to wrest power from the crown and the feudal aristocracy, sought to impose their own conceptions of 'natural' rights through laws that were 'man made' (see Chapter 1 and, for example, Thompson 1975). For precisely this reason, conservatives in the mould of Edmund Burke have been mistrustful of any extension of human rights, since the only common right that they would recognise is the 'right to adjudication'; that is the right to be governed by the decisions of established authority with the power to translate imagined rights into realities (see Scruton 1991: 16–18). Rights are an explicit challenge, not only to traditional paternalistic authority, but also to newer forms of administrative authority. Fabian academics such as Richard Titmuss (1971), for example, have expressed themselves to be in favour of 'creative' or 'individualised' justice administered by compassionate experts, rather than the crude 'proportional' justice bestowed by rights that are legally prescribed. There are therefore those on both the left and right of the political spectrum who would question the need for rights that might impair the exercise of benevolent authority in the interests of the welfare of the people.

The history of the welfare state had been a story of transition from relief based on charity and discretion to benefits based on legislation and entitlement. Though conservatives resisted the welfare state and Fabians championed it, the common ground they shared was an attachment to the value of discretionary decision making. The compromise which both were prepared to strike with the liberal ideal of 'rights' can best be understood when it is realised that rights need not extinguish the scope for discretionary decision making. Dworkin (1977) makes the point that administrative institutions in advanced capitalist societies function in a discretionary 'void', surrounded like the hole in a doughnut by legal rules and principles. Rights created by legislation require the exercise of administrative discretion for the interpretation and application of those rules. The creation of rights to welfare extended rather than diminished administrative power, and the expansion of the discourse of rights into the realm of welfare has generated new theoretical and practical concerns about the relationship between state authority and the individual citizen.

In Chapter 10 I shall discuss the extent to which recent thinking about rights has sought to pay more attention to the responsibilities as well as the rights of citizenship. Behind this idea lies an assumption that, as a result of global forces, society has been changing and that we now inhabit a 'risk society' (Beck 1992). Class has been superseded as an organising principle and displaced not as T.H. Marshall foretold by citizenship with its attendant rights and guarantees, but by risk: the risk that is generated by unrestrained global markets and revolutionary technologies. The task of the welfare state is increasingly to do with the management of risk (Giddens 1994) and the promotion of responsible behaviour (Dean 2000). In so far that the contemporary inheritors or interpreters of traditional conservatism and Fabianism would both seem to have been embracing elements of a new communitarian agenda that is more sceptical about the efficacy of state intervention (e.g. Putnam 1993; Etzioni 1995; Tam 1998), the consensus about the role of the state and the scope of welfare rights may well be changing. None the less, that consensus still strongly supports the idea that dispensing welfare rights provides a means of regulating or influencing individual behaviour. Instances of this will be demonstrated throughout Part II of this book.

Challenges to the nature and effects of welfare rights have come from the radical wings of both the political Right and the political Left and from a range of radical new intellectual and social movements. These disparate challenges, albeit for quite different reasons, are concerned about the association between social rights and social control.

The neo-liberal challenge

In seeking to recapture and revitalise the classical doctrines of economic liberalism, so-called 'neo-liberals' would seek to restrict the rights of citizenship to civil and political rights, and primarily to the negative liberties by which the free play of market forces may be guaranteed. Though the distributive outcomes of impersonal market forces may be unequal, this is neither intended nor foreseen and cannot therefore be unjust. According to Hayek (1976) the very idea of social justice and of social rights that might compensate for such injustice is no more than a mirage. If the rich and successful have moral obligations, how and to whom these may be discharged is a matter of choice: such obligations are not enforceable and give rise to no implication that those who fail to prosper have rights against those who succeed. Translating wants and needs into rights was once described by the late Enoch Powell as 'a dangerous modern heresy' (1972: 12).

Among the things that neo-liberals condemn has been the substantive development since the Second World War of welfare states in countries such as Britain and, for example, the United Nations' Universal Declaration of Human Rights, which has been discussed in previous chapters. The significance of the latter, as we have seen, was that it encompassed not only civil and political rights (the right to life, freedom of movement, right to a fair trial, universal enfranchisement, etc.), but also social and economic rights, including the right to social security, to work, to education and even to leisure.

At the level of rhetoric at least, welfare rights enjoy internationally recognised status as basic human rights (see Watson 1980: ch. 10). This gives rise to two kinds of objection, the first characterised by Nozick, who claims that welfare rights violate property rights; the second from Cranston, who claims that welfare rights do not meet the conditions necessary to qualify as basic human rights.

Turning first to Nozick (1974), his argument is based upon a contentious interpretation of Kant's alternative formulation of the 'categorical imperative', namely that respect for other persons depends upon their being regarded as ends in themselves and not as means. This he uses to build a case against any form of social rights requiring redistribution. For Nozick, the inviolability of the individual is synonymous with the inviolability of the property in which her rights are vested. To redistribute any portion of that property to another is to treat that person as a means and not an end. We may not violate persons for the social good because, says Nozick (in words remarkably similar to Margaret Thatcher's infamous 1988 declaration that 'there is no such thing as society'), 'there is no *social entity* with a good which undergoes some sacrifice for its own good. There are only individual people with their own individual lives' (1974: 32). Individuals may choose to undergo some sacrifice for their own or somebody else's benefit, but they should not be compelled to do so in the name of some other person's 'right'. Such compulsion does not create social rights but rights of the state over the property of its own citizens; rights that violate the principle of respect for persons.

Second, there is Cranston's denial that social rights can be human rights (1973 and 1976). Drawing upon the traditions of legal positivism that have long been associated with classical liberalism, Cranston returns to the distinction discussed in Chapter 1 above between legal rights (which are 'positively' defined) and human rights (which are 'morally' defined). Human rights pertain to a human being by virtue of her being human and, according to Cranston, they have three tests of 'authenticity': practicability, paramount importance and universality. Civil and political rights by and large meet these criteria in so far that they are relatively easily secured by appropriate legislation, they are fundamentally necessary to the just functioning of capitalist society and they may be applied genuinely to everybody. Social and economic rights, however, are of a different order. The resources required for a social security system, for example, may be beyond the command of governments in the poorest 'developing' countries; social services and economic security may represent an ideal, but they are not essential; and the needs which social rights address are relative, not universal. Therefore:

> the effect of a Universal Declaration which is overloaded with affirmations of so-called human rights which are not human rights at all is to push *all* talk of human rights out of the clear realm of the morally compelling into the twilight world of utopian aspiration. (1976: 142)

Objections to these views are rehearsed elsewhere (e.g. Plant *et al.* 1980: ch. 4; Watson 1980: ch. 10). The two points which need to be drawn out are that what is here characterised as the neo-liberal case against social rights rests, first, upon the costs of achieving social rights and in particular the role this affords to the state and, second, that social rights do not supplement but undermine the liberties necessary to the perpetuation of capitalism.

The neo-Marxist challenge

From the opposite end of the ideological spectrum comes a contrasting set of arguments, but arguments that can be just as sceptical about the value of social rights. First, there is a group of academic writers who have sought to interpret Marxist principles in relation to the role that social rights play in regulating labour and sustaining rather than undermining capital. Second, there are theorists who have developed the Marxist critique of the form of individual legal rights in order to demonstrate the capacity of social rights for ideological mystification and control.

Turning to the first of these approaches it is necessary to be clear that there are different strands of thought within neo-Marxism. There is an *intrumentalist* strand that adopts from Marx's earlier writings the idea that the state under capitalism acts as no more than 'a committee for managing the common affairs of the whole bourgeoisie' (1848: 69). There is also a *structuralist* strand deriving from Marx's later writing and which analyses state forms as an expression of the immanent logic of the capitalist system and its class antagonisms. When neo-Marxists have come to analyse the twentieth century welfare state and the significance of the development of social rights, both these strands have become to some extent intertwined.

The first kind of critique was developed by writers such as Saville (1958), O'Connor (1973) and Gough (1979). They began to forge an account of how the welfare state had developed, claiming in essence that it was the product of three interacting influences. The first of these influences was the struggle by the working class for better living conditions. The social policy reforms obtained in this way had the effect of increasing levels of social consumption and general living standards; but they also benefited capital by furnishing an element of 'quantitative regulation' over labour power – partly by reducing the direct costs of labour, and partly by having the state look after people whose labour was not required. The second influence was capital's growing need for an efficient environment and a productive workforce. The reforms resulting from this influence amounted to the investment by the state of human capital and the necessary modification of labour power through the provision of health and education services so as to produce better workers. The third influence was a concern for political stability. The policies resulting from this influence involved the discharge of the social expenses necessary for the 'qualitative regulation' of labour power; or, more crudely, for the production of contented workers through the provision of those benefits and services required to secure social order and a degree of ideological control.

The neo-Marxist writer to engage most directly with the idea of social rights was Claus Offe. One of his central arguments was that 'the owner of labour power first becomes a wage labourer as a citizen of a state' (1984: 99). Industrial capitalism required more than the passive compulsion of economic forces in order to get people to accept the burdens and risks associated with wage labour and a market economy. To make people actively participate it was necessary to have what Offe described as 'flanking sub-systems', namely systems of political–administrative and normative control. Social policy is 'the state's manner of effecting the lasting transformation of non-wage labourers into wage labourers' (*ibid.*: 92). This is the basis upon which Offe challenges T.H. Marshall's account of social rights (see Chapter 1). Social rights were not some optional extra or final refinement to citizenship under capitalism; they are, according to Offe, a necessary part of it. Without such rights citizens would not 'muster the *cultural motivation* to become wage labourers' (*ibid.*: 94). Within Offe's account, social rights were necessary, first, as a precondition for the suppression of begging and modes of subsistence that might undermine the wage labour system; second, as the medium through which to justify the provision of facilities for improving the quality of labour power (in ways of which individual self-seeking capitalists are incapable); third, as a mechanism by which potentially or conditionally to exempt certain parts of the population from labour force participation (mothers, children, students, disabled people, old people). Social rights are as important as civil rights as a device for articulating labour power with the market.

Turning now to the second kind of neo-Marxist critique, this is concerned less with the substance or effects of social rights as with their form. Marx himself argued that law and state apparatuses are no more than 'superstructural' phenomena, supported and indirectly shaped by the economic 'foundations' upon which they are constructed (1859). In *Capital* (1887), however, he went further and sought to demonstrate that the form of individual rights within bourgeois liberal ideology is a logically necessary consequence of capitalist production and market exchange. Because under market conditions goods must be exchanged as commodities, the producers and owners of such commodities must recognise in each other the rights of private proprietors and relate to each other on the basis of legal and contractual rules. Under capitalism it is not only materials and products that are traded but, following the destruction of feudal land tenure, real estate and even human labour are 'freed' to enter the market as commodities. Rights in ownership – of goods, land or labour power – become the universal foundation of human relationships. Unlike Hegel (whose account of rights was similar – see Chapter 1), Marx dismissed rights in ownership as an illusion, a 'fetishised' form that obscures the fundamentally exploitative substance of the social relations of production under capitalism.

In the course of the twentieth century these ideas have been taken up by other writers, foremost of whom was Pashukanis (1978). Writing in the 1920s Pashukanis argued that, since it is the exchange of commodities that forms the very basis of social life under capitalism, even such fundamental legal concepts as equity, restitution and entitlement are all derived from the commodity form. Just as 'value' is a concept which fundamentally defines our understanding of the nature and capacities of commodities, so 'right' is a concept that fundamentally defines our understanding of the nature and capacity of human beings. The individual juridical subject or citizen, as the bearer of rights, is the 'atom' – the simplest irreducible element – of legal and administrative theory. Pashukanis argued that this private form of possessive individual right has been rendered universal by being appropriated into the sphere of public and administrative law. This abstract line of reasoning has been developed by later theorists (see Holloway and Picciotto 1978) who have claimed that the form of the state – and the form of welfare rights and social legislation – is 'derived' from capitalism's characteristic commodity form and from the nature of the wage relation as the most exploitative expression of that commodity form (see Dean 1991: 14–16). The challenge here is that social rights are not all they seem. To cloak human welfare in an ideological discourse of 'rights' conceals the fundamental nature of relations of power under capitalism. It is nonsense to suggest that civil rights will guarantee that individual employees may bargain on equal terms with corporate employers, and it is nonsense to suggest that social rights will guarantee unemployed people, pensioners or disabled people power to negotiate their claims with departments of state. Social rights give expression to the ultimate dominance of capital over labour and serve to extend or permeate that dominance beyond the immediate sphere of the wage relation, into the sphere of state–citizen relations, and into everyday life.

Once again, objections to these views are rehearsed elsewhere (e.g. Campbell 1983 or, more generally, Hall and Held 1989). However, in spite of differences between them, the essence of the neo-Marxists' case against social rights is, first, that in ameliorating the exploitative impact of capitalism they help ensure its survival; second, that social rights provide a powerful mechanism for state/ideological control.

The challenges of 'postmodernity'

As we have entered the twenty-first century it is tempting, if perhaps facile, to suppose that we have attained a new age of 'postmodernity'. In Chapter 3 it was noted that the global trends which allegedly characterise postmodernity are, first, the exhaustion of 'grand narratives' such as liberalism and Marxism; second, far-reaching cultural changes resulting from technological, economic and social changes; third, political pluralism and the growth of new social movements. Such trends, it is claimed, pose a threat to the notions of universalism and progress upon which democratic-welfare-capitalism is founded (for succinct accounts see Williams 1992 and Hewitt 1994). Against such views theorists like Habermas (1985) and Giddens (1990), albeit in different ways, argue that modernity continues to evolve and that the great Enlightenment project is not yet complete.

With regard to the first of the abovementioned trends, Taylor-Gooby (1994) has retorted that the world is witnessing not a global disillusionment with all grand narratives, but the ascendancy of just one of them. The spreading influence of New Right thinking in the capitalist world, the collapse of communism and the far-reaching effects of the monetarist policies of the IMF and World Bank in the 'developing' world signal a near global triumph of a classical or neo-liberal version of the capitalist project and of the patterns of poverty and inequality which such an ideology is prepared to tolerate. The full significance of this, says Taylor-Gooby, is obscured by the 'ideological smokescreen' (*ibid*.: 385) of postmodernism.

None the less, the second and third of the trends attributed to postmodernity are of undeniable importance, not least because they have fomented alternative insights, theories and critiques concerning the nature of *modernity* rather than 'postmodernity'. To the extent that these bear upon the 'modern' notion of social rights, it is to these that this chapter now turns. I shall first discuss what are sometimes called post-structuralist critiques of modernity, second, I shall examine 'emancipatory' critiques associated with new social movements (specifically, feminism and anti-racism) and, finally, I shall touch upon some of the 'defensive' critiques emanating from the new political pluralism (the distinction between emancipatory and defensive social movements is drawn from Habermas 1987b: 393).

Post-structuralist critiques

Theorists of postmodernity have called into question whether the eighteenth-century Enlightenment that gave birth to 'modernity' was ever a dispassionate quest for truth and reason. On the contrary, according to Bauman, it was an exercise in two parts:

> First, in extending the powers and ambitions of the state, in transferring to the state the pastoral functions previously exercised by the church, in reorganising the state around the function of planning, designing and managing the reproduction of social order . . . secondly, in the creation of an entirely new and consciously designed mechanism of disciplinary action, aimed at regulating and regularising the socially relevant life of the subjects of the teaching and managing state. (1987: 80)

Bauman is echoing here the arguments of Michel Foucault, whose claim had been that modernity was based not on scientific reason and rationality but the 'will to power'; that the legitimacy of modern governance was an effect of power and not truth or justice; that the reality behind the veil of democratic-welfare-capitalism is that of an inherently 'disciplinary society' (see especially Foucault 1977). These arguments have influenced some particular critiques of the disciplinary aspects of social policy (Squires 1990; Dean 1991). The basis for such approaches has been a re-examination of the history of the welfare state and of the increasingly sophisticated surveillance and disciplinary processes associated with the administration of welfare rights and social legislation. These approaches invoke a relational theory of power that holds that the shift from feudalism to capitalism was associated with a shift from coercive to adminis-trative (welfare) state power. Administrative state power has had as much to do with the regulation of human behaviour as the 'dull compulsion' of economic forces. The development of state welfare and social rights has involved new *technologies of power* and pervasive new *disciplinary techniques*. The characteristic of these technologies and techniques is that, unlike class power, they bear upon *individual difference*. In place of the uncontrollable mass is the controllable individual subject.

My own account (Dean 1991) has concentrated upon three intersecting processes by which citizens of the modern welfare state have been constructed. First, there has been an historical process of transition 'from begging bowl to social wage' (*ibid.*: 37). In place of the indiscriminate giving of alms to the anonymous poor there has been erected the complex panoply of the welfare state which scrutinises and documents each individual 'client' or 'case'. In place of careless humanitarianism there has been inserted meticulous paternalistic control. Second, there has been an historical process of transition 'from corporal to pecuniary sanctions' (*ibid.*: 43). In place of such practices as the public whipping and branding of vagrants there have emerged more discreet and gentle forms of coercion based on benefit penalties and disqualifications. In place of an explicit Malthusian desire to punish the poor there have developed more subtle forms of containment. Third, there has been an historical process of transition 'from oppression to discipline' (*ibid.*: 51). In place of crude processes of classification and surveillance associated with the workhouse and the Poor Laws there have been constructed administrative systems based on legal definitions and regulations to which citizens must submit in order to exercise their 'rights'. In place of the prying concern and moralistic edicts of philanthropists and utilitarians there has emerged a voluntaristic discourse based on the idea that citizens of the welfare state are juridical subjects with the freedom to exercise their rights and a responsibility to abide by the rules.

The history of the welfare state is therefore seen not as a story of progress towards the development of universal social rights, but as a story of developing state power and increasingly sophisticated methods of social control. It is additionally argued that, far from dismantling state power, recent policies of welfare retrenchment have often involved subtle refinements to the disciplinary mechanisms that underpin our rights to welfare (*ibid.*: ch. 7; Dean 1988/9, 2000).

Feminist critiques

In the sphere of social rights – as in the sphere of civil and political rights – women are 'second-class citizens' (see, for example, Lister 1990). Past generations of feminists have campaigned against limitations upon property rights (not redressed until 1882) and voting rights (not fully redressed until 1928), yet women remain by and large economically and politically disadvantaged. In the 1940s feminists campaigned for social rights (Dale and Foster 1986) and against the limitations upon women's social rights that the Beveridge Report portended (see Abbott and Bompas 1943).

Feminism's most recent 'wave', however, has challenged, in ways that previous generations did not, the underlying form as well as the substance of their 'rights'. The problem with the universalistic liberal conception of equal rights is that, even where it acknowledges that men and women should be treated the same:

> treating people as though they are the same is quite different from treating them as equals. This approach neglects crucial differences, for example, the fact that in a market economy being a parent means being less 'free' and hence less 'equal' in the labour market than a single person; a mother is significantly less free and equal than a father. (Langan and Ostner 1991: 139)

Though there remains a liberal feminist strand whose concern is to promote equal opportunities legislation (Williams 1989: 44–9), the 1970s and 1980s witnessed the birth of socialist and radical strands of feminism whose resistance to women's oppression is founded in an analysis of patriarchy. Patriarchy is regarded as a structural characteristic of human society and, in spite of important differences between the newer strands of feminism, their central theoretical insight relates to the distinction that may be drawn between society's public and private spheres (see especially Pascal 1986/1997). The public sphere is where civil and political rights reside; it is the domain of the market and the state; it is the site of productive and administrative activity that is dominated by men. The private sphere, in contrast, is not inhabited by rights; it is the domestic domain of hearth, home and family; it is the site for the reproduction of social life, a process to which women are confined. The public/productive sphere is separated from, yet dominates, the private/reproductive sphere. Social rights have been immensely important to the articulation between the two. As Pascal puts it, the welfare state was created 'in the void between the factory and the family' (1986).

Welfare rights and social legislation have succeeded in redistributing resources from men to women but, for all that, the development of the social rights of democratic-welfare-capitalism has failed women on two counts: first, because they have been instrumental in the supervision and enforcement of women's dependency in the private sphere; second, because they have not compensated women for their disadvantaged position in the public sphere.

Women and the issue of women's dependency have been ignored and rendered invisible in most mainstream (or 'malestream') analyses of social rights. Certainly, this was true of T.H. Marshall (see Lister 1990: 56). While social rights may have ameliorated the effects of class differences, their effects on gender differences were not even considered. Such architects of the welfare state as Beveridge were so inured to patriarchal ideology that it was explicitly assumed that married women would be financially dependent upon their husbands. While such directly discriminatory features have since been removed (albeit in Britain largely as a result of Equal Treatment Directives from the EU), the structure of social security benefits, for example, remains indirectly discriminatory. In practice it is predominantly male heads of household who claim benefits on behalf of predominantly female dependants. As Lister puts it, for such women 'rights mediated by their partners cease to be genuine rights' (*ibid.*: 58).

Similarly, the systematic disadvantage of women in the public sphere, and particularly in the labour market, has been ignored. For example, Esping-Andersen's influential account of the role of social rights in 'de-commodification' (which I outlined in Chapter 1) has been criticised by Langan and Ostner (1991) because, although it recognises the importance of women and families at the empirical level, it fails to confront their theoretical significance.

> Men are commodified, made ready to sell their labour power on the market, by the work done by women in the family. Women on the other hand, are decommodified by their position in the family. Thus men and women are 'gendered commodities' with different experiences of the labour market resulting from their different relationship to family life. The role of social rights in decommodification differs according to gender, in general protecting men's position in the labour market while disadvantaging women by restricting their access to certain areas of employment.
> (1991: 131)

Once again, the issue is not only one of direct discrimination (though the strategies of employers for excluding women from higher paid men's jobs are important), but also of the failure of social rights to redress the unequal burden of (unpaid) caring and domestic work which women carry. As Smart has put it, 'the acquisition of rights in a given area may create the impression that a power difference had been "resolved"' (1989: 144). Social rights, especially in countries such as Britain, have not done enough in terms of guaranteeing care provision (for example, for pre-school children or disabled relatives) fully to allow women independent access to the labour market; and they have done nothing at all to guarantee a more equitable sexual division of labour within the ideologically constructed family. Additionally, some feminists advance arguments similar to post-structuralists and point out that, historically, seeking refuge in claims to 'rights' has resulted for women in their being subjected 'to more refined notions of qualification . . . more centralized knowledge of sexual relationships, child care organisation, and so on . . . the possibility of greater and greater surveillance' (Smart 1989: 142).

More recently, feminists such as Sevenhuijsen (1998; 2000) have challenged the fundamental ethical premise that underpins welfare citizenship by arguing for a 'democratic ethic of care' that 'starts from the idea that everybody needs care and is (in principle at least) capable of care giving' (2000: 15). Inclusive relationships, it is argued, are achieved in the context of specific social networks of care and responsibility and cannot be created by ascribing rights and responsibilities. The citizen must first be understood not as an abstract individual or 'equal rights holder', but as a 'self-in-relationship'. On the one hand, Sevenhuijsen argues, 'vulnerability is part and parcel of ordinary human subjectivity' (*ibid.*: 19), while on the other hand care is a daily practice. There is a resonance between this line of reasoning and the argument I advanced in Chapter 2 when discussing 'interpreted needs'. A feminist ethic of care, potentially, displaces the discourse of welfare rights in favour of an understanding that human freedom is built upon interdependency: it is our need for and our capacity to care that precede and shape our rights and responsibilities. This is an important line of reasoning to which I shall return in Chapter 11.

Anti-racist critiques

Like the feminist critique, the anti-racist critique of social rights claims that members of minority ethnic groups in countries such as Britain remain 'second-class' citizens (see Lister 1990: 52). As a social movement (rather than as an intellectual critique) anti-racism has not had the same profile as feminism, but just as contemporary feminism is organised around a theoretical critique of patriarchy, so anti-racism has been organised around a theoretical critique of racism. There are differences between anti-racist theorists concerning the degree to which racism is autonomous of other forms or dimensions of oppression (Williams 1989: ch. 4), but what distinguishes the anti-racist critique from 'liberal' concerns about racial discrimination is that it regards racism as an ideology. Racism is seen not as a set of attitudes held by 'white' or majority ethnic groups about people from minority ethnic groups, but as a set of outcomes arising from a system of legal, policy, institutional and discursive practices. Just as the sexual division of labour is rooted historically in the ideological construction of 'the family', so there is a racial division of labour that is rooted historically in the ideological construction of 'the nation' and, in Britain's case, its rise and fall as an imperial power (Miles and Phizacklea 1984).

The rights of citizenship enjoyed by minority ethnic British citizens have not prevented their being twice as vulnerable to unemployment as 'white' citizens (Oppenheim 1993) and, when in employment, having lower average earnings (see, for example, Breugal 1989). The incidence of poverty is higher among Britain's minority ethnic population than among the 'white' population (Amin and Oppenheim 1992) and yet there is evidence that the take-up of social security benefits is lower among the former than the latter (see, for example, NACAB 1991; Cook and Watt 1992). Inclusionary notions of citizenship and the rhetoric of universal social rights are contradicted by exclusionary practices towards people from minority ethnic groups and their differential access to welfare. The 'racialisation' of politics in post-war Britain has revolved around two contradictory moments: on the one hand, the extension of immigration control and restrictions upon the definition of citizenship; on the other hand, the development of race relations legislation and measures supposedly to guarantee the civil rights of minority ethnic groups (see, for example, Solomos 1989). The former has had both real and symbolic significance for the extent to which people from minority ethnic groups can become or consider themselves to be British citizens; the latter has been limited in its effects and has failed to secure substantive equality of access to welfare benefits and services. Both moments have a common fulcrum. As was pointed out by Cranston in his polemic against social rights (see above), civil and political rights are relatively easy to secure, but social rights do not come cheap. To guarantee employment, social security or housing requires resources. If such resources are constrained (whether for economic or political reasons), one way to limit demand is to adopt a restrictive definition of who shall be a citizen; another is to ration public resources and, while it is possible formally to guarantee equality of opportunity for *individual* citizens, administrative rationing may tend substantively to exclude those *groups* of citizens who are already subject to systemic disadvantages.

Since the first Aliens Order of 1905, the preoccupation of British immigration controls has been to prevent poor racial minorities from obtaining any right of citizenship that might entail an expenditure of public funds. The original legislation had been fuelled by anti-Semitic sentiment following an influx in the late nineteenth century of Jewish migrants from Eastern Europe. Its effect was to exclude from Britain any 'alien' not having adequate means of assistance and to provide for the expulsion of aliens found to be in receipt of poor relief. This precedent has informed all subsequent immigration controls, including those introduced in the 1960s and early 1970s to restrain Commonwealth immigration. The latter controls had been fuelled by racist sentiment directed against African-Caribbean and South Asian immigrants from former British colonies who had been enticed to Britain during a period of labour shortage in the immediate post-war period. The principles upon which such immigration controls were built were enshrined in nationality law in 1981, effectively excluding from citizenship all but those with a link by direct descent to the UK. As recently as 1988, the right of British citizens to be joined by a non-European spouse was made subject to the condition that they must be able to maintain that spouse without recourse to public funds. It is people from minority ethnic groups (especially those of African-Caribbean and South

Asian ethnic origin) who have been most systematically excluded from British citizenship and, to the extent that social rights are synonymous with 'recourse to public funds', it is from the social rights of citizenship that they are most rigorously excluded (see Craig 1999). The most dramatic illustration of this has been witnessed in recent years with the imposition of draconian restrictions on the rights of asylum seekers (see Chapter 5).

Because access to social security benefits, housing and other forms of welfare provision can therefore be conditional upon immigration status, 'it has become legitimate for a range of officials to question claimants and others about their status and thus to act as agents of immigration control' (Gordon 1989: 7). This can act as a deterrent, even for people from minority ethnic groups who are legitimately settled in Britain. What is more, access to social rights is often dependent upon citizens' capacity – in terms of knowledge and linguistic skills – to exercise their rights, and/or upon their past employment record (in the case of state pensions, for example). Race relations legislation, which provides a somewhat circumscribed right of individual redress, is unlikely to be strong enough to guarantee equality of access for all. It will be of little value to those whose difficulties relate to a lack of information or language skills and no value at all to those who are excluded from rights by the structural features of state provision.

The emancipatory claims of feminism and anti-racism are based upon an analysis of relations of power or oppression other than class and upon dichotomies other than those between the market and the state. Fiona Williams (1989 and 1992) emphasises the importance of the intersections between class, gender and 'race' and argues for social policies that can resolve the tensions between universal prescription on the one hand and the recognition of social diversity and difference on the other. Rather than argue on the basis of universal or general conceptions of need, emancipatory critics argue from particular needs (of women and minority ethnic groups) to general needs. There is a sense in which they attempt on behalf of particular constituencies to redeem the universal promises offered by the 'liberal' conception of rights (see Hewitt 1993).

Defensive critiques

The 'defensive' critiques to which I finally turn offer a different kind of challenge to the Marshallian conception of social rights. The examples that will be cited, while not necessarily representative of new social movements, have in common the two-fold characteristic attributed to such movements by Alan Scott (1990) in that they are concerned both to promote an expansion of citizenship and to insert excluded groups within the polity. I propose very briefly to outline three complementary lines of argument in favour of a democratisation of the welfare state and a rethinking of the basis for social rights. What links the three approaches is that they are (or tend to be) anti-statist. However, their scepticism of state intervention is more radical in character than the essentially conservative communitarianism to which I alluded in the opening section of this chapter.

First, perhaps a seminal formulation of the pluralist critique of the welfare state was that provided by Hadley and Hatch (1981). It was a critique informed in some respects by the community development movement of the 1970s and prefigured in others by the writing of Illich *et al.* (1977) and Lipsky (1976). Hadley and Hatch's quarrel was with the centralised nature of the welfare state and the character this afforded to the administration of social rights. Unitary government, they claimed, is an inheritance that has suited parties of both left and right and has now become entrenched by virtue of its own internal momentum. The result is bureaucratic, unaccountable and inefficient. It gives to professionals and officialdom unwarranted power to control the behaviour of clients and service users. The solution which Hadley and Hatch recommended was a shift to welfare pluralism with a greater role for the voluntary and informal sectors (a demand that was readily colonised as part of a neo-liberal reform agenda) and the development of 'participatory alternatives' to centralised social services (an objective that was just as readily subverted to the cause of welfare consumerism). The nature of such participatory alternatives, as Hadley and Hatch conceived them, would have been such as to give clients or service users the right to an active role in negotiating the nature of the services they received. The performance of such services, what is more, would be judged with reference to outputs, rather than inputs.

This emphasis on results, rather than resources or 'rights', represents a theme espoused in common with my second example, namely Waltzer (1983). Waltzer has contended that *justice* is more important than 'rights', since distributive justice or equality represents outcomes (which can be assessed) rather than objectives (which cannot). Justice itself, however, 'is a human construction, and it is doubtful whether it can be made in only one way' (*ibid.*: 5). Equality, Waltzer argues, does not require the elimination of difference and what justice must entail is egalitarianism 'without the Procrustean bed of the state'. The bed in the Procrustean legend was one to which victims were fitted by being forcibly stretched or butchered and Waltzer's case is that human beings need not be so manipulated; it is social goods, not citizens, that should be controlled or made to fit. What is required is not universalism, but a form of 'complex equality'. In a broadly similar vein, writers such as Keane (1988) advocate a form of 'civil society socialism' in which human co-operation would be governed neither by the compulsion of market forces, nor by the administrative power of a *dirigiste* state. In some respects the argument is more anarchistic than socialist (see my further discussion in Chapter 11 below). However, to the extent that the state would still exist, it would be accountable to civil society (the sphere of voluntary co-operation) and would act as guarantor of social needs, and only, for example, to the extent that such needs could be identified or generated in the course of ecologically sustainable production and consumption.

There is therefore some potential overlap between this and my final example, namely that of ecologism (see Fitzpatrick 1998). Though there is a 'deep Green' strand within the ecology movement that is not concerned with social rights (Ferris 1991), ecological modernisers, social ecologists and eco-socialists clearly are (Dean 2001). The ecological critique of welfare rights is premised upon an objection to the way in which social policy is contrived to sustain a 'productivist' regime: a regime that is dependent not only upon the exploitation of wage labour and the marginalisation of other socially necessary human activities, but upon the wasteful and damaging mis-appropriation of natural resources and an unsustainable commitment to economic growth. Such thinking had in part been influenced by Claus Offe, the neo-Marxist theorist, who is mentioned above. Offe had been a prominent member of the German Green Party and latterly became a convert to the idea of a Basic Income (a universal cash benefit which would replace all existing social security benefits and tax allowances) (1992). Basic Income is supported (but was not conceived) by some ecologists, because it would supposedly guarantee the autonomy of the citizen – both from the market and the state (see, for example, Kemp and Wall 1990). The existing pattern of welfare entitlements, which seek for example to maximise work incentives, is tied to the logic of capitalist production. Eco-socialists and social ecologists seek an alternative role for social rights in facilitating more diverse, yet more sustainable patterns of human existence that are cognisant not just of the needs and claims of current generations, but future generations as well.

The common theme of these defensive critiques is a rejection of the generality of the centralised state and social rights based on prescription; and an insistence on the particularity of civil society and the importance of participation in need satisfaction.

Summary/conclusion

This chapter has considered several critiques of the ideological notion of welfare rights and of the practical consequences of social legislation. These critiques are diverse. The element that they have in common is a recognition that social rights of citizenship must inevitably involve some propensity for social control. Where the critiques differ is in the reasons that they regard such a propensity to be problematic.

The neo-liberal objection is that rights involving the redistribution of income or property are corrupting. They are not rights at all; on the contrary, they are an infringement of real (i.e. property) rights or a distraction from properly enforceable (i.e. civil and political) human rights. The neo-Marxist objection is that social rights, in spite of the advantages they have brought the working class, are exploitative. They are a necessary component in the process by which labour power is reproduced and articulated with the capitalist market system and they are a source of ideological mystification. The post-structuralist objection is that the extension of social rights is constituted as an extension of administrative state power, based on an increasingly sophisticated array of disciplinary techniques for the definition and control of individual subjects.

Feminist and anti-racist critics of social rights complain that women and minority ethnic groups are systematically excluded from social rights. Social rights function to the advantage of men and 'white' society. There are also related defensive critiques whose concern is with the undemocratic nature of social rights and their capacity to impose conditions of social uniformity and/ or to reinforce ecologically destructive behaviour.

Inevitably, this complex spectrum of arguments has been somewhat simplified, but the purpose of this chapter has been to demonstrate that social rights are controversial. In Part III I shall return to some of these controversies and put them into a broader context. First, however, it is important that the theoretical approach adopted in Part I of this book should be grounded in some practical accounts of welfare rights in a specific context, namely Britain. It is to this task that Part II of the book now turns.

Part II

Welfare rights in practice

Chapter 5

Rights to subsistence

The Universal Declaration of Human Rights speaks of a right to social security (UN 1948: Article 22) and, more particularly, a person's 'right to security in the event of unemployment, sickness, disability, widowhood, old age or other lack of livelihood in circumstances beyond his control' (Article 25). In different parts of the world and at different moments in human history people have achieved social security by different means. Human subsistence may after all be sustained by more than one form of social organisation. Social security may be ensured through the simple exchange of goods and services, or by the organised distribution of benefits in kind or in cash. A defining feature of democratic-welfare-capitalism is that everyday subsistence is conditioned by a cash nexus. However, cash benefits can be organised in accordance with a variety of principles, not all of which provide the same degree of security. This chapter will be concerned very specifically with what in Britain is called the social security system, though the rights which that system provides are in fact qualified rights to income maintenance. These are rights guaranteed by legislation, but whether they provide social security will be left to the reader to judge.

Carried with any right to social security are also conditions and duties. Social policy in the area of income maintenance is driven as much by the conditions and duties that it imposes upon the recipients of cash benefits as by the rights which it creates. With or without a welfare state, the social organisation of human subsistence requires that individuals co-operate. Social guarantees of income maintenance are therefore based on particular normative assumptions about the way that individuals should behave. In democratic-welfare-capitalist societies this entails assumptions about individuals' liabilities to maintain themselves through paid employment and to maintain each other within families. As has been discussed in Chapter 4, social rights are inseparable from the enforcement of socially constructed duties.

The chapter is divided into five sections. The first outlines the changing structure of the British social security system and its relationship to tax and occupational systems, not least because this will be necessary to aspects of both Chapters 6 and 7. The second section considers what has been the main subsistence benefit provided by that system, while the third discusses the ways in which the welfare state enforces the responsibilities of family membership. Finally, the fourth section will examine the specific rights of older people, and the fifth those of disabled people and their carers.

A hybrid system

The unusual complexity of British income maintenance arrangements reflects the fact that they constitute a hybrid system, combining elements of at least three different principles of social security: social assistance principles, social insurance principles and contingency or categorical principles. Additionally, as Titmuss (1958) remarked in a seminal essay, such income maintenance arrangements co-exist with parallel systems of fiscal and occupational welfare. The social security system has complex and changing inter-relationships with the tax system on the one hand, and with the system of occupational pensions and benefits and regulated private pension schemes on the other. Not all these complexities can be satisfactorily encompassed within this chapter, but it is important to set the explanation that follows in the wider context illustrated in Table 5.1. The income maintenance system may be understood as being composed of three systems – the social security system, the tax system and the occupational system – although these systems now overlap and interact in more complex ways than had applied when Titmuss was writing. Although the rest of this section will focus upon the three principles that inform the three main limbs of the social security system, it also addresses the ways in which certain kinds of provision have either spilled over to become a part of the tax system or else, in the case of benefits and pensions based on employment, have become enmeshed with the occupational system.

Social assistance

The modern British social security system has its origins in the Elizabethan and Victorian Poor Laws (de Schweinitz 1961; George 1973; Novak 1988; Dean 1991: ch. 3; McKay and Rowlingson 1999). The underlying principle of relief under the Poor Law has provided the basis of what is now called social assistance. Poor relief was never a right. The local parish, the Poor Law Unions and the Public Assistance Committees that succeeded them were charged with responsibility for controlling vagrancy and relieving destitution. The means by which they did so was left in part to their discretion, though such discretion became subject increasingly to central government direction. Social assistance emerged from the Poor Law as a result of two developments: first, a gradual erosion of the infamous nineteenth-century workhouse test in favour of 'out-relief' (money payments to paupers in their own homes); second, the development of systematic means-testing (standardised methods of calculating relief by comparing people's subsistence needs with their assessed means).

Nationally administered means-tested benefit schemes were developed separately from the Poor Law for old people (in 1908) and for uninsured able-bodied unemployed people (in 1934). The final repeal of the Poor Law came in 1948 as part of the post-Second World War Beveridge reforms. Those reforms retained a nationally administered, weekly paid, means-tested benefit called national assistance as a residual safety-net for those who might not be adequately provided for by new social insurance and categorical benefit provisions

Table 5.1 The British income maintenance system(s)[1]

Social security system				Tax system	Fiscal benefits (tax allowances/exemptions)	Occupational system — Employment-related benefits		
'Universal'/contingent or categorical benefits (non-means-tested/non-contributory)	Social insurance benefits (contributory)	Social assistance benefits (selective/means-tested) — Regulated schemes	Social assistance benefits — Discretionary schemes	Tax credits		Statutory	Non-statutory	Private (contracted out)[3]
Child benefit	Retirement pension and second state pension (or formerly SERPS)	Income support/Disability and Pensioners' minimum income guarantees/Pension credit		Working families' tax credit/Disabled person's tax credit/or, from 2003, Working tax credit	Personal allowances	Statutory sick pay	Occupational sick pay/maternity or paternity pay/health insurance benefits	Personal pension plans
Disability living allowance/Attendance allowance	Jobseeker's allowance					Statutory maternity/paternity pay	Occupational pensions	Stakeholder pensions
Carer's allowance (currently Invalid Care Allowance)	Incapacity benefit[2]	Social fund		Child tax credit (from 2003)	Exemptions on pension contributions			
Industrial injuries and war pensions schemes	Bereavement benefits	Housing benefit	Discretionary housing payments					

Notes:

1 The table illustrates the relationship between different delivery systems and different categories of benefit – including the emerging overlap between the tax system and social assistance provision.

2 Incapacity benefit can in effect be a categorical benefit in the case of people who were or became incapable of work when they were young, or a partially means-tested benefit in the case of people who receive payments from private, occupational or public service pension schemes.

3 Although such schemes are also open to people who are not employed, they are in effect a part of the occupational system because they entitle people who are employed to contract out of the state second pension scheme and instead to make contributions out of their wages/salaries to a private pension provider.

(see below). In the event, national assistance became anything but residual and was itself reformed in 1966 to become supplementary benefit. The new benefit retained a means-test which was in principle no less selective than that which had applied before, but the legislation which introduced it contained a symbolic declaration that people who satisfied the means-test conditions were entitled to their benefit as a 'right'. In 1988 the supplementary benefit scheme was in its own turn reformed to become income support (IS). Subsequently, while still bound to the structure of the IS scheme, the form of IS that is payable to unemployed people was recast in 1996 to become income-based jobseeker's allowance (JSA – see Chapter 6); the form that is payable to retirement pensioners was recast in 1999 to become the pensioners' minimum income guarantee (MIG), which from 2003 is for some pensioners to be supplemented by a pensioner credit (see below); and the form that is payable to disabled people was recast in 2001 to become the disability income guarantee (DIG).

There are, in addition to IS, two other kinds of regular benefit that function in accordance with social assistance principles; that is to say, which are selective or 'targeted' through the use of a means-test. First, there are 'in-work' benefits that may be claimed by certain low-paid employees in order to boost their incomes to subsistence levels. These are working families' tax credit (WFTC) and the disabled persons tax credit (DPTC), which will from 2003 be incorporated into a new working tax credit scheme (WTC) (see Treasury 2001). These will be discussed in Chapter 6. Second, there are housing benefit (HB) and council tax benefit (CTB), local authority administered benefits that may be claimed by people on low incomes in order to help meet their rent or council tax liabilities. Local authorities are also empowered to make certain discretionary housing payments (DHPs). All these housing-related benefits will be discussed in Chapter 7.

Recipients of means-tested benefits are also entitled in certain circumstances to make applications to the social fund (SF). The fund was created in 1988, replacing provisions which had previously been made under the national insurance scheme (see below) for maternity and death grants, and under the supplementary benefits scheme for single payments or grants to meet exceptional need. The SF has two distinct elements. For claimants who are already in receipt of specified means-tested benefits the regulated SF provides:

- modest payments, now called Sure Start maternity grants, towards maternity expenses, provided the claimant has received health and welfare advice from a health care professional;
- payments towards funeral expenses, subject to strict conditions and set maxima;
- cold weather payments to members of certain vulnerable groups in the event of sustained cold weather.

The regulated SF also makes a modest annual winter fuel payment to all pensioner households.

The discretionary SF provides, on a strictly rationed basis, community care grants (intended to assist people in leaving or avoiding institutional care), budgeting loans and crisis loans. Community care grants and budgeting loans are available only to claimants in receipt of IS (including income-based JSA, MIG and DIG), though crisis loans are available in theory to assist anyone in an emergency that is facing an immediate short-term need. The discretionary SF, together with DHPs (see above and Chapter 7 below), functions according to quite different principles to other modern social assistance benefits: first, because the nature, extent and urgency of need is determined by officials upon an entirely discretionary basis; second, because the scheme is budget limited and officials must prioritise applications in accordance with available resources; third, because in the case of the SF much of the expenditure is made by way of loans which applicants must repay (for a fuller discussion see, for example, Craig 1992 and, for recent statistics, DSS 1999b).

While the discretionary SF and DHPs are forms of social assistance that appear to hark back to principles of the Poor Laws, other elements of contemporary social assistance would appear in the twenty-first century to be entering an entirely new phase, albeit a phase that has been informed by relatively recent policy innovations in the USA. I have already briefly mentioned the means-tested in-work benefits that have lately been recast as 'tax credits' administered by the Inland Revenue and which from 2003 will be incorporated into the WTC. At the same time, the specific components of all social assistance benefits (including tax credits) that had been payable to families in order to support children will be incorporated into a new child tax credit (CTC), administered once again by the Inland Revenue (see Treasury 2001). I shall discuss the CTC again later in this chapter. The change is significant, however, since it is part of an important attempt to shift responsibility for the administration of those elements of social assistance that are payable for working adults on the one hand and for children on the other from the government department responsible for the social security system (which, since 2001, has been the Department of Work and Pensions) to the Inland Revenue. It is not clear at the time of writing how far-reaching the administrative consequences might be – although it has been suggested, for example, that WTC and CTC may be based on annual assessments rather than paid as a week-by-week entitlement (Inland Revenue 2001) – but the development is symbolically important since it signals a shift away from the traditional mode of means-testing and creates a new form of social assistance that will function as part of the tax system under the direct control of the Treasury.

Finally, the recipients of social assistance may be entitled to a range of incidental benefits in kind, including exemption from certain health service charges, including charges for prescriptions, dental treatment and spectacles (see Chapter 8). IS and income-based JSA claimants are entitled to free school meals for their children.

Around a third of all social security spending in Britain currently goes on social assistance benefits, but this by itself does not reflect the central place which means-tested or selective benefits have in the UK, where social assistance criteria are the ultimate determinants of the living standards of nearly one in every six people. This compares with fewer than one in ten in countries like Japan and the Southern European countries, but one in four in the most heavily means-tested country, New Zealand (Gough *et al.* 1997).

Social insurance

Social insurance may be remembered as one of the big ideas of the twentieth century. The concept has exerted considerable influence over social policy (Gilbert 1966; Peden 1991), yet by the turn of the twenty-first century in Britain it has been largely eclipsed, leaving behind within the social security system some obsolete and arcane administrative features. Insurance is concerned with the management of risk. Yet, in spite of arguments that the role of the state is to facilitate the management of individual risks (e.g. Giddens 1994), the prevailing political consensus is shifting away from social or collectively organised insurance, in favour of individual self-provision and a social safety-net.

The principle of social insurance is that all workers compulsorily contribute to a national insurance fund and, in the event of sickness, unemployment or retirement, they are entitled to claim upon that fund. The attraction of such a scheme in a democratic-welfare-capitalist society is obvious. It creates social rights based upon a collective sharing of risks, but it does so without undermining the free play of market forces or the responsibility of individuals to provide for themselves. In so far that insurance-based social security benefits give to their recipients a sense of entitlement, it has been a popular concept. Unfortunately, however, the practical and political difficulties of maintaining a national insurance fund in accordance with actuarial conventions have never been surmounted and the popular credibility of the concept has progressively been undermined by fears about its alleged unsustainability. Unfortunately too, social insurance schemes protect workers as employees, not citizens. Social rights based on insurance principles are enjoyed by those who 'earn' their entitlements in the labour market, while citizens who have been excluded from the labour market can benefit only as dependants of those who have contributed or, alternatively, if the insurance principle is broadened (some might say compromised) so as to admit those who are excluded by giving them 'credits' or notional contributions. In particular, as will be discussed below, social insurance has systematically disadvantaged women.

The first National Insurance Act of 1911 provided limited unemployment and sickness insurance, schemes that all but collapsed during the 1920s and 1930s. The National Insurance Act of 1946, however, represented the centrepiece of what Beveridge had intended should be a comprehensive social security system. The 1946 Act provided that all workers should pay a flat rate weekly contribution in return for which there would be an entitlement to flat rate weekly benefits, pensions or grants covering sickness, invalidity, unemployment, maternity, widowhood, retirement and death. It was believed that – together with family allowances (see below) and free health care (see Chapter 8) – such a scheme would supersede the need for stigmatising forms of social assistance. In the event, successive governments failed to underwrite national insurance at a level that would have made this possible.

In the course of the 1960s and 1970s the flat rate principle was abandoned in favour of graduated national insurance contributions and earnings-related benefits and pensions. In this way, it was hoped, benefit and pension levels for the majority could be raised above poverty levels. In the 1980s, however, a radical Conservative administration effected a number of changes that have relegated social insurance as a principle to the sidelines. Earnings-related additions to short-term benefits were abolished and the value of pension additions under the state earnings-related pension scheme (SERPS) were halved. The convention by which the basic retirement pension (RP) was uprated annually in line with general earnings was also abandoned, so as to link pensions only to price inflation, the effect of which will be to render the value of the RP in the twenty-first century 'nugatory' (Portillo 1993). Instead, the Conservative government at this time initiated a process by which provision for pensions beyond the declining state minimum would be extended principally through occupational and private provision. Certain short-term national insurance benefits – sickness benefit and maternity allowance – were similarly displaced into the occupational welfare system through the introduction of statutory sick pay (SSP) and statutory maternity pay (SMP) (see Chapter 6). The widow's benefit scheme was 'streamlined'. In the 1990s, incapacity benefit (IB) and contributory jobseeker's allowance (JSA) have been introduced: the former replaced the sickness and invalidity benefit schemes and reduced their scope though the application of stricter medical tests; the latter merged the administration of contributory unemployment benefit with that of means-tested IS.

Since 1997, the New Labour government has not moved to reinstate social insurance. SERPS has been replaced by what is likely to become a flat rate second state pension (S2P) that will provide a modest enhancement to the contributory pension for people on the lowest incomes, although the main thrust of policy has been the promotion of stakeholder pensions (SHPs) – a specially regulated private arrangement for lower earners. The reform of widows' benefits has been consolidated with a revised bereavement benefit scheme for widows and widowers. IB, as we shall see, has been further reformed and no longer functions entirely as a contributory benefit.

Although the proportion of social security spending attributable to social assistance and categorical benefits overtook that spent on contributory benefits in the early 1990s (McKay and Rowlingson 1999), what remains of social insurance is not inconsiderable. The cost of the basic RP is still the biggest single charge on the social security budget. None the less, the application of the insurance principle has been effectively hobbled. It is no longer supposed that the basic RP, bereavement benefits and the IB scheme should provide adequate replacement incomes. Benefits such as maternity allowance (which may still be claimed by a small number of women who have paid national insurance contributions but are not currently employed) and a range of abolished benefits to which contributors may still be entitled until they are phased out remain as an anomaly.

At the core of any social or national insurance scheme lies the contributory principle: the idea that people must pay something in before they can get anything out. If social insurance is to survive as a credible component of the British social security system, it will be necessary to modify the contributory principle so as more fully to recognise the various kinds of non-monetary and social contributions that citizens may make to national well-being (e.g. Webb 1994; CSJ 1994). Limited concessions have been made so as to credit people with insurance contributions when they have been unable to pay them and in some instances this erodes the distinction between contributory and non-contributory benefits. It also means that the contribution rules have become thoroughly arcane. Detailed accounts are provided elsewhere (for example, in CPAG's *Welfare Benefits Handbook*) and what follows is a bare outline. Members of the national insurance scheme may establish a contribution record in the following ways:

- Employees contribute a percentage of their earnings (subject to an upper and a lower limit) and their employers are separately liable to pay a percentage of each employee's earnings (subject to a lower, but no upper, limit). Employees and employers pay reduced contributions if the employee 'contracts out' of the S2P (which replaced SERPS in 2002) in order to contribute to an occupational, stakeholder or private pension scheme.
- Low-paid workers who earn less than the lower earnings limit for national insurance purposes, but are in receipt of in-work tax credits, also receive national insurance 'credits' towards their national insurance records. Additionally, since 2001, employees who earn more than the prescribed lower earnings limit – but less than a slightly higher 'primary threshold' – do not have to pay contributions, but also receive credits (i.e. they are treated as if they had paid such contributions).
- Self-employed persons, provided their incomes exceed a certain minimum, pay a flat rate contribution and they must additionally pay a percentage of any profits falling within set limits.
- People who are neither employed nor self-employed may make voluntary contributions at a flat rate, though these give rise to limited entitlements.
- People who are registered as 'jobseekers' (i.e. as unemployed), who receive incapacity benefit or invalid care allowance or who are on approved training courses receive credits towards their national insurance records.
- Since 1977 limited forms of 'starting credits' have been available for young people staying on at school after the minimum school leaving age.
- Since 1978 a limited form of home responsibilities protection or credit has been available for people who have spent periods looking after dependent children or adult invalids.

Entitlement to social insurance benefits depends upon having established a contributions record before any claim is made. The only exception to this at present relates to a small number of people who have been incapable of work since they were young and since 2001 have been able to qualify for IB without meeting any contribution conditions. In spite of the various concessions by which people can be 'credited in' to the national insurance scheme, those in low-paid, part-time and intermittent work may still be excluded or may fail to achieve a complete contribution record in the course of their working lives.

To qualify for national insurance benefits, contributors (or, in certain circumstances, their spouses) must have paid and/or been credited with contributions to a specified level for a requisite period of years. The precise rules for each benefit are different, but there is a requirement that certain of the contributions giving rise to an entitlement must have been actually paid, rather than merely credited: once again, this can penalise many who are wholly or partly excluded from the labour market, especially women.

'Universal', contingency or categorical benefits

A universal social security benefit, if such existed, would represent a social right in its purest sense. In so far that there are benefits payable to parents for their children and to disabled people to meet additional living costs without the imposition of either a means-test or contribution conditions, these are sometimes referred to as universal benefits. However, the term is in one sense a misnomer. Such benefits are conditional on claimants' circumstances or status and are properly defined as either contingency benefits (because they are intended to meet particular contingencies) or categorical benefits (because they are intended to meet the needs of particular categories of people). (Incidentally, the term 'universal' is occasionally, if even more misleadingly, used in relation to the basic retirement pension, which, although it is received virtually, but not entirely, universally by people of pensionable age, remains in reality conditional upon claimants' insurance contribution records.) For the purposes of the discussion that follows, my preferred term is 'categorical' benefit, since this signals the extent to which such benefits are conditional not precisely upon a person's actual social situation or needs, but upon criteria by which certain categories of persons may be more or less arbitrarily defined.

The first categorical benefit in Britain was family allowance. The family allowance scheme was introduced in 1948, though it was further developed in 1978 through the effective incorporation of child tax allowances so as to produce the child benefit (CB) scheme, which provides a weekly non-taxable benefit, payable to parents (almost invariably mothers), for each co-resident dependent child. (There is a parallel guardians allowance scheme that makes provision for orphaned children.) When family allowance was first introduced it was not payable for a first child, only for second and subsequent children. CB has always been payable in respect of each child up until she leaves school or until the age of 19 if she remains at school or in full-time further (not higher) education, or more recently, until the age of 18 if she is registered unemployed but not receiving benefits. Since 1991 CB has been payable at a higher rate for the first child in a family than for second or subsequent children.

The level at which family allowance and subsequently CB was paid was never intended to be sufficient to meet the actual subsistence needs of a child. It symbolised none the less a contribution by the state on behalf of the wider community towards the costs of bringing up children and to the needs of the next generation. It was also regarded as a key component of the 'social wage'; that parcel of state benefits which can function to reduce the extent to which 'real' wages must include provision for workers' families (Land 1975 and 1992). CB is often ridiculed because it is paid to all parents, even the most affluent (Boyson 1971; Dilnot *et al.* 1984). From 1987 until 1991 the value of CB was deliberately frozen, on the explicit premise that resources should be diverted from inefficient and expensive categorical provision to means-tested benefits such as family credit which is 'targeted' on the families who most need help (DHSS 1985). Thereafter the Conservative government of the day relented and restored the uprating of CB and a New Labour government in 1999 went so far as to boost its real value. Despite this, it is not clear that CB will always be retained in its present form. In 2001 the government temporarily replaced the somewhat anachronistic married couples tax allowance with a children's tax credit – an income-related fiscal benefit not dissimilar from pre-1978 child tax allowances – that would from 2003 be rolled in to the new CTC (see above) and so enhance its scope: CTC will pay variable amounts to different families, depending on their circumstances. The government had rejected suggestions that the abolition of the married couples tax allowance should finance further enhancements to CB and once again priority for reform would seem to have been given to means-tested forms of provision – albeit through the tax system – and there is speculation at the time of writing that although categorical CB is to be retained it may yet, for example, be made taxable (Barnes 2000), a move that would compromise its universality. It has also been suggested that CB for young people over 16 may be replaced by education maintenance allowances (see Chapter 8 below).

Between 1978 and 1997 a small additional categorical benefit, lone-parent benefit, was paid with child benefit to lone parents. This represented a partial if belated concession to the Finer Committee's recommendations for a 'guaranteed maintenance allowance' (Finer 1974), but it was eventually scrapped purportedly in favour of across the board enhancements of benefits for children in all kinds of family.

Categorical provision within the Beveridgian social security system was limited in scope precisely because the system was primarily informed by social insurance and not strictly universal principles. However, a non-contributory industrial injuries scheme was also incorporated into social security to provide benefits and pensions for people who were injured and/or disabled in the course of their employment, whether as a result of an accident or an industrial disease. The scheme replaced the provisions of the Workmen's Compensation Act of 1897, under which injured employees were obliged to seek compensation from their privately insured employers. The original scheme of 1946 has since been heavily modified, but the main benefit under the scheme is disablement benefit, the amount of which is determined on a tariff basis in accordance with the extent of disablement incurred and which may be supplemented with various allowances. A very similar war pensions scheme survives to provide benefits and pensions for service personnel and others disabled in the course of war or armed conflicts.

In the post-Second World War social security system, therefore, categorical provision was made for children until such time as they could become social insurance contributors (and/or – in the case of females – until they could obtain dependency on a social insurance contributor through marriage) and for people whose capacity as a social insurance contributor was impaired through disablement in the course of their employment or in war. No provision was made for people who might never become (or might never marry) a social insurance contributor. People who were disabled from birth or since child-hood, people with severe learning difficulties, and people who provided full-time care for dependent adult relatives might never obtain membership of the national insurance scheme. For these people, the only provision that existed was through means-tested benefits. From the 1970s onwards, to remedy this omission, a range of new benefits was developed for disabled people and carers and, as we have already seen, other changes have been made quite recently. Although these will be described in greater detail later in this chapter, it is important to note that certain of the benefits – attendance allowance (AA), mobility allowance and, later, disability living allowance (DLA) – were intended to provide for the additional living and mobility costs that disabled people incur and that these were categorical; that is, they were not subject to either means-testing or a contribution condition, although they were strictly contingent upon disability as defined by medical tests and criteria. In this way categorical benefits have come to play a significant, but not central, role.

The traditional means-test

Depending on one's view, means-tested social assistance benefits represent either the 'safety-net' of the social security system, or its most efficient compon-ent. This section will outline the workings of income support (IS), the main British social assistance benefit. (Note: unless otherwise stated, references to IS may be taken also to apply to income-based JSA, the MIG and DIG.) As we have seen, IS can trace its roots all the way back to the Poor Laws and, in spite of the often bewildering complexities of the scheme, its essential principles are both simple and traditional. It may be that the more sophisticated forms of means-testing that have been emerging – such as the WTC and the CTC – will in time upstage the traditional form of means-test that is embodied in IS. For the foreseeable future, however, IS retains a pivotal role. The object of a traditional means-test is to guarantee a minimum standard of subsistence. In practice, however, IS guarantees different standards for different groups of people and some groups it excludes from any right to subsistence.

The details and even the terminology used in connection with social assist-ance schemes are subject to continual revision by governments. However, at the heart of any means-test lies a comparison between a claimant's needs and her means; a calculation which in its simplest form 'tops up' a person's means to meet her needs (see Figure 5.1). Translating this principle into practice requires elaborate processes of definition (for a full account see, for example, CPAG's *Welfare Benefits Handbook*).

Under IS, a person's needs are determined with reference to an 'applicable amount'; the weekly amount of money that is deemed under the legislation to

NEEDS	–	MEANS	=	ENTITLEMENT
(applicable amount)	(minus)	(income)	(equals)	(benefit payable)
		(subject to 'disregards'		
		and to disqualification if		
		capital exceeds a ceiling)		

Figure 5.1 'Top-up' means-test calculation

be needed for a person and her family to live on. The applicable amount has up to three components:

- A personal allowance, which varies according to the claimant's age, whether she resides with a partner, and (at the time of writing) the number and ages of any children in her family. The monetary values of personal allowances derive from scales that are reviewed annually but which owe their origin to subsistence standards originally defined by Rowntree (see Chapter 2 above), albeit that these ought never to have been interpreted as standards for social adequacy (Veit-Wilson 1992). Since these scales were first applied in 1948, they 'have been uprated on the basis of historical precedent, opportunism and political hunch' (Bradshaw 1993: xiii). The basic personal allowance for a single person aged 25 or over currently stands at rather less than one seventh of average male earnings, while provision made through personal allowances for children, in spite of recent improvements, will still fall short of the standard required for maintaining children even on a 'low cost' budget (Oldfield and Yu 1993; Parker 1998). However, personal allowances for dependent children will from 2003 disappear from IS and be included in the CTC.
- A premium which will apply only if the claimant (and/or a member of her family) is a member of a particular 'client group'. The client groups which attract premiums are: families with dependent children; people who are caring full-time for an invalid; people who are disabled and in receipt of other 'qualifying' benefits; and pensioners. Higher-level premiums apply if the claimant's family includes a disabled child; if a severely disabled claimant or family member has no one to look after them; for pensioners who are above certain ages and/or who are also disabled. The rules that govern eligibility for premiums are often complex, and in the case of disability-related premiums often depend upon a claimant or family member's eligibility for some other qualifying benefit.
- Housing costs, but only in instances where these are not met by housing benefit. Generally, this will apply to the cost of mortgage interest payments faced by homeowners and this is discussed in more detail in Chapter 7.

For IS purposes a person's means are assessed with reference to her income (including income from other social security benefits) and her savings or capital. Certain income may be disregarded in whole or in part, though these 'disregards' are limited. The disregards that apply in the case of income from child maintenance or disability benefits are discussed later in this chapter, while those that apply to income from earnings are discussed in Chapter 6. Certain savings, investments or capital may also be disregarded, including the value of the claimant's own home. Unless it is disregarded, the possession of savings or capital that exceed a certain modest value will disqualify the holder from income support, although in the case of people of pensionable age the 'pension credit' to be introduced in 2003 will provide a different set of rules. Pensioners will be means-tested not on their capital, but on the income from their savings. If their savings and second pension income exceed a certain threshold they will have no MIG entitlement, but if it falls below that threshold they will receive a tapered 'credit' in addition to their basic MIG entitlement. The calculation of a claimant's means requires the claimant to disclose exhaustive details, not only of her own personal resources, but also (as will shortly be seen) of any person(s) who are deemed to be members of her 'family'.

The form of this means-test is such that, relatively speaking, it privileges certain groups in the population at the expense of others. This results partly from the effect of premiums. The premium applicable to an ordinary pensioner couple is worth four times as much as that for a working-age couple with children. The personal allowance for young people aged 18 to 24 is around one-fifth less than that for those aged 25 or over. Personal allowances for 16- and 17-year-olds are even lower, though most 16- and 17-year-olds in fact have no entitlement to income support at all: they represent just one of a number of groups who are subject to special rules or who are excluded from entitlement altogether. The social security system at present assumes that people aged 16 and 17, if they are not in employment, should be in full-time education or training and usually it is only if they are lone parents, if they are sick or disabled, or if exceptionally they might otherwise suffer hardship that they may claim.

In general, no one may receive IS if she or her partner is in full-time employment (currently defined as employment for more than 16 hours per week). People who are employed for more than 16 hours per week may be entitled to other means-tested benefits or tax credits (see Chapter 6). People who are employed but are on strike or locked out as a result of a trade dispute may claim IS, but subject only to special rules. People who are unemployed must claim income-based JSA rather than IS which, although it is in other respects identical, is subject to additional conditions concerning the claimant's jobseeking and availability for work, matters that will be discussed in Chapter 6. Otherwise, the only people who may claim IS without being subject to such conditions are those who satisfy the incapacity for work test (also discussed in Chapter 6) or who are mentally or physically disabled, and those who are over 60 years of age or who are lone parents. Special rules apply to IS claimants who are in residential care or nursing homes, to people going in or coming out of hospital or prison, to students and to people with no settled accommodation.

Special rules also apply to 'persons from abroad'. These rules are especially significant because of the wider implications they have for social citizenship. Although these or similar rules apply to all benefit entitlements, it is most usually in relation to claims for IS that the fundamental issues arise. In this regard, entitlement to IS (and related means-tested benefits) is subject to three tests. The first, the immigration status test, excludes from benefit anyone who under immigration law has entered or remains in the UK illegally or subject to a condition or an undertaking that they shall have no recourse to public funds. The second, the residence directives test, relates to nationals from European Economic Area states, and excludes them from benefit unless they are economically active, so excluding students, retired people and lone parents, but giving certain rights to workseekers (who may none the less be directed to leave the UK after 6 months). The third, the habitual residence test, was introduced in 1994 to prevent alleged 'benefit tourism' (Lilley 1993) and denies benefits even to EU and returning UK nationals if they cannot establish that they are habitually resident: the test may take account of a claimant's past residence, employment and family ties, but also their future intentions and prospects. Those who fail the above tests may in certain limited circumstances be able to claim reduced benefits, for example, pending the outcome of immigration appeals or applications for asylum. However, in the specific case of refugees entering the country and making claims for asylum since the introduction of new rules in 2000, they are – unless and until their claims to refugee status are accepted – entirely precluded from claiming benefits and must depend on assistance from the National Asylum Support Service. At the time of writing, this provides support principally by way of food vouchers, rather than in cash, but an alternative system has been promised for the Autumn of 2002.

The arena of immigration and asylum law lies beyond the scope of this book and the specific issues associated with the rights of migrants to claim subsistence are both complex and fluid (but see, for example, CPAG's *Migration and Social Security Handbook* and JCWI's *Immigration, Nationality and Refugee Law Handbook*). From the bare outline above, however, the scope for discriminatory application will be self-evident. One particular effect is to implicate the social security system in the application of immigration policies that are inherently racist (Amin and Oppenheim 1992; Bloch 1997). What is more, the additional checks entailed in administering such tests engender a climate of suspicion and uncertainty which deters many claimants from minority ethnic groups from claiming benefits to which they are legally entitled (see NACAB 1991). IS and the tradition it embodies functions not only as a safety-net to catch those who fall, but also as a boundary screen to exclude or deter those whose claim upon the right to subsistence may be put into question.

Enforcing family responsibilities

Earlier in this chapter it was remarked that social security provision rests on assumptions about people's liabilities to maintain each other within families. This has consequences for the mutual interdependency of adults, as well as for the basis upon which financial support for children may be secured. Although the British government has declared that it is committed to supporting families (see Home Office 1998), it has never had an explicit family policy and many of its objectives remain implicit: this is particularly so when it comes to the limitations that are imposed upon rights to subsistence. This section will firstly consider the particular significance of social insurance and social assistance regimes for women, before turning to the issue of child support maintenance.

The Beveridgian model of social security assumed that married women would (and should) by and large be dependent upon their husbands. The nature of a social insurance-based system of social security is such as to make entitlement conditional upon labour market ties in a context in which labour markets systematically disadvantage women. This continues to be the case in spite of the introduction of equal opportunities provisions within employment law and equal treatment provisions within social security law (Glendinning and Millar 1992). Female labour force participation has risen dramatically and continues to do so, yet women tend to remain in less well-paid, less secure employment and remain less likely than men to establish national insurance records that will entitle them independently to benefits and pensions. Feminists argue that this reflects more than a failure of the labour market; it is also a failure of the social security system to redress the unequal burden of unpaid caring and domestic work which women carry in their families (see discussion in Chapter 4).

With social insurance benefits, assumptions about family dependency are implicit, but with social assistance benefits they become quite explicit. Contribution tests are applied on the basis of an individual worker's insurance record; means-tests, on the other hand, are applied directly to households or families. In the jargon of the old supplementary benefit scheme, a claimant and the members of her/his immediate household were referred to as a 'unit of assessment'. The IS scheme uses the cosier term 'family'. The assumption, none the less, is that the needs and means of a cohabiting man and woman and any children for whom they are responsible should be shared or 'aggregated'. The computation of 'applicable amounts' and of income resources extends so as to include a claimant's 'partner' and child dependants. In so doing means-tested schemes pay no regard to the dynamics of family relationships and the ways in which these are in practice negotiated (see Finch and Mason 1993). Instead, such schemes impose their own rules and definitions.

For social assistance purposes the rule is that people must claim as a 'couple' and will be treated as 'partners' if they are married and living in the same household, or if they are not married but 'living together as husband and wife'. This, the so-called 'cohabitation rule', has several implications and effects:

- It assumes the normality of heterosexual relationships and marriage. The relationships of gay and lesbian couples are not recognised and stable heterosexual relationships are characterised in terms of their semblance to marriage.
- It compels men and women who share a household and have a stable relationship to be financially interdependent whether or not they may choose to be so.
- It seriously prejudices the position of a non-claiming partner in situations where 'family' resources are not equitably shared in practice.
- It excludes from benefit anybody whose partner's resources are adjudged sufficient for her 'family' as a whole, so depriving that person of any independence she may have previously enjoyed.

- Because the applicable amount for a couple is less than that for two independent adults, it reduces the income potentially available to the 'family' as a whole.

It is women rather than men who are most likely to be disadvantaged. So far as women in two-parent families are concerned, they are likely to exercise less control over 'family' income than men (Pahl 1989) yet it is usually they who must bear the burdens of daily household management and the brunt of the sacrifices entailed in doing so on a low income (Bradshaw and Holmes 1989). Additionally, aggregated means-tested entitlements stand to be reduced on account of any part-time earnings belonging to a claimant's partner, which may outweigh the advantage of the partner continuing in such employment: it is characteristically women in families on benefit who are obliged to surrender the independence that part-time work may have given them (McLaughlin *et al.* 1989). So far as lone parents are concerned, 90 per cent of whom are women (Burghes 1993), the existence of a cohabitation rule subjects them to a degree of surveillance, whether actual or implied. Elements of the rule also apply to the receipt of bereavement benefit. Lone parents lose their particular independent entitlement to benefit if they should take a 'partner'.

Over and above the aggregation of needs and means within families for the purposes of social assistance, social security law also imposes a specific duty to maintain one's spouse and/or children so long as income support is being paid for them. This applies regardless of whether one lives with one's spouse or children, though it ceases to apply following divorce and/or when children reach the age of 16 (or in some circumstances 19). A similar provision applies in the case of anyone who under immigration law is a 'sponsor' of a 'person from abroad' who may have had recourse to IS. The government has power to pursue 'liable relatives' for the recovery of benefits paid for their legal dependants and to enforce or seek court orders for periodic maintenance. In the case of maintenance for children, such powers were enlarged and passed in 1993 to the Child Support Agency (CSA).

The assumption that underlies the child support scheme administered by the CSA is that biological parents have an inviolable duty to support their children financially, regardless of any changes or breakdown in family or living arrangements. The scheme provides a formula (for full details see CPAG's *Child Support Handbook*) by which to calculate the liability of 'non-resident parents' (mainly fathers) for the maintenance of dependent children with whom they do not co-reside and machinery by which to enforce the payments of such maintenance to the 'parents with care' (mainly mothers) of the children concerned. The scheme is therefore concerned to guarantee the subsistence needs of children, but it seeks to do so by defining rights for parents with care. What it creates, however, are not strictly social rights, but personal rights that are mediated by the state. The CSA assumed powers as to the making of maintenance orders which had previously been vested in the courts and which had for the most part been exercised only in the course of legal proceedings between private individuals. The intention had been generally to increase the level and consistency of maintenance payments by absent parents (DSS 1990), but specifically thereby to diminish the cost of social assistance benefits for lone parents (see Garnham and Knights 1994b).

Because child support maintenance payments count as income for the purposes of certain means-tested benefit entitlements, the effect can be to substitute a private entitlement for a social entitlement. Although child support maintenance is not taken into account for the purposes of calculating WFTC (or, from 2003, WTC – see Chapter 6) it does count, subject only to a modest disregard, in the case of IS, HB and CTB. The provision of the disregard for IS has only recently been conceded. While some parents with care of a qualifying child under the child support scheme may choose whether to avail themselves of the CSA's services, any such parents who receive IS (including income-based JSA) have no choice. They are required to make an application for child support and, unless they can show 'good cause', they are subject to a 'benefit penalty' (a reduction in benefit entitlement) for failing to co-operate.

The original child support formula was Byzantinely complex (Garnham and Knights 1994a), but it has since been radically simplified: the intention, none the less, was that 'no-one should be allowed to duck their responsibilities for their families and their children' (DSS 1999a: vii). In essence the formula stipulates the percentage of the non-resident parent's net income that should be paid in child support maintenance, taking into account the responsibilities he (it usually applies to fathers) might have for children in a second family. Non-resident parents on low incomes or who are themselves receiving benefits are required none the less to pay a nominal minimum contribution. Provision exists for the CSA not only to assess an absent parent's liability to child support, but also to collect payments on behalf of parents with care, for which purpose they are equipped with potentially quite draconian powers, including the power to attach earnings or to seek to have the driving licences of non-compliant non-resident parents revoked by way of a penalty. Where the enforcement of rights and responsibilities in relation to subsistence collide with the private sphere of family relationships, the consequences can be far reaching.

Security in old age

Old age is relative. In the mid-nineteenth century average life expectancy in England was around 40 for men and 42 for women. In the late twentieth century, it was 74 for men and 79 for women (Jackson 1998). Retirement in old age, however, is a recent phenomenon. The proportion of men aged 65 or more who were retired from the labour force increased from around a half in the 1930s to well over 90 per cent in the 1980s (Walker 1987). Townsend has argued that, as longevity increases and labour markets tighten, retirement is 'a kind of mass redundancy' (1991: 6). While social security in 'old age' may be a fundamental human right, most people over the age of 65 are not yet frail or physically dependent. The socially manufactured expectation of retirement represents a form of 'structured dependency' (*ibid.*).

Pensionable age in Britain was set in 1946 at 60 for women and 65 for men (although, in order to equalise pensionable ages, between 2010 and 2020 there will now be a phased increase in the pensionable age for women from 60 to 65). Prior to 1989, social security law also specified a 'retirement age' (65 for women and 70 for men) and between pensionable age and retirement age people were obliged to retire in order to receive a state pension. More recently, retirement has not been a condition of entitlement for the basic state pension and any earnings that a pensioner continues to receive will not affect her/his pension, though the RP is itself taxable. None the less, the basic contributory pension is still called a retirement pension. Its value by itself is no longer sufficient to provide subsistence by contemporary standards. It has been estimated that at the end of the twentieth century it was worth 15 per cent of male average earnings and that by 2050 it will in real terms be worth just half this amount (DSS 1998b). Nor, save for an age addition of literally a few pence per week for people over 80, does the value increase as people become older, when they are in fact more likely to be frail and vulnerable (Henwood and Wicks 1984). Though retirement pension is received by the vast majority of people of pensionable age, for most it is supplemented by other benefits (SERPS/S2P, disability benefits and/or means-tested benefits), by SHPs or by occupational or personal pensions.

To qualify for basic RP, a claimant or her late spouse must in the course of a year at some time have actually paid the equivalent of a year's worth of minimum level national insurance contributions (i.e. a sum equivalent to the national insurance 'lower earnings limit') and she must have paid or been credited with a year's worth of minimum level contributions for a 'requisite number' of years in the course of her 'working life'. There are limited circumstances in which divorced people can rely on a part of an ex-spouse's contribution record. Additionally, the requisite number of years' contributions can be reduced by the home responsibility protection provisions, but only up to a certain limit. The system is such as to disadvantage women and indeed anyone with a discontinuous employment record or who has worked in part-time employment at wages beneath the national insurance minimum (below which no contributions are paid). It is possible for people to defer their claim for retirement pension for up to five years after reaching pensionable age and so earn a slightly increased pension. As with most contributory benefits, increases in pension are payable for dependants. Married women who do not qualify for a pension on the basis of their own contributions may claim a reduced pension (at 60 per cent of the basic rate) provided both she and her husband are of pensionable age and her husband is in receipt of a basic pension, and this entitlement substitutes for a husband's entitlement to an increase for his wife as a dependant. For pensioners aged 80 or more who do not qualify for a basic pension, there is a non-contributory pension (paid at 60 per cent of the basic rate).

In addition to the basic RP, pensioners currently receive a nominal Christmas bonus and have the cost of their annual television licence met. More significantly, they may also receive a small amount of 'graduated retirement benefit' (based on contributions paid under a scheme which was in place between 1961 and 1975) and, if they have not been 'contracted out', an additional pension either under SERPS (which operated from 1978 to 2002) or the S2P. When SERPS was introduced in 1978 it was intended that, when the scheme had been in operation for a full 20 years, contributors should expect to retire with an additional pension equivalent to one quarter of the average earnings they had enjoyed during the 20 best earning years of their lives (revalued for inflation). After 10 years a Conservative government reduced this provision so that pensioners in the scheme who retired in or after 1999 could expect an additional pension of only one fifth of their revalued average earnings, calculated over the *whole* of their working life. The New Labour government elected to replace SERPS in 2002 with S2P, which is expressly designed only for the lowest-paid workers. While S2P is to be an earnings-related scheme until 2007, the expectation is that thereafter contributions under the scheme will provide only a flat rate addition to the basic RP and, although the government claimed that this should raise pensions above the level of the pensioners' MIG, this now seems unlikely (Piachaud 1999; Ward 2000). The significance of the S2P is that it is possible for those caring for pre-school children or disabled relatives and for disabled people themselves to be credited in to the scheme: they will be assumed to have made contributions as if they had been receiving a set qualifying level of earnings.

The policy makers' expectation, however, is that most pensioners will not have contributed to SERPS or S2P, but will have contributed instead either to an occupational pension scheme operated by their employer, an approved form of personal pension scheme operated by an insurance or investment company, or an SHP. SHPs are specially regulated private pension schemes that are intended to be better suited to employees with lower to middle-range earnings than the personal pension schemes that had been promoted (and subsidised through direct contribution rebates) by the Conservative government in the 1980s and 1990s. The funds operated by occupational, personal and SHP schemes benefit from tax exemptions on income and capital gains and to qualify as 'contracted out' schemes they must meet certain minimum standards. It remains the case, however, that although many 'defined benefit' occupational schemes (that guarantee retiring employees a proportion of their final salary) offer significant security, many other occupational schemes and all personal pension and SHP schemes are 'defined contribution' or 'money purchase' schemes. The eventual proceeds from the latter provide an annuity on retirement, though the value of this will be determined by the performance of investment markets and will not be guaranteed or index linked. Additionally, the value of personal pensions plans in particular can be eroded by charges for fund management. It should be emphasised that rights to occupational, 'personal' and stakeholder pensions are individually based rather than social rights and, though they are governed to an extent by social legislation, they do not purport to guarantee social security.

The extension of occupational pension provision in the decades following the Second World War undoubtedly did much to alleviate poverty in old age but coverage reached a plateau at around 50 per cent (McKay and Rowlingson 1999). Access to better-quality occupational schemes is often denied to women

because of the hours, the grade or the type of the jobs they characteristically fill (Groves 1992: 205). Although the contracted out personal pensions
developed in the late 1980s and early 1990s were taken up by around 28 per
cent of male employees, they attracted only 19 per cent of female employees
(although around a third of those joining such schemes will have ceased contributions within three years – see Waine 1999). Similarly, because of the
gendered structure of the labour market, it is anticipated that two-thirds of
the employees that will be attracted to SHP schemes after 2002 will be men
(DSS 1998b: 49). Although the S2P will be of benefit to women workers,
Falkingham and Rake (1999) have argued there is a risk that women will be
ghettoised into this, the least privileged part of the pension system.

In spite of Britain's complex pensions policy, it remains the case that those
who are most disadvantaged in the labour market are least likely to be able to
exercise a right to security in old age.

The rights of disabled people and carers

Excepting the specific case of industrial injuries benefits and war pensions,
social rights that are directed to the special subsistence needs of disabled
people have lagged behind the development of other rights. Benefits that are
dependent upon a test of incapacity for work or which assist disabled people
who are able to work will be considered in the next chapter. This section will
describe a clutch of benefits that were first introduced in the 1970s in order to
supplement benefit provision for severely disabled people. These were never
intended to be earnings replacement benefits, so much as categorical benefits
to meet the additional living costs incurred by disabled people. The benefits
originally introduced were called attendance allowance (AA) and mobility
allowance. These were reformed in the 1990s and, although AA still exists for
people aged 65 and over, a benefit called disability living allowance (DLA) has
incorporated mobility allowance and provision for the attendance or 'care'
needs of younger disabled people.

DLA and AA are both non-contributory, non-means-tested benefits, which
are not taxable and may be paid in addition to means-tested benefits (except
under the special rules applying to claimants living in residential care and
nursing homes). They are subject, however, to stringent eligibility rules.

DLA has two separately assessed components: the care component and the
mobility component. The care component is payable at three different rates:
the highest rate is equivalent currently to around three-quarters of the basic
RP for a single person, the middle rate to around a half and the lowest rate to
around a fifth. The mobility component is payable at two rates: the higher
rate is equivalent to just over a half of the basic RP for a single person and the
lower rate is the same as the lowest rate for the care component.

The care component may be claimed by or on behalf of people from birth
to the age of 65, provided they have met the relevant 'disability conditions' for
three months (unless they are diagnosed to be terminally ill) and are likely to
do so for at least a further six months. The disability conditions establish the

three levels of disability appropriate to the three rates at which the care component is payable. The conditions define circumstances in which a person is so severely disabled physically or mentally that she requires attention in connection with her bodily functions or supervision to prevent substantial danger to herself or others. If the attention required is frequent and/or the supervision required is continual and it is required both day and night, or if the claimant is terminally ill, she will qualify for the highest rate of benefit. If such attention or supervision is required throughout either the day or night, or if in certain circumstances the claimant is a home renal dialysis patient, she will qualify for the middle rate of benefit. If the attention required is 'limited', being required for only a period or periods within the course of the day, or if the claimant (provided she is aged 16 or over) is unable to prepare a cooked main meal for herself, she will qualify for the lowest rate of benefit. The scope for dispute regarding the interpretation of conditions such as these is considerable. The bodily functions to which the attention condition relates include such things as going to the lavatory, getting in or out of bed, getting dressed or undressed. The supervision condition extends to include supervision that is merely precautionary, such as might be required by a person who suffers from fits, or who is liable to behave violently or unpredictably.

The higher rate mobility component of DLA may be claimed by people aged between 3 and 65 and the lower rate by people aged between 5 and 65, provided they have met the relevant disability conditions for at least three months, they are likely to continue to do so for a further six months, and provided they would benefit from enhanced mobility (which might not apply if they are in a coma or cannot safely be moved). To qualify for the higher rate mobility component a claimant must be unable or virtually unable to walk as a result of a physical disability; or both blind and deaf, or have no feet; or severely mentally impaired and suffering from severe behavioural problems such that she already qualifies for the highest rate care component. To qualify for the lower rate mobility component a claimant, though she can walk, must be so severely disabled, physically or mentally, that she cannot usually walk outdoors without guidance or supervision.

AA is administered in the same way as the care component of DLA, save that it is claimed by people over 65 and with the important difference that it is not available at the lowest rate.

The introduction of the original AA scheme in 1971 involved a recognition of the care needs of severely disabled people but it was not until 1976 that a benefit expressly for the carers of disabled people was introduced. The benefit is currently called invalid care allowance, it is paid at barely 60 per cent of the level of the basic single person's retirement pension, and it is a non-contributory, non-means-tested benefit. It has been proposed (DWP 2001) that the benefit will be renamed carer's allowance (CA) and, although this has not been confirmed at the time of writing, that is what I shall call the allowance. Although it is a categorical benefit like DLA and AA, CA is taxable and it is taken fully into account for the purposes of means-tested benefit entitlements. The level of subsistence achieved by many carers, therefore, is determined not by CA, but by IS (within which provision is made for a carer's premium, the additional value of which stands at just over a quarter of a single adult's weekly personal allowance). In spite of this, CA does represent a symbolic recognition of carers as citizens and is valued by those that receive it (McLaughlin 1991). However, when first introduced the allowance was not made available to women caring for a spouse or male partner, upon the assumption that such women would have been available to care in any event. The legality of this discriminatory provision was successfully challenged in the European Court (see Chapter 9). Similarly, CA has been denied to carers who first claim it after reaching the age of 65, although it has been proposed that this restriction will be rescinded. CA should therefore be available to anybody over the age of 16 who is providing regular and substantial care for a person who is in receipt of DLA at the highest and middle rates or AA (or the constant attendance allowances available under the industrial injuries and war pensions schemes). Claimants must demonstrate that they are not gainfully employed and that they are not in full-time education.

DLA, AA and CA represent an ambiguous group of benefits. They are partly concerned with the right to subsistence and in this respect they need to be understood in the context of other benefits that may compensate disabled people for their exclusion from the labour market, and these I discuss in Chapter 6. They are partly concerned with establishing the right to social care, an issue to which I shall return in Chapter 8.

Summary/conclusion

Any concept of social rights will include a right to the means of subsistence. In advanced capitalist societies this requires the provision of cash benefits. This chapter has discussed the British system of cash benefits. The system is complex because it employs three different principles of provision. First, the social assistance principle provides for benefits upon demonstration of need by means-testing. Second, the social insurance principle provides for benefits upon the payment of contributions from earnings and in the event of a particular contingency. Third, what is sometimes called a 'universal' principle that provides for benefits, with neither means-tests nor contribution conditions, but as a response to some generally defined contingency or for a particular category of persons. The peculiarity of the system as a whole also arises because the main social security system that has embodied these principles exists in increasingly close juxtaposition with the tax system and the occupational benefits system.

Though elements of social insurance and categorical provision remain important, it is the social assistance principle that has regained ascendancy as we enter the twenty-first century. At the centre of the social security system is a means-tested benefit, IS, which continues to employ a traditional form of means-test based on a calculation of the shortfall between a citizen's needs and her means. This form of means-test may arguably be being upstaged by a more complex form (details of which I shall discuss in the next chapter) often now framed as tax credits. None the less, the nature of the traditional means-test has ensured that the needs of different groups are assessed differently and the needs and means of individuals are 'aggregated' with those of their families.

The state continues, through the categorical benefit CB, to make a partial contribution towards the cost of bringing up children, although the significance of this contribution may arguably change as the CTC is introduced. What does not change is the assumption by policy makers that families have a role in providing or guaranteeing the subsistence of their adult members as well as children. Such assumptions are reflected both implicitly in the case of social insurance and explicitly in the case of social assistance. The consequences are such as to amplify the disadvantages of women and to enforce particular patterns of dependency within families. At a time when patterns of family formation have become more fluid, the child support scheme is imposing permanent responsibilities for the subsistence needs of children upon biological parents, rather than the state.

This chapter has also paid particular attention to benefit provision for older people and disabled people. Though still based on social insurance principles, basic pension provision for older people has become increasingly inadequate to the subsistence needs associated with the socially constructed status of 'retirement'. Basic state provision must be supplemented. For a minority this must be done by way of the S2P. For most it is achieved privately, through SHPs, personal or occupational pensions paid for in the course of their employment. However, women and disadvantaged groups may have limited access to additional pensions and some may even be denied independent rights to a basic pension: in such circumstances people must fall back on social assistance. Certain categorical benefits are available for people who are severely disabled, though such provision is addressed to their special needs, rather than their basic subsistence needs which will usually still be met from within other parts of the social security system. A categorical benefit is also available to those who care for severely disabled people, though at such a level and on such terms that many will also require social assistance.

This chapter has focused on the basic structure of the British income maintenance system and on provision that is made for those who are, by and large, excluded from the labour market. The next chapter turns to the social rights of people who are actually or potentially economically active.

Chapter 6

Rights and work

The Universal Declaration of Human Rights states that 'Everyone has the right to work, to free choice of employment, to just and favourable conditions of work and to protection against unemployment' (UN 1948: Article 23[1]). In practice, however, no right to work exists in British law. The availability and choice of employment are subject to market forces and, although macro-economic and local development policies may aim to create jobs, employment for all is not and never has been guaranteed. Rights *at* work are not, strictly speaking, social rights in the sense that previous chapters have given to that term, but primarily civil or contractual rights. None the less, contracts of employment are subject to legislative regulation and where workers' rights are guaranteed by statute they are often referred to – particularly within the European Union – as social rights. In Britain limited protection exists, for example, against unfair dismissal, but ultimately there *is* no protection against unemployment. To the extent that social security provision exists for the protection of people during unemployment, the rights afforded by such provision are clearly tied to a *duty* rather than a right to work.

It was observed in the last chapter that rights to social security are generally predicated upon assumptions about people's duties to maintain themselves. This is implicit, not only in British social legislation, but in the UN declaration itself, which also says, 'Everyone who works has the right to just and favourable remuneration ensuring for himself and his family an existence worthy of human dignity, and supplemented, if necessary, by other means of social protection' (Article 23[3]). While the right to work has not been translated into British social policy, the assumptions of this last mentioned clause have been:

- The existence of individuals and families is assumed normally to be ensured through remuneration obtained by 'work'.
- 'Work' is synonymous with employment. It does not encompass such activities as caring for children and disabled relatives, domestic labour, or voluntary effort expended in the interests of the community. However important these activities may be to the maintenance of 'human dignity', they need not and do not attract 'just and favourable remuneration'.
- Where remuneration from employment is insufficient some form of 'social protection' may be afforded. Economic rights may therefore be supplemented, though they will not be supplanted, by social rights.

In Britain the New Labour government has declared that its aim is to 'rebuild the welfare state around work' (DSS 1998a: 23). In the pursuit of this aim the government is committed:

- To a policy of 'welfare-to-work'. The intention is to promote an active rather than a passive welfare state that insists upon 'work for those who can' (*ibid.*: iii). The government also promises 'security for those who cannot [work]' through the kinds of rights discussed in Chapter 5, but the centrality of 'work' was nowhere more clearly expressed than following the 2001 General Election when the re-elected Labour government transferred key functions in relation to employment from what had been the Department of Social Security in order to create the Department of Work and Pensions (DWP).
- To making work pay. This is to be achieved partly through a national minimum wage (NMW), partly through a system of means-tested 'in-work' benefits or 'tax credits'.
- To making it easier to combine work and family life (see Home Office 1998). This is to be achieved partly through a national childcare strategy (NCS), partly by promoting 'family-friendly' employment practices.
- But also, none the less, to maintaining 'the most lightly regulated labour market of any leading economy in the world' (DTI 1998: 1).

This chapter will examine the relationship in Britain between 'work' (narrowly defined as paid employment) and 'rights' (where these are specifically defined in social legislation). The chapter focuses, first, upon the protections which employees have at work and, second, upon the rights, penalties and duties to which people of working age who are not in employment may be subject. Attention then turns to two forms of social protection: first, the in-work benefits or tax credits available to low-paid employees and, second, the benefits available to employees and others prevented from working by 'incapacity'.

Employment protection

Employment protection is a complex area of law and what follows is but the briefest resumé. (For a more detailed treatment see, for example, Jefferson 2000.) I shall discuss the broad context in which workers' rights have been framed; the question of pay, working hours and holidays; the rights of working parents; protection against sexual, racial and disability discrimination; and, finally, dismissal and redundancy.

The context for 'social' protection in employment

The origins of social protection for workers may be traced back to nineteenth-century Factory Acts that had sought, for example, on paternalistic grounds to prevent employers from exploiting women and children. However, when it came to establishing the rights of workers, before these were ever enshrined in statute they were articulated and defended by trade unions. For much of the

twentieth century there was a broad consensus that workers' interests were
best served by collective bargaining between industry and organised labour
(Kahn-Freund 1977). The right to form and to join trade unions is one of the
'universal' rights declared by the UN (1948: Article 23[1]). The position
under British law is that nobody may legally be refused work, dismissed or
victimised for being or for *not* being a member of a trade union. However,
Conservative governments during the 1980s and 1990s had sought to erode the
power of trade unions (see Johnson 1990: 30–1) and trade union membership
has dramatically declined from around 58 per cent of all employees to less than
30 per cent (Machin 2000). Although the 1997 New Labour government did
legislate to enhance trade union recognition rights, it did not repeal many of
the restrictions that the Conservatives had imposed on the unions and, in
comparison to those continental European countries in which trade unions
are acknowledged as key 'social partners', the influence of British trade unions
in the industrial relations and policy making arenas remains extremely limited.
In spite of this the services of a trade union are often an effective means of
enforcing individual rights in employment.

The political trend in Britain towards the curtailment of trade union power
reflects a deeper tension concerning social protection in employment, which
in recent years has been the subject of contradictory pressures. On the one
hand, the European Union (EU) has been concerned to promote what it calls
a 'social dimension' to the process of European economic integration and
development (CEC 1993). To this end the EU Charter of Fundamental
Social Rights of 1989 and the Social Protocol – or 'Social Chapter' – to the
1993 and 1997 Maastricht and Amsterdam Treaties have sought to build
upon earlier measures under the Treaty of Rome relating to freedom of movement, health and safety at work and the equal treatment of men and women.
These measures belatedly bring a limited degree of enforceability to certain of
the principles contained in the Council of Europe's purely declaratory Social
Charter of 1961. In the event, the Council of Europe's Social Charter was
revised in 1996 so as to provide not a right of individual redress, but of
Collective Complaint by trades unions and non-governmental organisations
to a European Committee for Social Rights. Elements of the revised Charter
have been incorporated by the EU in a Charter of Fundamental Rights pro-
claimed in Nice in 2000 but not in a directly justiciable form. The outcome
has been a programme of reforms focused primarily upon workers' rights, the
harmonisation of employment protection measures and some more general
proposals for enhanced protection for socially excluded groups. On the other
hand, British governments have been seeking in various ways to curtail the
body of legislative protection by which a 'floor of rights' had been established
for employees since the Second World War, claiming that the costs of such
protection were making British industry uncompetitive. For these reasons,
Conservative governments had refused to sign up to the EU Social Chapter
(even though this could not insulate Britain entirely from the effects of social
directives enacted under earlier EU powers). The New Labour government of
1997 restored or created certain important rights for employees and it moved

swiftly to sign the EU Social Chapter. However, New Labour has been keen to be 'business friendly' and so to place certain limits upon employee protection measures. In Europe New Labour governments, like their Conservative predecessors, have sought to constrain the development of social initiatives and, when translating EU social directives into domestic law, have tended to interpret them in a restrictive or minimalist way.

The essential context for recent employment protection policy has been the effect – both real and imagined – of economic globalisation (see Chapter 3) and the quest by business to promote 'flexible' working practices. One of the principal challenges to social security and employment protection policy has been the emergence of what would once have been regarded as 'atypical workers' – employees whose jobs may be part-time, impermanent or irregular (Blackwell 1994) – many of whom had been excluded not only from social insurance schemes, but also from formal employment protection. As a result of recent EU directives part-time workers in Britain do now enjoy broadly the same level of statutory protection as full-time workers. However, full protection is still denied, for example, to 'self-employed' workers (though the distinction between the status of an employee and an independent contractor is fraught with difficulty) and in relation to some matters to people over pensionable age (who are subject to the expectation that they may retire – see Chapter 5). Also the level of protection available to people working for small employers (those with fewer than 15 or 20 employees, depending on the provision in question) may be less than for those working for large employers, notwithstanding that small businesses employ a substantial and increasing proportion of the labour force (Watson 1995).

Most workers' rights, even statutory rights, arise because they are implied or imposed within a contract of employment (whether it be written or unwritten) and employers are required within a specified period of time to provide employees with a written statement of their main terms and conditions of employment. Protected employees are therefore entitled to be informed, both of their contractual rights and of their rights in matters that may be governed by statutory regulation (including sick pay and pension arrangements). This applies whether or not the provision that the employer makes is more generous than the statutory minima laid down. The entitlements of protected employees to information also extend, for example, to a right to receive itemised pay slips and, in the event of dismissal, to a written statement of the reasons for dismissal. Disputes over terms of employment and in relation to such matters as discrimination, dismissal and redundancy may be resolved by the Employment Tribunal (see Chapter 9).

Pay, working hours and holidays

Until the introduction of the NMW in 1999, Britain had been the only major industrialised nation not to have minimum wage legislation. Even the limited protection once afforded by statutory Wages Councils had been abolished by a Conservative government in the 1980s. The NMW, which requires employers to pay a minimum hourly rate for all adults (with a reduced rate for young people aged 18–21), was therefore a major landmark. In spite of dire warnings from the business community, the initial introduction of the NMW resulted in an increase in the national wage bill of just 0.5 per cent and had no adverse effects on the British economy (Exell 2001). However, although the government has chosen periodically to uprate the level of the NMW, at the time that it was introduced it declined to legislate for such upratings and there remains a risk that subsequent governments could allow the real value of the NMW to decline. Additionally, the level at which the NMW is set is low: whereas the Council of Europe has recommended a 'decency threshold' equivalent to around two-thirds of average full-time earnings, at the time of writing the level of Britain's NMW is barely half that level. In its attempts to minimise the effect on employers the government has limited the effectiveness of the NMW in abating poverty and has been obliged, in order to make work pay, to supplement the wages of low-paid workers through in-work benefits (see below).

Although it had been forced upon the UK by EU directives, the other major innovation to be introduced since New Labour was first elected relates to the regulation of working time. The 1998 Working Time Regulations ostensibly imposed a maximum working week of 48 hours and rules relating both to rest periods and to night-shift working. In practice, however, a wide range of professionals, transport and emergency service workers are exempted from the regulations and, at the time of writing, employees may in any event enter agreements with their employers not to be bound by the regulations. Once again, therefore, the practical effect has been minimal. The one area in which the Working Time Regulations have made a difference relates to holiday entitlement: the Regulations established for the first time in British law a right to a minimum period (currently 4 weeks) of paid holiday.

The minimum rights of employees to sick pay are discussed later in this chapter.

Legislating for 'family-friendly employment'

In its bid to promote family-friendly employment the New Labour government was able to build upon a limited legacy of maternity rights, consisting of statutory maternity pay (SMP) and maternity leave provision.

Although it is not a benefit for incapacity, SMP was originally modelled closely on statutory sick pay (SSP – see below). It has substantially replaced an earlier short-term national insurance benefit, maternity allowance (MA), and is now administered by employers (although, unlike SSP, it is still partially financed by the government). Pregnancy does not necessarily imply incapacity for work, though it is treated for social security purposes in a similar way. SMP is payable during the period of ordinary maternity leave (OML) to which employees are statutorily entitled (and which is to be extended from 18 to 26 weeks in 2003 – see below). For the first six weeks of that period, SMP is payable at 90 per cent of the claimant's normal earnings and, for the remainder of the OML period, at a lower rate (currently set at the same level as SSP). The entitlement is 'earned' after six months' employment with the same employer, providing earnings exceed the national insurance minimum. For women who have been self-employed or who changed or left a job just before or during pregnancy, an adapted form of MA, paid by the government, has been retained. From 2003 statutory paternity pay (SPP) will be introduced and this will entitle the fathers of newborn babies to two weeks' leave that will be paid at a level equivalent to the lower rate of SMP.

As already indicated, pregnant women, in addition to SMP, are entitled to maternity leave and may reserve the right to return to their jobs at the end of that period. OML is a right of all women employees, but women with at least a year's continuous service with the same employer are also entitled to additional maternity leave (AML) amounting, from 2003, to a further 26 weeks. Employers are not required to pay employees during AML. The effect of the change proposed for 2003 is to extend from 29 to 52 weeks the period during which a woman may, after having a baby, return to her previous job. In addition to the statutory minimum maternity and paternity leave provisions, in compliance with an EU directive, mothers and fathers with more than a year's continuous service and who have children under the age of 5 years have, since 1999, been afforded the right to unpaid parental leave, which may be taken up to a maximum of 13 weeks per child, in blocks of up to a week or more at a time, but subject to a minimum period of prior notice having been given and the right of the employer to postpone the requested leave. Employees have also since 1999 enjoyed a right to have a reasonable amount of time off – on an unpaid basis – in order to attend to *bona fide* domestic emergencies. It is also proposed that, from 2003, the parents of young children may be entitled not to demand, but to request flexible working hours. The rights described above may also apply, in an appropriate form, to the parents of adopted children.

Recent extensions to the rights of working parents have been significant, but in this respect Britain still lags behind many of its European partners and New Labour remains reluctant to legislate in ways that employers may regard as unduly onerous (DTI 2000). The government prefers to encourage the development of good employment practice through the promotion of a 'Work-Life Balance' campaign directed to employers. Many of Britain's best employers have been responding voluntarily, but others have not and it remains the case that it is more highly paid staff that are benefiting, while low-paid workers often feel too insecure in their jobs to demand rights of this nature (Dean 2002). The ability of parents – and especially mothers – to benefit from such rights will depend not only on the extent to which the worst employers can be regulated, but also on the extent to which effective rights to childcare provision may be developed (see Chapter 8).

Protection from discrimination

British anti-discrimination legislation extends to three areas – sex, race and disability – but does not directly address discrimination on the grounds of either age or sexuality (though claims in respect of the latter may be sustainable under the Human Rights Act and/or the European Convention and there are regulations to prevent discrimination against persons undergoing gender reassignment). The principal items of legislation extend to cover discrimination in spheres other than employment, but because they are most often invoked in relation to the rights of workers, they will be discussed in that context.

General legislation to outlaw sexual discrimination was preceded in Britain by the Equal Pay Act of 1970, which imposes on all contracts of employment the condition that the employer shall not provide less favourable pay or conditions on the grounds of sex. However, because labour market practices often result in segregation between women's jobs and men's jobs, it is often difficult to prove that women are being paid less for work that is the same as or that is of equal value to that performed by men. Subsequently, the Sex Discrimination Act of 1975 and the Race Relations Acts of 1976 respectively also provided redress before the Employment Tribunal should employees be directly or indirectly discriminated against in the course of their employment upon the grounds of sex, 'race', colour, national or ethnic origins. The only exceptions that are permitted relate to circumstances where gender or race represent a 'genuine occupational qualification'. Unlike other employment rights, these extend to all employees, regardless of length of service and even apply to job applicants. In practice, however, it may once again be difficult to prove that less favourable treatment has resulted from gendered or racial motives, or that the imposition of particular criteria necessarily bear unequally upon different sexes or ethnic groups. The legislation creates procedures by which employers may be formally questioned about discriminatory practices and it created two independent bodies, the Equal Opportunities Commission (EOC) and the Commission for Racial Equality (CRE), that are charged to promote equality of opportunity and prevent discrimination and which have powers to conduct investigations and to advise and support individual complainants.

The more recent Disability Discrimination Act of 1995 created a broadly similar legal framework, but only after the New Labour government introduced additional legislation in 1999 to create the Disability Rights Commission (DRC) to function as the direct counterpart to the EOC and CRE. Disability under the Act is defined as physical or mental impairment that has a substantial and long-term adverse effect on a person's ability to perform necessary tasks, but unlike the sex and race discrimination legislation, employers may be permitted to discriminate if they can establish a 'justifiable reason' for treating a disabled person less favourably than other workers. While employers are required to provide such 'reasonable adjustments' as may be necessary in the workplace so that a disabled person should not be disadvantaged, various kinds of employer are exempted from the requirement and the cost, in relation to the state of the employer's finances, is relevant to whether or not such adjustments may be adjudged reasonable.

Unfair dismissal and redundancy

Employment law also provides protection against involuntary unemployment since it defines the circumstances in which employees may be 'fairly' dismissed. The right *not* to be *un*fairly dismissed is heavily qualified. At the time of writing it is only available after one year's service with the same employer. To dismiss unprotected workers, employers need have no reason. Otherwise, they may rely on one of five possible causes:

- reasons relating to the employee's capability (because, for example, she is no longer fit to do her job);
- because of misconduct;
- redundancy (because the employee's job has ceased to exist);
- because of some legal constraint (as would apply, for example, if a driver was disqualified from driving); or
- for some other substantial reason.

It must additionally be reasonable to dismiss for the reason upon which the employer relies and the employer must act reasonably when deciding to dismiss somebody. It may be reasonable in certain circumstances for an employer to offer alternative employment rather than to dismiss. In practice, the Employment Tribunal – which considers complaints of unfair dismissal – makes this test of 'reasonableness' a test of the employer's conduct, rather than an objective test of 'fairness'. For example, an employee who is dismissed for misconduct but has subsequently been proved innocent of an alleged offence at work may still be held to have been fairly dismissed, provided her/his employer acted reasonably at the time and genuinely believed the employee to be guilty. Employment Tribunals have the power to order employers to reinstate or re-engage unfairly dismissed employees, though it is more usual for employers to be ordered to pay compensation. Similarly, protected employees who are dismissed on the specific ground of redundancy must, in any event, be paid compensation subject to a statutory minimum based on their length of service with the employer concerned. If it can be shown that an employer had to make redundancies but that the selection of a particular employee for redundancy was unfair, then the employee may be compensated for unfair dismissal as well as redundancy. When it is available, compensation may represent a remedy in the legal sense, but it does not of course prevent unemployment.

The working-age benefits regime

Protecting against the consequences of unemployment has been one of the central tasks of the social security system, the basic structure of which was outlined in Chapter 5. In the past that protection stemmed partly from social insurance (the national insurance unemployment benefit scheme) and partly from social assistance (most recently, IS). Cash benefits for unemployed people have always been conditional upon some test of their willingness to work. In recent years, however, the introduction of jobseeker's allowance (JSA) has redoubled the rigour with which that test is applied in the case of those who are registered as unemployed and, through the development of the New Deals, the scope and reach of the test have been extended so that elements of it may touch anybody of 'working age' who is not in employment but who is in receipt of a social security benefit.

Jobseeker's allowance

JSA is a social security benefit (introduced in April 1996) for people who are unemployed. The name of the benefit announces its primary purpose: it is a benefit providing social protection to unemployed people only if they are seeking employment. What is more, the rules of the JSA scheme function to penalise people who may have become voluntarily unemployed.

The JSA is in fact two schemes in one (DE/DSS 1994). It includes a short-term contributory benefit, which prior to 1996 was called unemployment benefit, and a means-tested or income-based benefit, which is a form of IS. What they have in common is that both are payable subject to the terms of a Jobseeker's Agreement, into which claimants are required to enter. The benefits were initially administered by the Social Security Benefits Agency and Jobseeker's Agreements by the government's Employment Service: at the time of writing, these two agencies are about to be combined into a single government agency, which was originally to be called the Working Age Agency but will now go by the name of JobCentre Plus (JC+). Contributory JSA is payable only for the first six months of a spell of unemployment and on condition that the claimant meets stringent contribution conditions which exclude those who have not recently been in employment. (The requirement is that the claimant must within the preceding two years have actually paid employees' national insurance contributions equivalent to half a year's worth of minimum-level contributions and she must have been paid or been credited with a year's worth of minimum-level contributions in each of the preceding two years.) Though it is not fully means-tested in the way that IS is (in so far that the claimant's savings and the resources of her partner, if any, are not taken into account), contributory JSA is means-tested in respect of any part-time earnings that claimants might obtain and any occupational or private pension that they might have as a result of early retirement. Income-based JSA is subject to the same means-test as IS (see Chapter 5), albeit with a rule which permits the partners of claimants to work up to 24 hours per week – rather than 16 hours per week – without disqualifying the claimant (though the partner's earnings are still taken into account). Both forms of the allowance are subject, after three months, to special earnings disregard rules which allow claimants to 'roll up' a proportion of deducted part-time earnings above the standard disregard level and to have these deductions repaid (subject to a maximum) as a lump sum 'back to work bonus' when the claimant leaves benefit for full-time employment.

The rates (or 'applicable amounts') for income-based JSA are the same as IS and the rates of contributory JSA are aligned with those of a single person's personal allowance for IS purposes (so that young people are paid less than older people). Claimants who qualify for contributory JSA but who have dependants (assuming their partner, if any, is not working full-time and they do not have significant income from other sources) will also have to claim income-based JSA. After six months' unemployment, all claimants are entitled only to the income-based JSA.

Claimants of JSA are required to register or 'sign on' at a jobcentre and to declare not only that they are unemployed, but also that they are actively seeking work. They must declare their willingness to take full-time employment (defined for these purposes as up to 40 hours per week, though claimants may be expected to accept employment for fewer hours per week if it is offered). Since unemployment benefit was first introduced in 1911 it had always been subject to a condition that its recipients should be available for work and at various times additional conditions were imposed requiring that claimants should be 'genuinely' or 'actively' seeking work, with provision for benefit to be withdrawn if claimants should fail without reasonable excuse to take up a job offer or a place on a government retraining scheme. The same rules were applied to unemployed people who claimed social assistance benefits. The latest device, the Jobseeker's Agreement, requires the claimant to agree, as a condition of entitlement, to a programme of activities in order to find or return to work. Only during an initial 'permitted period' (currently 13 weeks) are claimants allowed to seek employment in their former occupation, after which they must agree to look more widely for jobs. Allowances are withdrawn if agreements are not 'honoured'. Explicit obligations are defined and enforced for each claimant and the terms of Jobseeker's Agreements are periodically reviewed. JC+ 'advisers' have power to make Jobseeker's Directions requiring claimants, for example, to attend workshops or courses in jobseeking skills or to improve their acceptability to employers in other ways. Claimants who fail to meet the 'labour market conditions' for benefit (by not proving they are available for and actively seeking work and/or by failing to complete and sign a Jobseeker's Agreement) receive no benefit. Claimants who flout Jobseeker's Directions are disqualified from benefit for a fixed period. The explicit intention is that it should be possible for 'benefit to be stopped where the unemployed person's behaviour is such that it actively militates against finding work' (DE/ DSS 1994: para. 4.13).

Not only are the claimants of JSA coerced into 'jobseeking' upon terms imposed by the JC+, they may also be penalised depending upon the circumstances in which they come to be on benefit. Rules of this nature have applied since unemployment benefit was first introduced and have functioned as a deterrent to unemployment. The penalties involved take the form of a disqualification from benefit (currently, for up to six months), with provision for hardship payments (a reduced level of benefit) if it can be demonstrated that a member of the claimant's household will suffer hardship as a consequence of the sanction. The sanction applies if a claimant is deemed to have given up their previous employment (or a place on a government approved training scheme) without 'just cause', or if they have been dismissed from their employment (or a training scheme) for misconduct. The effect is to ensure that employees should cling to their jobs, however unsuitable, and to inflict a double punishment upon anyone who is sacked from a job (for a fuller discussion, see Dean 1991: 104–7).

JSA is also denied to people who are on strike or who are prevented from working as a result of a trade dispute. The dependants of such people may be eligible to claim IS, although their entitlement is reduced by a set amount on account of assumed income from strike pay (whether or not any strike pay is received). This provision was originally applied to unemployment benefit in order that the government should not be seen to give succour to one side in a trade dispute, though in practice the rules relating to social assistance for dependants were made more stringent in the 1980s and it is difficult to construe the effect as anything other than the punishment of strikers and their families.

In some ways, the advent of JSA under a Conservative government made the nature of benefits for unemployed people more transparent. The White Paper which preceded its introduction openly declared that the benefit regime proposed represented an 'important step' in the government's labour market reforms (DE/DSS 1994: para. 1.2) and was noted by some commentators to be 'soaked in the language of labour deregulation and the free market' (CPAG 1994b: 7). Arguably, such benefits have always been extended not so much as a social right as an incentive to remain in, to enter, or to re-enter the labour market. The conditions attaching to benefit have implied a certain reciprocity between citizens' rights to benefit and their obligation to work. The introduction of the Jobseeker's Agreement has translated such reciprocity from a general principle to an explicit requirement. It has turned social rights and obligations sanctioned by general rules into individual rights and obligations sanctioned by an individual agreement.

The New Deal

This approach has been extended by New Labour governments with the very clear aim of ensuring that rights and responsibilities should go together (Labour Party 1997 and 2001). The centrepiece of New Labour's welfare-to-work policy was the New Deal. The New Deal built upon elements of the various kinds of training and work-welfare schemes that had been developed by previous governments (Ainley 1993; Gardiner 1997), but it was more systematic and more far reaching. There were six main New Deal programmes – introduced at different times during New Labour's first term of office and in a variety of pilot areas, all of which have, from 2002, been consolidated and rolled out nationally in the form of the 'single gateway' claims process administered by the JC+ (which was itself piloted as the 'ONE' initiative), to create what amounts to a permanent New Deal (see Millar 2000; Trickey and Walker 2001).

The original New Deal pilots were aimed at getting key groups of benefit recipients – young unemployed people, long-term unemployed people, lone parents, the partners of unemployed people, disabled people and unemployed people aged 50 and above – into employment. There was an important distinction between the schemes for young and long-term unemployed people in which participation was compulsory and where the object was to enhance employability and the other schemes which were voluntary and where the object was to 'enable' participants. The 'gateway' concept was developed to refer to participation by claimants in job-focused interviews with Personal

Advisers or a period during which working-age claimants receive tailored advice and intensive support with their jobseeking and to prepare and assist them to (re)enter the labour market.

JSA claimants are required to enter the gateway if they have failed to obtain employment after a certain period of time (originally set at 6 months for young unemployed people and 18 months for 25–50-year-olds). If they should not have obtained employment by the end of the gateway process they are then required to take up options on temporary six-month subsidised employment or training placements. In the case of the original New Deal for young people, which had been funded by a windfall tax on the private utilities, there were additional options involving trial periods in self-employment or placements in voluntary sector or environmental task force placements. However, the application of JSA sanctions (see above) may be applied to ensure that claimants are not allowed the option of remaining on benefit. At the end of the six-month option period claimants that have not obtained permanent employment return to receive further jobsearch assistance.

Older JSA recipients, lone parents in receipt of IS, the partners of unemployed people and disabled people receiving benefits had been invited to participate voluntarily in the New Deal pilots. New Deal initiatives have included the provision of employment credit payments to unemployed people aged 50 or over who re-enter the labour market, discretionary assistance with childcare costs for lone parents who agree to work part-time and a provision that automatically treats the childless partners of jobseekers – if they are beneath a certain age – as joint claimants. The intention under the new regime for working-age claimants is that all these groups be required to attend compulsory work-focused interviews as a condition of receiving benefits, although they will not necessarily (at the time of writing) be compelled to take up specific employment or training options. Pivotal to the effectiveness of the New Deal is the role played by Personal Advisers who advise, assist and support participants in relation to benefits and allowance (including in-work benefits) and the training and employment opportunities that are available. The risk foreseen as the New Deal moves beyond its pilot stages and as caseloads increase in scale and diversity is that certain tensions would be exacerbated: between claimants' and employers' expectations, between the welfare and control functions of the Personal Advisers, and between the need for flexible responses and the ability to deliver forward planning to meet individual circumstances (Millar 2000). The New Deal has given birth to a new 'active' benefits regime for those of working age that is at best paternalistic and at worst coercive. It is a regime that in one sense promotes the right to work (although it does not create permanent jobs – see Peck 2001), while undermining the rights of those without work.

In-work benefits

One of the fundamental assumptions of the Beveridgian social security system had been that, subject to the availability of universal health care and family allowances, wages from employment would always be sufficient to ensure against poverty. Whether or not such an assumption was ever justified, it has been completely invalidated by employment market trends and, since the 1970s, growing wage inequality with downward pressure on wage levels at the bottom of the earnings distribution (Goodman and Webb 1994). The persistence of low-paying forms of employment together with the expansion of 'atypical' employment patterns have necessitated (and have to an extent been facilitated by) the introduction since the 1970s of means-tested in-work benefits.

A precedent for such benefits had been established, albeit briefly, in the eighteenth century by the Speenhamland system of poor relief (see George 1973), though for a century and a half the idea that the state should intervene to subsidise low wages had been shunned by governments of all political persuasions. The eventual reintroduction by a Conservative government of a benefit by which to top up the wages of working families was justified as a preferable alternative to any extension of universal family benefits. The benefit, originally called family income supplement, was revised in 1988 to become family credit and promoted, again by a Conservative government, as a benefit that – unlike child benefit – was accurately 'targeted' on those working families in greatest need. In 1999 the New Labour government replaced family credit with working families' tax credit (WFTC) which, as has been explained in Chapter 5, will be replaced in 2003 by a combination of the working tax credit (WTC) and the new child tax credit (CTC).

At the time of writing the precise details of the WTC and CTC have still to be announced and I shall therefore use a brief description of the WFTC scheme in order to illustrate the basic principles of the means-test on which in-work tax credits in general (and also housing benefit – see Chapter 7) operate. WFTC is payable to lone parents or to couples with dependent children, where the lone parent or either member of the couple are in full-time employment (defined as employment for more than 16 hours per week). It is not therefore available to part-time employees, who may only claim IS (if they are lone parents) or income-based JSA (where they are one of a couple and if they can establish their availability for employment of 24 hours or more per week). Where the claimant herself is in employment, payment of the WFTC is made through her pay packet on behalf of the government by the employer: this arrangement was intended to make WFTC seem less like a social security benefit and to allow claimants more readily to associate the income they were receiving with work. In two-parent households, however, where the claimant is the man, the effect may be to deprive women of independent income and/or to perpetuate the norms of the 'traditional' male breadwinner household (Goode et al. 1998; Land 1999). It is possible, none the less, for women in couples to be the claimant and, if they are not in employment, to receive payment of WFTC directly from the Tax Credit Office. The calculation of WFTC (and related benefits/tax credits) is a 'taper' calculation. It is a more complex form of 'needs minus means' calculation than the income support calculation described in Chapter 5 (for a more detailed explanation see CPAG's *Welfare Benefits Handbook*):

If **NEEDS**	>	**MEANS**	*then*	**ENTITLEMENT**	=	MAXIMUM
(applicable amount)	(is greater than)	(income) *(subject to 'disregards' and to disqualification if capital exceeds a ceiling)*		(benefit payable)	(equals)	(maximum credit/ allowance/ benefit)
If **NEEDS**	>	**MEANS**	*then*	**ENTITLEMENT**	=	MAXIMUM –
(applicable amount)	(is less than)	(income) *(subject to 'disregards' and to disqualification if capital exceeds a ceiling)*		(benefit payable)	(equals)	([NEEDS – MEANS] $\times$ n%) (maximum credit/ allowance/benefit *minus* a proportion of 'excess income')

Figure 6.1 'Taper' means-test calculation

- Needs are determined with reference, first, to a set 'applicable amount' (which is the *same* for all families, but is set at the level of the personal allowance for an adult couple on IS) and, second, to a *maximum* credit level, determined with reference to a scale of allowances for one adult (but with additional credit if an adult member of the family is working more than 30 hours per week) and for each child in the family (though, with the introduction of CTC, this will no longer apply).
- Means (taking into account both income and capital) are determined in the same way as for IS purposes, but with some differences as to income disregards (most importantly, child benefit and income from child support maintenance are not taken into account).
- The maximum credit is payable if a claimant has less than the permitted amount of savings/capital and her income is less than the 'applicable amount'.
- If the claimant's income exceeds the 'applicable amount', the maximum credit will be reduced by a proportion (currently 55 per cent in the case of WFTC) of that 'excess', so that the benefit 'tapers' off as a claimant's income increases (and as her need for the benefit reduces). A schematic representation of the calculation is set out in Figure 6.1.

Linked to WFTC (and to WTC from 2003) is the childcare tax credit (CCTC) that can assist working parents with the cost of registered childcare. This will be discussed in Chapter 8.

The other means-tested in-work benefit at the time of writing is the disabled person's tax credit (DPTC) that replaced the disability working allowance first introduced in 1993. Disability working allowance was modelled on family credit and the principles of DPTC follow those of WFTC, with which it will effectively merge in 2003. DPTC is available to disabled people – whether or not they have dependent children – who are in full-time work. To qualify it is necessary that the claimant should have a physical or mental disability that puts her at a disadvantage in getting a job and that she had previously been receiving incapacity benefit (see below) or a disability benefit (see Chapter 5). Entitlement is determined using a taper calculation.

Because they are intended to make work pay, in-work benefits are supposed to play a part in enticing various target groups (and in the past this has applied particularly to lone parents) into low-paid employment. However, the incomes that people can realise through in-work benefits remain relatively modest and the complex basis on which they are calculated is not widely understood. Uncertainty about entitlement may be compounded by the precariousness of the jobs that are likely to be available (McLaughlin *et al.* 1989; Dean 2002). While the take-up of in-work benefits for families grew during the 1990s, the take-up of in-work benefits for disabled people has remained minimal. However, in neither case is there strong evidence that the availability of such benefits is by itself a significant incentive for people to (re)enter the labour market (for a summary of the evidence see McKay and Rowlingson 1999). This is not to say that in-work benefits are not important to the survival strategies of low-income working families (Dean and Shah 2002). In-work benefits or tax credits have become a necessary part of a low-pay economy and a scenario in which social security and labour market policy are drawn ever closer.

Incapacity

This next section will consider the various forms of protection that are supposed to provide security for people upon the basis that they are incapable of work through illness or impairment. These benefits are distinguishable from disability benefits since they depend explicitly upon a test of a claimant's capacity in relation to employment and are intended to replace the income that people might otherwise have earned from work rather than to meet the additional costs that may be associated with disability (Berthoud 1998). It is possible for people to qualify both for a disability benefit – for example, DLA – and for a benefit because of incapacity for work. The legislation recognises two forms of incapacity: short-term (incapacity lasting less than a year) and long-term. For short-term incapacity different provisions apply during the initial period of incapacity (currently, the first 28 weeks) and the remaining part of the first year of incapacity. Additionally, there are three different mechanisms for providing benefits: benefits that employers are required to pay; a contributory benefit called incapacity benefit (IB); and IS, which may be paid in addition to or in lieu of any of the other benefits (see Chapter 5). The section will discuss: first, the incapacity for work test; second, statutory employer benefits; and, finally, incapacity benefit.

The incapacity for work test was remodelled and made more restrictive by a Conservative government in 1995 (see CPAG 1994a) and then reformed again in 2000 by a New Labour government (Thornton 2000). It in fact consists of two tests, an 'own occupation test' and a 'personal capability assessment'. The 'own occupation test' is applied during the initial period of sickness, provided the claimant has a recognised occupation (at which she has worked during not less than eight of the preceding 21 weeks). The test requires that the claimant must be incapable 'by reason of some specific disease or mental disablement' of carrying on such work as might reasonably be expected in the course of her usual job and, for most purposes, a certificate to this effect from the claimant's own doctor will be accepted as sufficient evidence.

After the initial period, or if the claimant has no usual occupation, a 'personal capability assessment' is required. The assessment determines whether the claimant is capable of performing prescribed activities and it is intended that the assessment will rest upon two reports prepared by a doctor from the DWP's medical service. The first, an 'incapacity report', invokes in effect what was once called the 'all work test' that applied before 2000. This requires that a claimant's medical condition be measured against a range of functional capacities, namely: walking; standing; sitting; climbing stairs; rising from sitting; bending and kneeling; manual dexterity; lifting and carrying; reaching; speech; hearing; vision; continence; fits; mental health. The severity of a person's impairment is assessed against each criterion according to a scale and, if her total score exceeds a set threshold, she is adjudged incapable of work. Claimants must declare the extent of their impairment using a questionnaire and be prepared to submit to medical examination. The test excludes consideration of non-medical factors, such as claimants' age, education, training or suitability for the jobs of which they might functionally be capable, or whether such jobs in reality exist. During long-term incapacity, the extent of incapacity may be periodically reviewed and benefits may at any time be withdrawn if claimants are considered to be capable of work. The second report is a 'capability report' that provides advice concerning the claimant's capabilities and potential for further treatment or medical rehabilitation. The capability report is provided to the personal adviser responsible for conducting the claimant's compulsory work-focused interview under the single gateway claims process and is intended to assist with efforts to get the claimant back to work. Certain severely disabled claimants, including, for example, those already in receipt of the higher-level care component of DLA (see Chapter 5), may be exempted from the personal capacity assessment.

If people in employment should become sick or disabled – unless they are over pensionable age or earn less than the national insurance minimum contributions level – they are entitled to statutory sick pay (SSP). SSP has effectively replaced national insurance sickness benefit and is both administered and financed by employers. It is payable only for the initial period (currently, 28 weeks) of sickness, after which an employee would normally claim IB. There are no contribution conditions attaching to SSP and, subject to the general rules of the scheme, claims procedures and payment arrangements are essentially a private matter between employers and their employees and the arrangements that are made for the management of sickness absence (see Dean and Taylor-Gooby 1990). Claims may be made after four days' sickness absence, and most employers require some form of self-certification for absences of up to a week and medical certificates thereafter. SSP is currently payable at a fixed rate, presently equivalent to about 90 per cent of the level of a single person's basic retirement pension (RP). None the less, it counts as wages and is taxable. Although responsibility for administering SSP rests with employers, the scheme is closely regulated and disputes over entitlement may be referred by employees to a tax appeal commissioner (see Chapter 8).

The burden of protection for employees during initial periods of sickness absence is effectively therefore borne by employers, rather than the state. The initial period coincides in length with the period to which the less rigorous own occupation test of incapacity relates. Employees who remain absent from work through sickness after that period, in order to claim IB, must meet the relevant contribution conditions and the criteria applied by a personal capability assessment. Claimants who are not currently in employment, provided they meet the contribution conditions, may be able to claim IB on the basis of the own occupation test for the initial period (28 weeks), after which they too must submit to a personal capacity assessment. The contribution conditions for IB are broadly similar to those for Contributory JSA, except there is a requirement that national insurance equivalent to half a year's worth of minimum-level contributions must have been actually *paid* within *three*, rather than two, of the years preceding the claim. Since 2001 it has also been possible for people who were or became incapable of work when they were young (in most instances, before the age of 20) to qualify for IB without meeting any contribution conditions. This provision replaces the severe disablement allowance scheme that had existed prior to 2001.

IB is payable at three levels: the lower short-term rate, which is currently set at a level equivalent to around three-quarters of a single person's basic state RP and applies during the initial period of sickness; the higher short-term rate is set at the same level as SSP and is payable after the initial period until the end of the first year of incapacity (i.e., currently, for the 24 weeks after the first 28 weeks of sickness); the long-term rate, payable only after a year of incapacity, is currently set at a level just beneath that of the state RP. As with RP, additions for dependants may be claimed with long-term IB, and for people who become incapable of work below a certain age (currently, 35 or 45) there are small age additions that can in fact bring the level of incapacity benefit just above that of the basic RP. Once entitlement to incapacity benefit has been established it will remain in payment so long as the claimant is adjudged to remain incapable of work or until the claimant receives a RP. After the initial period of incapacity, incapacity benefit is taxable. Additionally, from 2001 IB has been partially means-testable in so far that payments may be reduced by a sum equivalent to half the amount by which any payments the claimant receives from a personal, occupational or public service pension scheme may exceed a set threshold.

The level of the various benefits available to people adjudged incapable of work have been described in the past by at least one commentator as 'incredibly stingy' (Berthoud 1998) and, as a result, many recipients are also eligible for IS to 'top up' their income to subsistence level. Receipt of any of the benefits described in this section automatically entitles claimants to do so, provided they also meet the other conditions attaching to the receipt of IS. Additionally, claimants who cannot qualify for IB (because they do not meet the contribution conditions and do not qualify on the grounds that they became incapable of work when they were young) but who do satisfy the incapacity conditions are entitled to IS. There are special premiums for disabled people on IS and

the benefit itself has been 'rebadged' for disabled people – as it has for retirement pensioners – as a disability income guarantee (DIG). Though they are
by no means generous, both means-tested and non-means-tested benefits for
people adjudged incapable of work provide a slightly higher level of income
replacement than is available to 'able-bodied' unemployed people, and this
may in part reflect a historical tendency for long-term sick and disabled people
to be treated as if they were somehow more 'deserving' of state support. This
implicit, if parsimonious, paternalism is curiously at odds with the introduction of the New Deal for disabled people and the concept of the capacity
report which were intended to be more consonant with a social rather than a
medical model of disability (Thornton 2000). While it may be argued that
disabled people deserve to be compensated not for their loss of function, but
for the disservices done to them by society (Bolderson, cited in Thornton
2000: 123), the focus of recent reforms has been upon individuals' incapacity
for work rather than the barriers that exist to participation by disabled people
within society and the labour market.

Summary/conclusion

What this chapter has illustrated is that the conditional nature of individual
rights guaranteed by social legislation is calculated to underwrite the citizen's
status as a wage labourer (cf. Offe 1984: 99). Such rights function to limit
rather than defend the security of the citizen and so to ensure or to maximise her
complaisance *in* employment and her availability *for* employment. A complex
array of protections exists for employees in the course of their employment,
though the extent of such protection is often less than in other Western
countries; certain of the most peripheral employees may be excluded from full
protection; many rights, such as those arising under anti-discrimination legislation, are difficult to enforce; and protection against dismissal is in practice
limited.

Protection of income during unemployment is now provided through JSA,
a hybrid benefit with a vestigial contributory element and a predominant
means-tested element. The benefit is explicitly conditional, not only upon
claimants' availability for employment, but also their compliance with the terms
of individual agreements requiring them actively to seek work. The withholding
or withdrawal of jobseeker's allowance is used as a sanction by which to control
the behaviour of unemployed people and to deter voluntary unemployment.
JSA provided the foundations on which New Labour's welfare-to-work policies
have been built. Central to this has been the New Deal. Originally piloted
among a range of target groups, it has now been made permanent, giving rise
to the single gateway claims procedure to which all working-age claimant
groups are subject, including lone parents and disabled people.

New Labour has also perpetuated the use of in-work benefits or tax credits for
low-paid full-time employees. In-work benefits are means-tested, using a 'taper'
calculation, the complex nature of which renders the basis of entitlement less
than transparent to most recipients. In the context of a low-wage economy,

however, this form of wage subsidy has become an important feature of welfare-to-work policy because it is thought that it 'targets' help to the poorest working people and families, and that it provides incentives to disadvantaged groups to take low-paid employment.

When people are or become incapable of work through sickness or disability, social protection is provided, in the immediate term, by way of compulsory employer provision and, in the longer term, by a contributory IB, though people of limited means are often obliged to top up these benefits with IS and those who cannot qualify for IB may have to depend on IS in any event. These benefits are distinguishable from disability benefits because they are subject to a form of work-testing: the receipt of benefit is conditional upon claimants establishing, not illness or disability, but that they are medically incapable of the functions or activities required for employment. Recent changes mean that more concerted attempts will be made to assess the capacity and to enhance the willingness of long-term sick and disabled people to (re)enter the labour market.

In recent years labour markets have become increasingly polarised between a privileged core of relatively secure and highly skilled workers, to whom social protection may be of marginal relevance, and a vulnerable periphery of insecure low-paid workers, for whom the rights which social legislation affords are potentially contradictory. Arguably, social legislation is failing to alleviate their insecurity within the labour market, while simultaneously compelling them to seek employment.

Chapter 7

Rights to shelter

Like nourishment and raiment, shelter is one of the most elemental of human needs. Curiously, food, clothing and housing are recognised in the Universal Declaration of Human Rights quite incidentally: they are numbered among the components of an adequate standard of subsistence (see UN 1948: Article 25). A specific right to a home is nowhere declared. The assumption it would seem is that citizens may secure their homes at will, subject only to the means of payment, and that the primary source of protection lies in civil and not social rights. None the less, where British social legislation does relate to housing, it creates four kinds of rights.

First, and of increasing importance, there are rights to personal subsidies to assist with the payment of housing costs. Second, there are protections against exploitation and eviction of residential occupiers. Third, there are protections against unsatisfactory housing conditions. Fourth, there are protections against homelessness. This chapter will consider each type of provision in turn. It will become clear, however, that even the protection afforded to homeless persons falls short of guaranteeing an unconditional right to housing. The present government has declared that its aim is 'to offer everyone the opportunity of a decent home' (DETR 2000: 7), but to have an opportunity is not quite the same as having a right.

Paying for housing

This section will discuss three different ways in which people may be entitled to state assistance with housing costs. The first is housing benefit (HB), a means-tested cash benefit available to tenants with low incomes. The second is council tax benefit (CTB), a means-tested benefit closely aligned with HB, which is available to assist people of all forms of housing tenure with the cost of council tax bills. The third is the housing cost element of income support (IS), which may be available to some homeowners. In the recent past there had been a fourth form of assistance, namely mortgage interest tax relief, a fiscal benefit that provided a subsidy towards the housing costs of homeowners: this potentially valuable tax concession had benefited mortgage payers regardless of their income and at its peak was costing the exchequer some £7.7 billion per year (CSO 1992), but it was phased out during the 1990s and finally disappeared in 2000.

Housing benefit

The Beveridgian social security system did not make separate provision for housing costs, but had included in national insurance benefits a notional element sufficient to meet average housing costs (Parker 1989). A safety-net was provided to the extent that means-tested national assistance (later supplementary benefit) could take account of actual housing costs. As a result of considerable regional variations in rent levels and rapid housing cost inflation, this arrangement became increasingly unsustainable, partly because it pushed increasing numbers of pensioners and others on to social assistance benefits simply to have their housing costs met, and because this in turn generated considerable inequities, as between people outside the labour market with access to social assistance and those in low-paid employment who could receive no benefits. In the 1970s, therefore, during the period in which family income supplement was also introduced (an in-work benefit and the predecessor to family credit – see Chapter 6), rent and rate rebate and rent allowance schemes were instituted. These benefits were the predecessors of HB and CTB. HB and CTB are social security benefits and are subject to rules laid down by national legislation, but they are administered by local authorities rather than by the Department of Work and Pensions. Because prompt payment of HB in particular can be critical to tenants' ability to meet their rents, efficient and responsive administration is essential. Delays in the processing of claims can result in tenants being evicted for non-payment of rent (see below). Unfortunately, however, since HB was introduced the sheer complexity of the system coupled with poor standards of administration on the part of some local authorities have meant that it has, on occasions, been as much a part of the problem faced by low-income tenants as the solution to their lack of income (e.g. Robson 2001).

HB was first introduced in 1982, though its current form was not established until 1988. HB effectively unified provision for the housing costs of all tenants, whether they be the tenants of local authorities, of housing associations (now called registered social landlords or RSLs) or private landlords, and whether or not they are in receipt of other social security benefits and/or in employment. To do this HB combined the provisions of the rent rebate and rent allowance schemes and the housing cost element of the old supplementary benefit scheme. Other than for claimants who are also in receipt of income support (IS, which for these purposes may be taken to include income-related JSA, MIG or DIG – see Chapter 5 above), the means-test applied for the purposes of HB is based upon a taper calculation (see Figure 6.1 and for a full account, for example, CPAG's *Welfare Benefits Handbook*). The maximum benefit for the purposes of HB is the claimant's 'eligible rent'. Eligible rents do not include mortgage interest repayments, ground rents on long leases or payments under co-ownership and conditional sale arrangements (which may in certain circumstances be met by income support), but they do include payments that are not strictly 'rent', such as licence fees or payments made by a claimant who is not legally a tenant (such as the deserted partner of the original tenant), where payments are necessary for claimants to retain occupation of their present homes.

However, the eligible rent will not necessarily be equal to the actual rent payable, since deductions may be made from the actual rent if it includes provision for non-housing costs (such as water rates and charges for meals, heating, laundry or other services), or if the rent is subject to restriction. Prior to 1996 local authorities could impose restrictions if they thought the rent a claimant was paying was excessive or if it was adjudged that the accommodation in question was unsuitable or too large for the claimant's household. The Housing Act 1996 introduced a procedure by which rent officers – locally based central government officials with responsibility for registering 'fair rents' under the Rent Acts (see below) – assumed responsibility for determining a claim-related rent, being the maximum amount that a landlord might reasonably charge for particular accommodation of a size appropriate to the claimant's household; a 'local reference rent', being the average reasonable market rent for 'assured' tenancies (see below) within the local area and which may be lower than the reasonable rent determined for any particular dwelling; and a 'single-room rent', being a special reference rent based on the average cost of single-room lettings that may be applied to single claimants under the age of 25, regardless of the type of accommodation they actually occupy. This procedure is invoked by local authorities, which may refer tenancies to the rent officer for determination and, in practice, it applies primarily to the private rented sector; prospective tenants are also entitled to refer to the rent officer for a pre-tenancy determination, so that they may know in advance how much of their rent will be eligible for HB purposes. Eligible rents are determined on the basis of the 'claim-related rent' recommended by the rent officer or the appropriate local reference rent if this should be lower. The procedure may be seen as an indirect form of rent regulation (Partington 1997), since low-income tenants whose eligible rent for HB is lower than the rent demanded by their landlord are expected to negotiate a lower rent or move to cheaper accommodation.

Claimants who also receive IS automatically receive maximum HB (i.e. full payment of their eligible rent). Other claimants' entitlement is based on a taper calculation in which:

- needs are determined with reference to broadly the same applicable amounts as apply for the purposes of IS (but with some slight variations);
- means are also determined in the same way as for IS, but with some variations in relation to income disregards and a higher savings/capital limit (currently twice that for IS);
- the amount of eligible rent that is met is reduced by a proportion of the amount by which the claimant's income exceeds her applicable amount;
- the taper that is applied is currently (at 65 per cent) more severe than that applied for the purposes of working families' tax credit;
- the amount of benefit payable can also be subject to 'non-dependant deductions' – reductions on account of the contributions that any non-dependant adult members of the claimant's household are assumed to make towards the claimant's housing costs (deductions are related to the income of the non-dependant and reduced, or no deductions are made, for non-dependants who are themselves on low income or are receiving IS).

For local authority tenants, their HB is credited at source to their rent accounts (so reducing the net rent payable), while for private tenants, housing benefit is paid to the claimant, or, in certain circumstances, direct to the claimant's landlord.

As with IS, there are restrictions on entitlement for persons from abroad and special rules and restrictions for full-time students. Because the HB means-test aggregates the needs and means of families in the same way as IS, it also reinforces the same assumptions about family dependency, although it takes these assumptions a step further: first, through the imposition of non-dependant deductions (referred to above); second, through a rule that precludes the payment of HB in circumstances where the claimant is closely related to her landlord. It is explicitly anticipated, on the one hand, that claimants' adult offspring who continue to live in the parental home should contribute to the household costs but, on the other hand, that people who reside with close relatives should be accommodated without any sort of commercial arrangement between them. HB extends the use of 'selectivity' in other ways. The imposition of rent restrictions can rest upon judgements about what kind of accommodation is or is not suitable for a particular person or family and/or upon the availability of cheaper alternative accommodation that might be adjudged suitable. Tenants – especially those in the most vulnerable social groups – may in practice have few options open to them or may simply elect to endure a reduced standard of living rather than to change their living arrangements (see, for example, Kemp 2000). It has additionally been proposed (DETR 2000) that, in future, payments of HB could be withdrawn from tenants who are guilty of 'anti-social behaviour' and from landlords who fail to maintain their properties in a satisfactory condition. Not only, therefore, has the HB scheme evolved into an instrument for rent control at the most impoverished end of the private rented sector, but it is also possible at the time of writing that it may assume additional far-reaching functions in relation to the control of tenants' behaviour and the regulation of housing conditions.

In 2001 a discretionary housing payments (DHPs) scheme was introduced to replace a system of 'exceptional hardship' and 'exceptional circumstances' payments that had operated within the HB scheme. DHPs, like Social Fund payments, are wholly discretionary and are met from a cash-limited local budget allocated to local authorities. They may be made to help people meet their rent or council tax liability. They function in certain situations to mitigate the effects of HB rent restrictions and/or non-dependant deductions where these are especially severe, but they are not a part of the HB scheme and are not available as of right.

Council tax benefit

HB provides personal subsidy for only one kind of housing cost, namely rent. Closely related to HB is council tax benefit (CTB), which is administered by local authorities alongside HB. CTB provides personal subsidy to people on low incomes towards the payment of council tax, which, as a tax on occupancy, may be regarded as another kind of housing cost. The council tax is the successor to the community charge (or poll tax) and, before it, local general rates. For an explanation of the basis upon which liability to council tax is determined see, for example, CPAG's *Council Tax Handbook*. Entitlement to CTB is based on a taper calculation in which the maximum benefit is the full amount of the claimant's council tax liability and the taper (currently at 20 per cent) is gentler than for either working families' tax credit or HB. Like HB, CTB may be subject to non-dependant deductions. Reductions have also recently been introduced for claimants living in expensive properties that fall within the higher council tax bands. However, there is an alternative form of rebate, the 'second-adult rebate'. This rebate compensates council tax payers for the effect upon their tax liability of the presence within their household of any non-dependant adult whose status does not attract a council tax discount but whose income is such they cannot contribute to the council tax. Second-adult rebate is available to tax payers whose circumstances are such that they would not themselves qualify for means-tested benefits, but where their non-dependants' circumstances are such that they need assistance.

Income support for mortgage interest

Assistance with housing costs *not* met by HB or CTB may be obtained through IS, the main nationally administered social assistance benefit. As was explained in Chapter 5, the 'applicable amount' used to determine a claimant's and her family's needs for the purposes of IS may in certain circumstances include their housing costs. The most commonly included housing cost is mortgage interest repayments (including interest payments on loans and second mortgages previously incurred to meet the cost of essential repairs, improvements or adaptations). The scope of income support for mortgage interest (ISMI) has lately been significantly curtailed. First, an upper ceiling has been imposed on the size of the mortgages or loans upon which interest repayments may be fully met (this currently stands at £100,000). Second, an initial waiting period has been introduced at the beginning of a claim for IS during which reduced or no mortgage interest costs will be met. The precise extent of the assistance that is available will depend on when the claimant's mortgage was taken out. For claimants with mortgages taken out earlier than October 1995, no assistance is given for the first eight weeks of any claim and only 50 per cent of the interest payments due will be met for 18 weeks after that. For claimants with mortgages taken out since October 1995, no assistance is given for the first 39 weeks of their claim. Homeowners are expected increasingly to take out private insurance to meet the cost of mortgage repayments in the event of unemployment and sickness, although few feel able to do so (see, for example, Cebulla 1999). For low-income homeowners who are not eligible for IS because they are in full-time employment there is no form of assistance with mortgage interest repayments (this contrasts curiously with the position of tenants in low-paid employment who may obtain assistance with their rent through HB).

As with HB, IS is subject to non-dependant deductions where provision is being made for housing costs. Similarly, there is provision to restrict the amount of housing costs that are eligible to be met if such costs are adjudged to be 'excessive', because the claimant's accommodation is larger than required for her and her family and/or because there is cheaper suitable alternative accommodation available in the area in which the claimant lives. Claimants in receipt of IS are also generally prevented from increasing their housing costs: tenants who buy their homes while in receipt of IS may receive assistance with housing costs only to the extent of their eligible rent for HB purposes prior to the purchase; and homeowners who take out additional mortgages or who move house and take out a bigger mortgage while in receipt of IS will receive no additional assistance with housing costs (unless, for example, the loan was required to fund adaptations or the move was to a home specially adapted to meet the needs of a disabled person). To the extent that means-tested benefits guarantee a right to housing, it is a right that is conferred at the expense of a claimant's right to choose.

Under certain circumstances, tenants and homeowners are therefore entitled to various kinds of subsidy in relation to their housing costs. These are subsidies to the 'consumption' of housing rather than its 'production' (Ungerson 1994). The 1980s and 1990s witnessed a major shift away from production or 'bricks and mortar' subsidies, towards personal subsidy. Such subsidy may indirectly stimulate the supply of housing and, certainly, the right to mortgage interest tax relief helped to fuel the expansion of owner-occupation in the 1980s. Mortgage interest tax relief, however, has now disappeared. Other forms of consumption subsidy – HB and ISMI – are strictly conditional upon a means-test. These subsidies are 'targeted' selectively to people whose purchasing power in the housing market (whether in the rented or owner-occupier sector) would otherwise be limited or non-existent, but with strict controls intended to temper 'excessive' costs and expectations. By themselves, such subsidies are not best calculated to stimulate supply. Nor does the present system ensure equity between tenants and homeowners. The New Labour government had promised reform of the system and at one stage there was talk of a unified housing tax credit. In the event the government has tentatively floated the idea of a regionally varied flat rate system of HB that might in time replace the present scheme, while concluding that root and branch reform will have to await a restructuring of rents across the social and private rented sectors and enhancement of tenant choice in social sector allocations (DETR 2000, and see Gibb 2001). As a result, as Robson (2001: 325) has concluded, 'an unpopular and hugely complex system of financial support for which few have a good word to say appears likely to limp on for want of any other option being offered'. Rights to personal subsidy and, just as importantly, the stringent conditions that may attach to such rights have become, and are likely to remain, a central feature of housing policy.

Protection against exploitation and eviction

An earlier strategy for ensuring the availability of affordable housing was to legislate to prevent landlords from charging excessive rents and to restrict the circumstances in which people may be evicted from rented accommodation. This was one of the key strategies pursued in Britain during the earlier part of the twentieth century when renting was the dominant form of housing tenure. At the same time, governments of all political persuasions made a considerable investment in subsidising the provision of low-cost public rented housing by local authorities. By the latter part of the century, however, homeownership had become the dominant form of housing tenure and, in the 1980s, Conservative governments attempted deliberately to 'deregulate' what then remained of the private rented sector on the one hand, and to diminish the public rented sector on the other (see, for example, Johnson 1990). Believing regulation to be the cause rather than a bulwark against the contraction of private rented housing, the government legislated to diminish the controls on private landlords. Distrusting the role played by local authorities, the government gave the tenants of council housing the right to buy their homes at a discount, while local councils were at the same time subjected to a greater degree of regulation than hitherto.

As a result, there are now three main 'species' of tenancy with varying degrees of legislative protection: protected tenancies, which are private tenancies created prior to January 1989; secure tenancies, which are mainly public sector tenancies; and assured tenancies, which are private and RSL sector tenancies created since January 1989. Additionally, there are several other forms of tenancy that attract lesser degrees of legislative protection. What is outlined below is an incomplete and much simplified account of a highly complex field of law. For a fuller explanation see, for example, Cowan (1999).

Rent regulation

Protected or regulated tenancies, where they survive, are those that still enjoy 'traditional' Rent Act protection; specifically under the Rent Act of 1977. Protected tenants enjoy the right to have a 'fair rent' determined for their tenancy by the rent officer. Since this right would be valueless if tenants who availed themselves of it could be evicted by their landlords, the legislation also affords security of tenure (see below). Certain tenants with what were called 'restricted contracts' were excluded from full protection. Either tenants or landlords can apply to have a 'fair rent' registered for a letting and, once registered, that rent becomes the maximum rent that can legally be charged. Applications to review the registered rent can be made periodically. The rent officers who determine and register 'fair rents' are independent public officials employed in local offices. In registering 'fair rents' they are required to ignore the effect of market conditions and to assume that no scarcity value attaches to rented accommodation. The number of tenancies over which rent officers have jurisdiction is tiny and declining, though they now have an entirely new jurisdiction under which they are called upon by local authorities to determine 'reasonable rents' and 'reference rents' for the purposes of limiting the amount of HB payable (see above).

Prior to the 1980s, it was assumed that, because public sector landlords and charitable bodies such as housing associations did not seek to return a profit, it was not necessary for their tenants to have special legislative protection. The Housing Acts of 1980 and 1985, however, introduced the concept of the secure tenancy and gave the tenants of local authorities, and of other public bodies and housing associations, a form of security of tenure broadly similar to that enjoyed by protected tenants. However, no specific legal mechanism is available to local authority tenants by which to challenge the level of rents, though, because they are elected bodies, local councils remain in principle democratically accountable: a council tenant enjoys political as well as legal rights against her/his landlord. Additionally, local councils have been required since 1980 to establish consultation procedures and, since 2000, Tenant Participation Compacts, though such arrangements do not give tenants any control over rent levels. Rents for local authority tenancies have remained, in theory, at the discretion of councils, albeit with a requirement that rents should, in time, approximate more closely to the market rents charged in the private rented sector. The financial regime imposed on councils by the 1989 Local Government and Housing Act restricted the discretion of local authorities and in effect forced council rents to rise. Housing association tenancies had once been subject, like protected tenancies, to the 'fair rents' scheme, but housing association tenancies granted since the enactment of the 1988 Housing Act are no longer secure tenancies; they are assured tenancies and rents are governed in principle by the same rules as for other assured tenancies. None the less, housing associations and the expanding range of not-for-profit housing companies – that have together come to be known as registered social landlords (RSLs) – are partly dependent on public capital funding through the Housing Corporation, to which terms may be attached, and are expected by government to offer affordable rents, while still operating within a competitive commercial environment.

Assured tenancies are the creation of the 1988 Housing Act, and – subject to some exceptions – any private or RSL tenancy granted since that legislation came into force is an assured tenancy. Though assured tenants enjoy a broadly similar (though somewhat reduced) degree of security of tenure to protected tenants, they are not entitled to a 'fair rent'. They must pay a 'market rent'. Private landlords may let premises for whatever rent a tenant will agree to pay and they may stipulate express terms for future rent increases. If terms for the variation of the rent have not been agreed, it is possible for the landlord – and in some circumstances the tenant – to serve notice to vary the terms of the tenancy and for the proposed variation of terms, if it is not agreed, to be referred by either party to the rent assessment committee (a body which began life as a higher appellate tribunal to the rent officer). The rent assessment committee has power to determine and to impose upon the parties what it adjudges to be the market rent for the property.

Repossession and succession

Where tenancies are initially granted for a fixed contractual term, upon the expiry of that term the tenancies do not cease and, unless the tenancy is renewed by agreement, they become 'statutory' tenancies upon the same terms and conditions as the contractual tenancies that preceded them. Landlords cannot legally recover possession against their tenants unless they can establish permissible grounds for doing so. Such grounds are specified in the relevant legislation and are of two kinds: discretionary and mandatory. There is some variation between the different species of tenancy, but generally possession may be sought where the tenant is in arrears with her rent or is in breach of some express or implied term of the tenancy. In such circumstances the county court *may*, if it is reasonable, grant an order for possession against the tenant. In the case of assured tenancies, the court *must*, if requested by the landlord, grant an order for possession if a tenant is more than three months in arrears with her rent (or eight weeks in the case of weekly tenancies) both at the date the landlord served notice of seeking possession (see below) *and* at the date of hearing. Similarly, in the case of both protected and assured tenancies, the court must grant possession if the landlord is a former owner-occupier of the property in question and it was let to the tenant on the express basis that the landlord would at some time return to occupy the property; or where the tenancy had been an out-of-season holiday or student letting. In the case of secure and assured tenancies, the court must grant possession if the landlord seeks to redevelop or demolish the property, though – only in the case of secure (i.e. public sector) tenancies – the landlord must make suitable alternative accommodation available to the tenant. The court also has a general discretion to grant possession to private landlords under protected and assured tenancies if it may be shown that suitable alternative accommodation is available to the tenant. To recover possession landlords under protected tenancies must first serve a notice to quit to terminate the contractual tenancy and then apply to the county court for an order. Landlords under secure and assured tenancies must first serve a notice of seeking possession, since only the court has power to terminate the tenancy. The court has power to suspend or attach conditions to an order for possession, but once an order is made and becomes effective, it may be enforced by eviction.

The 1996 Housing Act introduced additional provisions to make it easier to evict tenants who are guilty of 'anti-social behaviour'. First, local authorities were empowered to grant 12-month introductory tenancies, rather than secure tenancies, at the end of which possession may be recovered without having to prove any grounds. Second, the specific grounds on which possession may be sought against secure and assured tenants for nuisance or illegal behaviour were made more extensive and easier to establish.

Upon the death of a protected, secure or assured tenant (provided she has not herself inherited the tenancy by succession), her spouse may succeed to the tenancy or, in certain limited circumstances, another member of the tenant's family may do so, though the provisions for succession are particularly restrictive in the case of assured tenancies. Except in certain circumstances (where, for example, the property is sheltered accommodation or has been specially adapted for disabled occupiers), secure tenants after two years' occupation have a right to buy the property they occupy. No such right extends to protected or assured tenants, although they may in some circumstances have a right of 'first refusal' if the landlord seeks to sell the property and tenants whose tenancies have been transferred from a local authority to a RSL may retain a protected right to buy.

In addition to the main species of tenancy, there are a number of forms of occupancy that attract a much lesser degree of protection. First, there are 'restricted contracts', a term that most usually applies to tenancies granted by resident landlords before 1988. The vestiges of a rather complex regulatory regime still applies to the handful of such tenancies that were created before 1980, but for tenancies granted between 1980 and 1988, no security of tenure applies, other than a provision that tenancies must be determined by notice to quit before repossession is sought and that the court has power temporarily to suspend a possession order. Second, there are 'shorthold' tenancies, of which there are two kinds: protected shortholds, that could only be granted between 1980 and 1988; and assured shortholds, which may have been granted since 1988 and which recently, under guidance from the Housing Corporation, have been developed by RSLs to provide 'starter tenancies' that operate in much the same way as local authority introductory tenancies under the 1996 Housing Act. Shorthold tenancies are granted for a fixed term and subject to notice from the landlord that possession may be recovered after the expiry of that term upon the special mandatory ground that it is a shorthold tenancy. Though tenancies may continue as statutory tenancies after the expiry of the original fixed term, the tenant remains vulnerable indefinitely to repossession upon the shorthold ground. Across the private rented sector in many parts of the country, the assured shorthold tenancy has become the most widely adopted form of tenancy. Assured shorthold tenants have the right to apply to a rent assessment committee for a market rent to be determined if they can demonstrate that their rent is higher than other rents for assured tenancies but their vulnerability in due course to retaliatory possession proceedings makes it unlikely (unless they have other accommodation to which to go) that they will avail themselves of such rights.

There are other forms of residential occupier with limited rights, including: people whose accommodation is 'tied' to their employment; people who are sub-tenants or the tenants of mortgagors; people who are boarders or lodgers; people who are 'licensees' (who may be obliged, for example, to share the occupancy of premises). One unintended effect of the Rent Acts was to spawn various attempts by landlords to devise ways of evading them and, through such ploys as bogus 'non-exclusive occupation agreements', to deny their tenants legal protection. In general, however, virtually all residential occupiers are protected from summary eviction and harassment by the 1977 Protection from Eviction Act, the effect of which is to make it necessary or advisable for any landlord to seek an order from the court before evicting a residential occupier. Criminal proceedings may be taken against landlords by or on behalf of tenants and other occupiers who are unlawfully evicted or harassed. Alternatively, affected tenants may seek injunctions and damages by way of civil proceedings for breach of their right to quiet enjoyment. There are, however, a small number of tenancies and licences excluded from such protection by the 1988 Housing Act. These excluded categories relate principally to arrangements created since the Act by resident landlords who share a part of their accommodation with their tenants/licensees: this removal of regulation had been intended to encourage people to let out rooms in their own homes, though it represents a significant breach of the only universal right to be enjoyed by all residential occupiers.

Even trespassers or 'squatters' have some limited protection against violent eviction. The traditional protection against forcible entry was repealed by a more limited form of safeguard under the 1977 Criminal Law Act, which made it an offence to use or threaten violence to gain entry to any premises upon which a person present is opposed to such entry. The only exception allowed is in the case of an actually displaced residential occupier who may use reasonable force to evict squatters who have taken up residence in their home. Characteristically, however, squatting occurs in unoccupied property and it behoves the owners of such property to obtain court orders using special expedited procedures in either the county court or the high court. Additionally, the Criminal Law Act of 1977 makes it an offence for a squatter to refuse to leave residential property if requested to do so by a 'protected intending occupier' (being an owner or prospective tenant who wishes to move in), and the Criminal Justice and Public Order Act of 1994 subsequently made it a criminal offence for a trespasser to fail to vacate residential property within 24 hours of service of an interim possession order. The implication of this last provision is that, in the case of squatters, possession orders may be enforced not by civil procedures involving court bailiffs, but by arrest and criminal prosecution.

Homeowners

The class of residential occupier whose rights have not so far been discussed is the owner-occupier. To the extent that homeowners have the greatest degree of security of tenure under civil law, their need for statutory protection is correspondingly less. The rights of freehold owners, provided their property is not mortgaged, can only be interfered with in exceptional circumstances: for example, by compulsory purchase or closing orders made by public authorities or by orders made in the course of matrimonial or bankruptcy proceedings.

However, some homeowners are in fact long leaseholders (i.e. they may have purchased a lease, or an unexpired portion of a lease, of more than 21 years' duration) and both long leaseholders and freeholders may well have mortgages on their property. The 'ground' rents that long leaseholders pay are characteristically small and are not subject to regulation. None the less, the service charges that must be borne by leaseholders living in blocks of flats can be substantial and non-payment can result in forfeiture. Although most long leases are in fact longer than a natural life span (99 or even 999 years), when they expire they may become assured tenancies. In practice, however, it is comparatively rare for the term of a long lease to expire without a leaseholder acquiring the freehold. Under the 1967 Leasehold Reform Act, long leaseholders of *houses*, provided they have been in residence for more than three years, can compel the freeholder to extend the lease or to sell the freehold to the lease-holder. Long leaseholders of *flats* have in certain circumstances a right of first refusal should the freeholders decide to sell their interest. People who buy their homes with mortgages or who borrow against the value of their homes for other purposes consent to a legal charge against the value of their home and, should they default upon the terms of their mortgage by failing to make repayments, the lender has the right to repossess the home in order to recover the borrower's debt. As any other residential occupier, an owner-occupier has the right not to be summarily evicted. If a mortgagor falls into arrears with repayments, the lender must first serve a formal notice requiring repayment of all capital and interest due and only thereafter, if the mortgagor does not comply, proceed to court for a possession order. The court has power to suspend possession if suitable terms for the repayment of arrears can be set.

The last century, therefore, was characterised by the rise and fall of rent regulation – in favour of personal subsidy on the one hand and the promotion of homeownership on the other, but, in overall terms, a modest but significant extension of security of tenure for all but a few kinds of residential occupier. None the less, the right of the British person to defend her home is by no means absolute.

Housing conditions

While the last section considered rights to security of tenure, such rights do not by themselves ensure that the conditions in which people live will be satisfactory. This section will therefore consider, first, the rights that tenants (and in some circumstances other occupiers) have to obtain repairs and improve-ments in their homes and, second, the rights that owner-occupiers (and in some circumstances tenants) have to financial assistance with essential repairs and improvements.

Enforcing repairs

This book is not concerned to elaborate upon the multifarious civil remedies (in contract and tort) that may be available under landlord and tenant law. There are, however, two important legislative provisions upon which tenants may rely in this connection, although it may in practice be risky for them to do so if they do not enjoy security of tenure and expensive if they neither qualify for legal aid nor have access to legal services (see Chapter 9 below). The first is Section 11 of the Landlord and Tenant Act of 1985, which makes it an implied term or 'covenant' within any periodic or short-term residential tenancy created since 1961 (being the date of the legislation by which the provision first originated) that the landlord is responsible for keeping in repair the structure and exterior of the dwelling concerned and such installations as may be provided for the supply of water, gas, electricity, sanitation and space/water heating. Tenants, conversely, are generally liable for minor internal repairs and decorations. The other provision is Section 4 of the Defective Premises Act of 1972, which imposes an explicit duty of care upon all landlords subject to a repairing obligation such that they may be held liable for any personal injury or damage to property arising from any defect occurring upon the premises for which they are responsible.

Of greater concern in the context of this discussion are two legislative frameworks conferring specific powers upon local authorities and specific rights of complaint upon individuals: the first has arisen under housing legislation and is currently to be found in consolidated form within the Housing Act of 1985; the second has arisen under public health legislation and is currently to be found in consolidated form in the Environmental Protection Act of 1990. The former is concerned to ensure the fitness of dwellings for habitation; the latter to prevent conditions that may be prejudicial to health.

Under the 1985 Housing Act (as amended), the environmental health departments of local authorities have power in relation to any dwelling that is unfit for human habitation to serve notices or orders upon the owners or the persons responsible. Prior to 1996 such notices could require – depending upon which was the most satisfactory course – either that repairs be carried out to make the property fit; or the closure or, in some circumstances, the demolition of the property. Since 1996, however, local authorities have been permitted to serve deferred action notices upon owners indicating what action *might* subsequently follow. Although local authorities must then re-inspect within two years, even if the property remains unfit, they may still renew the delayed action notice rather than take substantive action. Owners may appeal to the county court against delayed action notices or against the requirements of any substantive notices that follow, but, if they neither appeal nor comply with the requirements, the local authority technically has power to carry out works to the property in default and to recover the cost. Occupiers who are displaced as a result of closure or demolition orders are entitled to rehousing and to compensation. Additionally, local authorities may serve repairs notices upon landlords or managers of properties that are not technically unfit but which are in serious disrepair. Local authorities also have powers to institute group repair (or 'envelope') schemes or to declare renewal or (very exceptionally) clearance areas as a means of dealing with pockets or whole areas of unfit housing. Fitness for habitation is to be judged with reference to structural stability; freedom from serious disrepair and dampness; the adequacy of provision for lighting, heating (and hot water), ventilation, cooking facilities, water supply, drainage and sanitation. The government is considering replacing this fitness standard with a more flexible 'health and safety rating' (DETR 2000). Tenants or occupiers may make complaints to their local authorities if their housing conditions are such as to interfere with personal comfort and local authorities are obliged to act. Failure to act may be challenged by judicial review or, alternatively, by a complaint to a magistrate (under Section 606 of the 1985 Housing Act) who, if satisfied that a dwelling or dwellings may be unfit for habitation, must require the local authority to make an inspection and report.

Under the 1990 Environmental Protection Act the environmental health departments of local authorities are also responsible for ensuring the abatement of 'statutory nuisances', a term which includes any premises in such a condition as to be prejudicial to health or a nuisance. This additional power enables local authorities to serve an abatement notice upon the person by whose act, default or sufferance the statutory nuisance arises (or upon the owner of the property concerned) requiring that such repairs or other works as may be necessary be carried out. Such notices may be appealed against in the magistrates court, but if an abatement notice is neither appealed nor complied with, the local authority may prosecute the person(s) concerned in the magistrates court, and/or carry out works in default and recover the costs. Individuals who are 'persons aggrieved' by a statutory nuisance may complain to their local authority or may alternatively lay information before a magistrate (under Section 82 of the 1990 Environmental Protection Act) so as to institute a prosecution against the person(s) responsible for an alleged statutory nuisance. This last mentioned remedy may be especially useful or necessary for dissatisfied local authority tenants. While the environmental health and housing departments of a local council may be quite separate, a local authority cannot prosecute itself!

The environmental health departments of local authorities have a range of other powers in relation to housing conditions that may be invoked upon complaint by a citizen. Such powers relate, for example, to overcrowding, dangerous buildings, fire precautions, drains, sewers and vermin control. Of particular significance are local authorities' powers in relation to houses in multiple occupation (HMOs). These powers are potentially extensive and can include the operation of registration schemes, the issuing of overcrowding notices, the service and enforcement of works and repairs notices, the making and enforcement of management regulations and, in extreme circumstances, the making of control orders by which the local authority may itself assume management of premises. At the time of writing, the government is proposing that local authorities should be required to establish schemes for the licensing of HMO landlords (DETR 2000).

Owner-occupiers, of course, are responsible for their own repairs, although for younger homeowners with large mortgages but modest incomes, and for elderly homeowners who may be asset-rich but income-poor, the cost of maintaining their homes can be problematic. Additionally, tenants are entitled in certain circumstances to carry out repairs to their homes, if their landlord has failed to do so. Secure tenants have the right under the 1985 Housing Act to do this, subject to giving notice to their landlord, and to recover the cost, and other tenants have a right established by case law to effect essential repairs and to set off the cost against future rent. Protected tenants and secure tenants – but not assured tenants – also have the right to carry out improvements to their homes, subject to their landlords' permission (though such permission may not be unreasonably withheld). An 'improvement' in this sense (for example the provision of a bathroom where none existed before) is more than a repair and, if the tenant has improved a property, the rent which the landlord subsequently recovers ought not to reflect the value of that improvement.

Housing grants

It has been possible in the past for owner-occupiers, landlords or tenants to obtain grants towards the cost of repairs, conversion and improvements through statutory schemes administered by local authorities. Successive governments during the post-Second World War period have promoted the use of public funds for the renovation of private housing stock, including mandatory grants for the cost of rendering properties fit for habitation (Balchin 1995). However, in 1990 a Conservative government for the first time made all such grants subject to a means-test. Following the deregulation of the private rented sector, it was argued, most private landlords should be able adequately to recover the costs of repairs and improvements in rent, while only the poorest owner-occupiers should receive assistance with maintenance or essential improvement costs. Subsequently, the Housing Grants Act of 1996 further constrained the system by limiting the provision of mandatory individual grants to the provision of prescribed facilities required for use by a disabled person, so that grants for private sector renovation works, for repairs or improvements to the common parts of inhabited buildings or to HMOs, became discretionary. Provision was made for home repair assistance by way of discretionary grants (or the provision of materials) but only to individual homeowners who are elderly, disabled or in receipt of a means-tested benefit. In practice, restrictions upon capital expenditure imposed on local authorities have meant that few have been very active in awarding discretionary grants. A more extensive housing grants system has been introduced in Scotland and the Westminster government, at the time of writing, is discussing a reform of the grants system in England and Wales, by which they hope to facilitate the provision of loans for homeowners to be secured against the value of their homes, and the development of Home Improvement Agencies that would assist vulnerable homeowners to organise the financing and conduct of essential home repairs (DETR 2000).

Local authorities in Britain have considerable powers to police the conditions of the housing that their citizens occupy, but limited resources (Leather 2001). Housing standards at the beginning of the twenty-first century are generally considerably better than they were at the beginning of the last century (Holmans 1999), but there remain in England alone some $1^1/_2$ million dwellings that are officially unfit for habitation (DETR 1998). While individuals may have rights of redress against landlords and local authorities, those who do not possess the means to secure that the housing they occupy is maintained in an acceptable condition cannot easily enforce a right to such maintenance.

Homelessness and the rationing of social sector housing _____

Housing and public health legislation therefore provide some measure of protection against overcrowded and insanitary housing conditions. This is similarly reflected in a duty laid upon local housing authorities (currently, by Section 167 of the 1996 Housing Act) by which they are required, in the allocation of public housing stock, to give 'reasonable preference' to people living in such conditions, to families with dependant children or that include someone who is pregnant, to those living in otherwise unsatisfactory conditions or whose social and economic circumstances make it difficult to obtain settled accommodation, and to those to whom authorities may owe a statutory duty. Additional preference should be given to those with particular needs that arise upon medical or welfare grounds. Since the 1996 Housing Act local authorities have been required to maintain a single register of those in housing need within their area, from which certain categories of person can be excluded – including those, such as asylum seekers, with no legal right to public assistance and others whom councils might choose to exclude, such as those with histories of rent arrears or anti-social behaviour.

In practice, however, local authorities are not legally required to have any housing stock at all. Even where they have statutory duties to rehouse people they may achieve this by way of arrangements with third parties, such as RSLs or even private landlords. Since local authorities were first empowered to provide public housing, access to such housing has always been rationed. Characteristically, rationing has been by way of waiting lists and points schemes by which to prioritise the claims and needs of prospective tenants. Local authorities are obliged to publish the details of their allocations policies and to have regard to a ministerial Code of Guidance, but the determination of criteria for allocation remains ultimately at their discretion (although, at the time of writing, the government has advanced proposals by which housing applicants would be banded according to the urgency of their need and, within each band, waiting-time would become the principal criterion for priority – see DETR 2000).

The purpose of council housing – as to whether it is to meet the general needs of the population or the special needs of the poorest – has always been a source of political controversy (Short 1982). Since the 1980s, however, the status of public or 'social' sector housing has unequivocally been reduced to that of a residual housing tenure reserved for those without access to satisfactory private sector alternatives (Clapham et al. 1990). The introduction in 1996 of the single housing register was supposed to dispense with the idea that it was possible to distinguish between those in general need who could wait on a waiting list, and those whose circumstances were so dire that they could 'jump' the queue and enter social sector housing by way of an 'emergency' route as homeless persons (see, for example, Mullins and Niner 1998). In practice, the treatment afforded to these two groups continues to be quite different.

Access to public housing has never been acknowledged as a universal right, even for homeless people. State policy for the relief of homelessness has always been either deterrent or selective. In the fifteenth century, homelessness, or 'vagrancy', could be subject to such violent punishments as whipping and branding. Under the Poor Laws it could result in an enforced return to the parish of one's birth and quite possibly incarceration in a bridewell or workhouse. The Beveridgian welfare state may have put an end to the workhouse, but the relief of homelessness was a social service reserved primarily for people who were aged or infirm and for 'persons in need of care and attention' (which term primarily referred to homeless women and children for whom only temporary shelter might be arranged). This changed with the enactment of the Housing (Homeless Persons) Act of 1977 which ostensibly placed a duty upon local housing authorities to provide permanent, not temporary, accommodation to certain classes of homeless person. It may be seen, however, first, that the right to housing which this provides is strictly conditional and, second, that the right to permanent accommodation has since been significantly diluted.

Legislative provision for the protection of homeless persons is now to be found in consolidated and amended form in Part VII of the 1996 Housing Act. The definition that the legislation gives to homelessness is, potentially, quite widely drawn. A person is homeless if she has no accommodation that she, together with her family, has a legal right to occupy. The definition extends to include people who, though they have accommodation, may be at risk of violence from some other person residing there, or if the condition of the property is so bad that she might not reasonably be expected to continue to reside there. In practice, local authorities and the courts (see Chapter 9) have often interpreted this definition narrowly. People living in great insecurity whose sole right to accommodation may be the law which protects them from eviction without a court order (see above) may be held not to be homeless unless and until such an order has been made and a warrant for possession executed. Additionally, it may be held reasonable for people living in appalling physical conditions to continue living there if the conditions prevailing in the area of the local authority concerned are generally so poor that other people can be shown to be living in conditions which are worse or at least equally bad.

People who establish that they are homeless must additionally surmount two further hurdles if they are to obtain rehousing. First, they must establish that they are in 'priority need'. This condition perpetuates the selective nature of the state relief of homelessness. Excepting provision for those made homeless by fire, flood or natural disaster, only certain categories of person may receive substantive assistance (other than advice). Only households with dependant children (or households which consist of or include a pregnant woman) and households consisting of or which include someone who is 'vulnerable' by reason of old age, disability, learning difficulty, mental health problems or 'other special reason' will otherwise qualify. Second, people must establish that they did not become homeless intentionally. This provision enables local authorities to probe into the backgrounds of homeless people to establish the chain of causation resulting in their present circumstances and the degree of culpability that may attach to their present or indeed their past conduct. The government, at the time of writing, is thinking about lowering these hurdles: it is proposed that the definition of 'vulnerability' for the purposes of establishing priority need status might be made more inclusive and that homeless people in priority need who are adjudged 'intentionally homeless' might none the less be allowed temporary accommodation (although local authorities should still reduce their priority for permanent housing from the housing register) (DETR 2000).

A homeless person surmounting these hurdles is owed a duty by the local authority to which she has applied. That duty is qualified in three important ways. First, if the homeless person has a local connection with another local authority area, she may be referred for assistance to that authority. Second, if suitable alternative accommodation is available for the applicant and her family within the local authority's area, the authority's duty is discharged by assisting the applicant to secure that accommodation. Third, whereas the original 1977 legislation was assumed (until a House of Lords ruling in 1995) to have implied a right to permanent rehousing, the 1996 Act explicitly provided that the duty of a local authority was to provide only temporary accommodation for a period up to two years, during which it should fall to the applicant to seek her own accommodation. Although local authorities have discretion to extend temporary accommodation and may (following regulatory changes introduced by the New Labour government in 1997) in due course consider those whom they have temporarily housed for permanent rehousing from the housing register, homeless people can be temporarily housed in social housing stock for no more than two years in any three-year period (although a change to this rule is currently contemplated). It should also be noted that assistance under the homeless persons provisions of the 1996 Housing Act, like social assistance, expressly qualifies as 'recourse to public funds' for the purposes of immigration law (see Chapter 5) and it is a right which is not in practice exercisable by people whose immigration status is not secure.

Local authorities continue to have a key role in enabling access to housing, whether in their own diminishing housing stock or in other forms of 'social' housing provided by RSLs. Such accommodation, however, now represents little more than a fifth of the total housing stock in the UK (Wilcox 1999: 113) and the rules by which people may access it are both highly complex and rigorously selective. The highly differentiated nature of the rights by which people can access such accommodation may hardly be regarded as amounting to a 'prize of citizenship' (Mullins and Niner 1998).

Summary/conclusion

Inevitably, perhaps, within a democratic-welfare-capitalist state housing remains highly commodified (see Chapter 1 and, for example, Ball 1983). Dwellings and land, even when their use is regulated or they are actually owned by the state, are leased or rented out, bought or sold as commodities in the market place. To the extent that it is possible for social legislation to create rights in relation to housing, it is constrained by the nature of property relations and the character of real estate as a particular kind of commodity. This chapter has reflected on four rather different kinds of legislative intervention.

First, social legislation may be used to guarantee the position of citizens in the housing market by underwriting their capacity to pay for housing. The most privileged form of housing tenure, owner-occupation, had in the past benefited from a universal fiscal subsidy. In contrast, the less privileged forms of housing tenure, the private and public rented sectors, are assisted by a selective form of social security subsidy. With the ascendancy of owner-occupation at the close of the twentieth century, the indiscriminate subsidy that had been provided through mortgage tax relief has been belatedly curtailed. For people remaining in the residual rented housing sectors, and for those owner-occupiers who find themselves on social assistance, the selectivity of means-tested benefits encroaches to the point that it may even take account of the quality and size of a person's home in relation to her needs and the composition of her household. The principal framework of social rights is therefore one that supports only those at the margins of the market. It is a framework that requires a considerable degree of surveillance of individual citizens' housing arrangements.

Second, social legislation may be used to achieve stability in the housing market. In the past tenants in the private rented sector were given certain rights with regard to rent levels and security of tenure. This process, however, became increasingly complex over time and increasingly marginal as the public rented sector and, more particularly, owner-occupation became more dominant forms of housing tenure. Latterly, Conservative governments have rejected any form or rent regulation that might hold rents beneath their 'natural' market level, while New Labour governments have now accepted a role for private renting. This chapter has discussed the different regulatory regimes that apply to private sector tenants, to public sector tenants, and to other forms of residential tenure, some of which are subject to minimal or no legal protection. The nearest thing to a universal right to be achieved under modern social legislation is the right of a residential occupier (including owner-occupying mortgagors) not to be evicted without a court first making an order for repossession. It is a right that fetters the power of market forces, albeit in many circumstances only to a minimal degree, and it is a right which has been eroded by more recent legislation.

Third, social legislation may be used to guarantee certain standards of production; that is to say, to ensure that housing is provided to a standard that is habitable and reasonably conducive to public health. This chapter has discussed the rights of redress that tenants have against landlords in respect of disrepair; the powers that local authorities may exercise to compel repairs and improvements to unsatisfactory housing; and the rights that people have to grants towards the cost of repairs and improvements. It may be noted, however, that landlord and tenant law is primarily a matter of civil, not social, rights; that the citizen's right to invoke the protective powers of local authorities under housing and public health legislation are subject to the willingness and capacity of local authorities to respond; and that the right to financial assistance with essential repairs and improvements is not universal but selective, being conditional upon a means-test.

Finally, social legislation may be used to guarantee citizens' access to housing. Legislation relating to the direct provision of social housing has been largely permissive, however. Local housing authorities have never been able unconditionally to guarantee access to housing. The nearest thing to a right to housing is a right afforded only to certain categories of homeless persons; it is conditional upon their past behaviour and it does not guarantee access to a permanent home.

Citizens do enjoy certain rights in relation to housing, but they are complex and qualified rights. Where social legislation protects or creates such rights, it does so, by and large, selectively. In housing, as with 'work', though social rights may ameliorate the impact of market forces, it is the latter that generally take precedence.

Chapter 8

Rights in education, health and social care

Though these systems form a major part of the welfare state, the social rights provided through our education, health and social care systems are seldom spoken of as 'welfare' rights. The reasons for this are partly cultural and partly legal. On the one hand, 'welfare' is a term that has come to be associated either generally with the dispensation of cash benefits rather than services in kind, or more particularly (and pejoratively) with services thought to be reserved only for 'the poor'. This ought not to deflect us from speaking of education, health and social care as 'welfare' services, since clearly they are critically important for the welfare of the human subject. On the other hand, there really are surprisingly few legally enforceable rights in relation to such services. The language of rights tends to surface in four ways:

- In relation to rights of complaint or redress. It is possible to have a clearly defined right of complaint, even when the nature of one's substantive entitlement is not so clearly defined. I shall be discussing rights of redress separately in Chapter 9.
- As a declaratory device for the setting of performance targets for service providers, which do not in practice give rise to justiciable rights for service users (or 'consumers'). Of significance here are public documents like the Patient's or NHS Charter and the Parent's Charter.
- In relation to the special needs of particularly vulnerable groups, such as children with special educational needs and people with mental health problems.
- In relation to particular kinds of benefits that are incidental to the substantive provision of educational, health or social care, such as exemption from fees or charges or assistance with associated costs.

In this chapter, I shall discuss education and health services under each of these last three headings. For the purposes of my discussion of social care, I shall be including the care of children as well as the care of frail elderly and disabled people. The language of rights is at its most problematic in relation to the provision of protective 'care', as opposed to specialised or professional 'services'. There have been long and enduring disputes about how to define the boundary between childcare and education on the one hand (see, for example, Daniel and Ivatts 1998) and between social care and health provision or 'treatment' on the other (see, for example, Hudson 1999). I shall return to discuss the ethical significance of care in Part III of this book, but there are two points to be emphasised here. First, there is a controversial distinction that some would make between the juridically competent citizen/consumer who may consciously exercise her rights to services and the vulnerable subject who may not be a fully competent or autonomous citizen and requires general or protective care, rather than particular or specialist services. Second, if care is to be a matter of rights there are potential conflicts between the rights of, for example, children and their parents and between those who receive care and those who provide it.

The rights of vulnerable citizens have been positively asserted in a variety of United Nations documents, including the Convention of the Rights of the Child, the Declaration on the Rights of Disabled Persons and the UN Principles for Older Persons (see Ferguson 1999). Best known of these is the UN Convention on the Rights of the Child of 1989, which has major significance for social policy because of its insistence that children are people with inalienable rights. This claim, however, raises a host of issues – concerning, in particular, the extent of children's autonomy – that cannot be fully addressed within the limited scope of this book, let alone within a single chapter. None the less, I shall be illustrating the ambiguity of children's rights in relation to childcare provision, although I shall not be dealing with the highly specialised subject of child protection. Similarly, there are complex issues concerning the rights of disabled people raised, for example, by the Independent Living Movement (see, for example, Campbell and Oliver 1996) and a tension between demands for independence and the right to dependency or 'asylum' (in the original meaning of the word). My purpose in this particular chapter, however, is to focus on the rights of disabled people to have their needs assessed and their rights in relation to assistance with the costs of care.

Education

Probably the most authoritative statement of a right to education so far as British citizens are concerned is provided in the First Protocol (Article 2) to the European Convention on Human Rights, which has been incorporated into English Law by the 1998 Human Rights Act (and by parallel enactments into the law of the other UK jurisdictions). This states that 'No person shall be denied the right to education'. This curious form of words is more equivocal than that contained in Article 26 of the Universal Declaration of Human Rights ('Everyone has the right to education'). It implies that the state is not necessarily obliged to provide education to satisfy the rights of citizens, but that where provision exists, no one should be excluded. In the event, since the Education Act of 1870 first introduced compulsory elementary schooling, the purpose was not to satisfy the right of citizens to an education, but to underwrite the nation's industrial prosperity and 'the safe working of our constitutional system' (Forster 1870). The same purpose is reflected in current policy discourse. The Labour Party's Commission on Social Justice (CSJ 1994) and its subsequent manifestos (Labour Party 1997; 2001) stress that the provision of education is an investment on behalf of the wider society: education 'is not just good for the individual. It is an economic necessity for the nation' (Labour Party 1997: 7).

So far as children are concerned, there are two implications that flow from the view of education as a public good. First, as Daniel and Ivatts put it, although education policy is 'in effect . . . social policy for children', 'rather than children's needs being placed at the forefront of education policy considerations, a variety of adult concerns and perspectives determine the policy outcomes' (1998: 168). This is most evident in relation to early years provision, where according to the advocates of child-centred provision the needs of children may actually conflict with the educational aspirations of parents and politicians. But it also applies to older children who, under the regime created since the introduction of a National Curriculum in the late 1980s, are subject to what one critic has called 'a factory-farm model of education, in which each child, like a battery hen, is to assimilate as much as possible of the food offered to it' (Kelly 1994: 94). The second implication is that the implied 'rights' of children actually arise as a consequence of an enforceable duty imposed by legislation upon their parents, requiring parents to make arrangements for the education of their children. Education for children aged 5 to 16 is compulsory: parents are compelled to send their children to school (or to make satisfactory alternative arrangements) and may be prosecuted should they fail to do so.

So far as post-compulsory education and training go – whether it be in the further and higher education sector or with employers – because citizens who participate do so by choice, questions of rights are largely confined to the extent of the assistance that they should receive in order to be able to do so. (For a more extensive technical account than that which follows of rights in relation to education see, for example, Ford *et al.* 1999.)

The rights of parents

The principle of universal, free education for all primary and secondary school-age children had been established by the Education Act of 1944. Secondary school provision was based on a tripartite system that involved the selection of children according to their aptitude for either grammar, technical or secondary modern schools, but changes during the 1960s and 1970s had seen a shift towards comprehensive schools and more child-centred teaching practices. Critics of the system that was emerging were concerned, on the one hand, that its universal nature constrained parental choice and, on the other, that the school curriculum was not equipping children for the demands of the contemporary labour market. The response of Conservative governments during the 1980s and 1990s was a raft of legislation – most notably the Education Reform Act of 1988 – which fragmented the system in a way that was intended to extend parental choice, while introducing a centrally regulated National Curriculum.

A new right of parental choice was set out in a *Parent's Charter* (DES 1991). The right was supposed to flow from a series of reforms that had included the introduction of open enrolment, formula funding and a national testing and inspection regime. The intention was that schools should admit as many pupils as they could accommodate, that schools would be funded in accordance with the numbers of children they could attract, and that the publication of school league tables would enable parents to make informed judgements about the relative performance of the schools available to them. In practice, parental choice has been largely illusory for many parents since popular schools that became oversubscribed were in a position effectively to choose the pupils they would take (and specialist schools were even allowed to select a proportion by ability), while provision in unpopular schools could be put at risk as they lost pupil numbers and therefore funding (see, for example, Ball 1998). The New Labour government is broadly committed to maintaining the system put in place by its predecessors (see Muschamp *et al.* 1999) and at the time of writing it has proposals for further increasing the diversity of the schools from which parents may in principle choose (DfES 2001).

Parents have rights of appeal against school admission decisions and against decisions to exclude their children from school, and a right formally to complain about the operation of the school curriculum (see Chapter 9). They also have the right to withdraw their children from religious education lessons (which are not governed by the National Curriculum) and from acts of religious worship in school, and they have the right to request that their children be withdrawn from sex education lessons (although the granting of such requests is at the discretion of school governors). Parents have a right – to receive from the governors of any school their children attend information with regard to the school's policies; to attend an Annual Parents' Meeting; to take part and stand in the election of parent governors (though parent governors only ever make up a minority of the membership of a school's governing body).

The New Labour government has introduced arrangements for 'school–home agreements', quasi-contracts entered between parents and the schools their children attend. Notionally, such agreements give rise to rights in relation to the expectations that parents might have of a school, but their primary purpose is 'to promote a culture of responsibility for learning within the family' (Labour Party 1997: 8) in relation, for example, to the supervision of homework. They form part of a system of 'two-way surveillance' (Muschamp *et al.* 1999: 117), rather than rights.

Children with special needs

Prior to the 1980s children who were disabled, or who had learning difficulties, were most often educated in special schools. But following the recommendations of the Warnock Committee (DES 1978) attempts have been made to ensure that children with special educational needs should be provided for in mainstream schools. Warnock estimated that while 20 per cent of pupils might need some sort of special educational assistance at some time during their schooling, only 2 per cent will require separate specialised facilities. The Education Act of 1981 provided a right for pupils to be assessed and to receive a statement of their special educational needs from their local education authority. Such statements may indicate the adaptations to school buildings or to school timetables or routines that may be required to accommodate a particular pupil's needs; the additional teaching resources she may require; or they may provide, for example, that elements of the National Curriculum should be modified or disapplied in her case. Schools receive an additional funding allocation based on the number of 'statemented' pupils they have.

In practice, however, the segregation of children with special needs is still occurring both within and between schools and the trend towards their integration in mainstream schools may even have been reversed during the 1990s (e.g. Oliver and Barnes 1998).

Education benefits and assistance

Schooling may be free to all, but children attending school need to be clothed and to travel to school. They need to be fed while at school and sometimes their education might involve residential and extra-curricular visits or 'trips'. These may entail significant costs (see Smith and Noble 1995).

Local education authorities (LEAs) are empowered, but not obliged, to operate discretionary school clothing or school uniform grant schemes to provide assistance for the children of poor parents. Because such schemes are discretionary they do not give rise to enforceable rights, and eligibility criteria and the scope of schemes – where they exist at all – are subject to variation. In contrast, LEAs are legally required to provide free transport or to meet the travel costs of pupils who do not live within walking distance of their schools.

Similarly, the 1944 Education Act had required LEAs to provide a midday meal to every child in a maintained school who wanted one. From 1950 a fixed national charge applied for school meals, but meals for the children of parents on low incomes were free. In 1980, however, LEAs were relieved of their obligation to provide meals at fixed prices (or at all) except that free meals (which need not be hot) should still be provided for children whose parents were in receipt of means-tested benefits. Later in the 1980s further restrictions meant that only the children of parents receiving income support (IS) now qualify for free school meals. The New Labour government restored the obligation to provide meals for all pupils (i.e. not just free meals) and, in the case of secondary schools, has delegated the funding for free school meals to schools themselves, rather than to LEAs. Primary and special schools, if they choose, can still have the funding administered for them by the LEA. As a result, practice with regard to free meals provision can now vary enormously. The evidence suggests that considerable stigma can attach to the children who claim the right to a free school meal and that many who are entitled to do so do not (McMahon and Marsh 1999).

Following the Education Act of 1988 it has been permissible for maintained schools to request voluntary financial contributions from parents towards the cost of their children's attendance on residential and extra-curricular trips, but with remission of contributions for parents who cannot afford to pay. In practice this would appear to have led to the introduction of 'voluntary' contributions for a range of school activities, in circumstances in which charging is not necessarily legal. As with the provision of free school meals, there is evidence that children whose parents cannot afford to pay such contributions may be stigmatised or else, to avoid this, parents may pay when they cannot afford to do so, or may even prevent their children from participating in certain school activities (Smith and Noble 1995). In the case of curricular activities, however – whether residential or non-residential and whether during or outside school hours – it is quite clear that children whose parents are in receipt of IS are entitled to participate without payment.

Turning now to the rights of young people and adults above compulsory school age, we turn first to provision for young people who stay on at school or who go on to sixth form or further education college to undertake 'non-advanced' qualifications (i.e. non-higher education qualifications, such as A or AS levels or GNVQs). LEAs have been empowered, but once again not obliged, to provide discretionary means-tested education maintenance allowances (EMAs) or further education grants to the parents of such children. Although most LEAs have operated some such provision, the nature and extent of the provision has varied widely (Burghes and Stagles 1983; Smith and Noble 1995). At the time of writing, however, the New Labour government is piloting a new EMA scheme in 15 LEA areas and it is envisaged that this may be rolled out nationally (Maguire *et al.* 2001). While still administered by LEAs, the scheme would be nationally funded with allowances being paid – possibly directly to young people and possibly with bonuses for attendance and achievement – in respect of 16–19-year-olds whose parents' income falls below a set level: the scheme partly compensates for the withdrawal in the 1980s of other forms of means-tested support for 16- and 17-year-olds, but its principal purpose is to encourage young people from lower-income families to remain in full-time education.

So far as higher education is concerned, from 1962 until 1990 Britain had a system that afforded mandatory awards for all students in order to meet their tuition fees and pay a means-tested maintenance grant. From 1990 a Conservative government froze the value of maintenance grants and introduced a system of top-up loans so that students (or their parents) should themselves contribute to the cost of their maintenance while at college or university. In 1998, however, a New Labour government went further: it required students to contribute to tuition fees – subject to exemptions for poorer students – and it abolished maintenance grants, retaining only supplementary grants for students who were themselves parents. A new student loan scheme was introduced and a system of Access Funds that provided discretionary relief to students experiencing hardship. However, exercising its newly devolved powers, the Scottish Parliament adopted a different system for Scotland and emerging evidence in England and Wales suggested that the new arrangements were failing to meet the government's objective of widening participation in higher education (see Naidoo and Callender 2000). At the time of writing, therefore, it appears that the government is considering withdrawing the requirement to pay tuition fees, reverting to a system of maintenance grants and seeking to recover the costs through a new graduate tax (*The Guardian*, 4 October 2001).

As a general rule, students – whether they be in higher education or, in the case of people aged 19 or over, in *any* kind of full-time education – are not entitled to receive means-tested social security benefits throughout the duration of their courses (i.e. including vacation periods). There are exceptions. Students who qualify for (IS) because, for example, they are lone parents, or pensioners, or are disabled, are able to receive benefit and study at the same time. Young people under 19 who are in 'non-advanced' education may be able to claim IS if they are themselves parents, or are disabled, or are estranged from their parents. Part-time students may be able to receive income-based jobseeker's allowance (JSA), provided they can demonstrate that they remain available for work and that they are prepared to give up their studies if a job becomes available. Couples who are both full-time students and have children may be able to claim IS/JSA during vacations. Similarly, full-time students are not normally eligible for housing benefit (HB) or council tax benefit (CTB) and, although a similar range of exceptions applies, even those students whose special circumstances entitle them to claim receive a reduced rate of HB during term-time. The assumption is that, for the most part, adults and young people over compulsory school age should either support themselves during their studies or rely upon resources explicitly provided for educational purposes.

Finally, a very substantial part of the formal learning that people undertake after leaving school is employment based and described as 'training' rather than education (see, for example, Vickerstaff 1999). There is an extensive machinery of national vocational qualification (NVQ) bearing traineeships and 'modern apprenticeships' offered by employers and overseen by industrial training organisations and local training and enterprise councils. At the time of writing, the New Labour government is seeking to develop the 'Connexions' service which, through locally based partnerships involving schools, local government and employer organisations, will provide personal advice and support for 13–19-year-olds to enable them to maximise their education and training opportunities. The government had also sought to assist older people to access employer provided training and related educational opportunities through the development of 'individual learning accounts' (DfEE 1998), although the initial scheme was abandoned because of the alleged misappropriation of funds by certain training providers (*The Guardian*, 25 October 2001). Additionally, the subsidised training placements into which young people are directed under New Deal programmes (see Chapter 6 above) are supposed to lead to NVQ qualifications. However, the scale of Britain's commitment to industrial training compares poorly with that which had applied prior to the 1980s (Ainley 1993), while the quality of its present system of work-based qualifications compares badly with that in other developed countries (O'Higgins 2001). By and large, despite New Labour's rhetorical commitment to it, 'life-long learning' does not yet constitute a substantive social right.

Health

Health is arguably *the* most basic of human needs (Doyal and Gough 1991; and see Chapter 2 above). The 1966 International Covenant on Economic, Social and Cultural Rights declares that its signatories – which include the

UK – 'recognise the right of everyone to the enjoyment of the highest attainable standard of physical and mental health' (Article 12[1]). This is echoed in the Constitution of the World Health Organisation, which declares that 'the enjoyment of the highest attainable standard of health is one of the fundamental rights of every human being'. It has been argued that human health and human rights are interdependent and inseparable causes (Mann *et al.* 1999). There is, of course, a distinction to be made between measures that promote public health and provision for individual health treatment. Although the legislation that created the National Health Service (NHS) in Britain places a duty on the relevant Secretary of State to promote a comprehensive health service, this does not secure for any particular individual a right to any particular service or resource (Lenaghan 1997).

The NHS, which was established in 1948, provides a comprehensive service that is (mainly) free to all at the point of delivery. The service is funded directly from taxes rather than through personal or social insurance and it is accessible to all citizens. A right of access, however, is not the same as a right to treatment. Attempts to enforce such a right through the courts have failed on the grounds that the statutory duty imposed by the NHS Act appears to offer 'no direct right to health service resources and . . . should be considered from the perspective of local health authorities who must do their reasonable best with scarce resources' (Court of Appeal, cited in Lenaghan 1997: 71). As a result, '[d]ifficult and agonising judgements have to be made as to how a limited budget is best allocated to the maximum advantage of the maximum number of patients. That is not a judgement the court can make' (*ibid.*). NHS resources are rationed on the basis of utilitarian principles rather than on the basis of individual rights. Defenders of this arrangement might contend that to give people clearly defined and enforceable rights might benefit the articulate and the affluent (those with the 'sharpest elbows') at the expense of the powerless and the poor, and that it may undermine both the clinical freedom of the health professional and the inherent trust that is supposed to characterise the doctor–patient relationship. Against this view, however, it has to be said that the NHS has so far failed to ensure social equity in health outcomes (Townsend *et al.* 1988) and some would argue that it has perpetuated oppressive and disempowering medical ideologies (e.g. Doyal 1979; Campbell and Oliver 1996).

The universal nature of the NHS as 'an act of collective goodwill and public enterprise and not a commodity privately bought and sold' (Bevan 1952: 106), ought in theory to have guaranteed that health provision became a social right. In practice, the rights of service users are more ambiguous.

The rights of patients

An attempt to define the rights of patients was made in *The Patient's Charter* (DoH 1992). The exercise formed part of the Conservative government's *Citizen's Charter* initiative, by which it sought to redefine the citizen as a consumer of public services (see discussion in Chapter 1). At the time of writing, a new *NHS Charter* has been promised to replace *The Patient's Charter* (see DoH 2000a: ch. 10). However, the original charter set out the seven rights that the NHS has established:

- To receive health care on the basis of clinical need, regardless of ability to pay. As we have seen, this right has never extended to being able to specify the nature and extent of treatment. As a result of medical advances and demographic trends, demand for treatment had been running ahead of the capacity of the NHS ever since it was established (e.g. Butler and Calnan 1999). The Conservative government's belief in the 1980s and 1990s was that the creation of a cost-constrained internal market within the NHS (see Chapter 1 above) would render the basis on which resources were allocated more transparent so that patients could to some extent shop around for treatment – albeit that their 'rights' would no longer be constrained merely by the vagaries of clinical judgement, but by managerial controls over the contracting process.
- To be registered with a general practitioner (GP). A central feature of the NHS has been that access to services is provided primarily through local GPs and provision exists to ensure that patients can register with a GP of their choice and can, if they wish, change their GP, although registration can be difficult for homeless people and others without a permanent address.
- To receive emergency medical care at any time, through a GP or the emergency ambulance service and hospital accident and emergency (A&E) departments.
- To be referred to a consultant, acceptable to the patient, when her GP considers this to be necessary, and to be referred for a second opinion if the patient and her GP agree this is desirable. Access to hospital or other specialist treatment, except in emergencies, is obtainable only on referral. The Conservative government sought to enhance the role of GPs as gate-keepers within the NHS by making many of them 'purchasers' of treatment on behalf of patients and, to an extent, the creation by New Labour of Primary Health Care Trusts (PHCTs), which negotiate service agreements with hospitals and are controlled primarily by GPs, has taken this a stage further (Paton 1999).
- To be given a clear explanation of any treatment proposed, including any risks and any alternatives, before the patient decides whether she agrees to the treatment. This provision gives cognisance to NHS patients' civil rights and liberties rather than their social rights. They may, for example, sue the NHS or individual health professionals for negligence and it is necessary that health professionals ensure that they have the consent of the patient before performing any medical procedure. Patients have a right to refuse treatment. This can and does give rise to complex legal and ethical dilemmas in emergency situations or where relatives may withhold consent for treatment or demand its withdrawal on behalf of patients who are prevented from making decisions for themselves.
- To have access to the patient's own health records, and to know that those working for the NHS are under a legal duty to keep their contents

confidential. Once again, this is a provision that stems from civil liberty concerns. In practice, freedom of information within the NHS remains problematic (ACHC 1994).

• To choose whether or not the patient wishes to take part in medical research or medical student training.

To these rights, the Conservative government sought to add: a right to detailed information on local health services, including quality standards and maximum waiting times; a right to be admitted for hospital treatment within a set period of time after being placed by a consultant on the waiting list; a right to have any complaint about NHS services investigated; and outline 'National Charter Standards', a set of aspirations or performance targets for the NHS. These additional rights stemmed from the consumerist ethos of the government and, as Baggott (1998: 262) has put it, 'are really conventions rather than rights'. New Labour's *NHS Charter* will tell people about the standards of treatment and care they can expect of the NHS. It will also explain patients' responsibilities (DoH 1997). A report for the New Labour government by Greg Dyke praised the original *Patient's Charter* because it had begun 'to legitimise a more consumerist culture' (1998: 11), but criticised it for being 'a "rag bag" of unconnected rights and service aspirations' (1998: 17). Dyke has proposed a Charter 'package', consisting of a statement of NHS values, local charters worked up by individual NHS organisations and a series of disease-specific 'user guides'. The government has additionally indicated that it will, for example, give new entitlements to patients whose operations are cancelled, it will pilot and develop a new patient advocacy and liaison service (PALS), and change the basis on which patients may complain (see Chapter 9 below).

It is difficult at present to see that the new charter will achieve a clearer exposition of patients' rights. It may succeed in more clearly articulating and communicating the service mission of the NHS, but it is unlikely to specify many strictly enforceable rights; still less to address any of the deep ethical controversies that surround, for example, the 'rights' that patients may claim to abortion, fertility treatment, genetic screening or assisted euthanasia.

The point at which patients' rights are necessarily more specifically defined relate, first, to patients with mental health problems and, second, to those instances in which health provision is not completely free and it is therefore necessary for patients who are not able to pay to seek exemption from charges.

Patients with mental health problems

The issue of consent to treatment may be especially problematic in the case of people with mental health problems and the 1983 Mental Health Act contains provisions by which people who are adjudged to be a danger to themselves or to others as a result of mental illness may be compulsorily detained. The Act provides a variety of safeguards concerning the procedures for compulsory admission to hospital, the rights of patients in respect of various forms of treatment while detained, their rights to be discharged and their rights to appeal against detention to the Mental Health Review Tribunal (Cooper 1994). Since the 1980s, however, the development of policies for care in the community has meant that patients with mental health problems are increasingly cared for in community settings, rather than hospitals and, at the time of writing, the government has proposed far-reaching reform of the Mental Health Act provisions. It is likely that a new Mental Health Act will institute a three-stage process: the first stage will allow for preliminary examination by two doctors and a social worker or mental health professional and, if required, urgent treatment under compulsory powers; the second for an assessment leading to a formal care plan, provided that assessment and initial treatment under compulsory powers shall not continue for more than 28 days unless authorised by a newly constituted Mental Health Tribunal (MHT); the third that the MHT may make a care and treatment order for a period for up to six months in the first instance, with power to make another six-month order thereafter and for further orders lasting up to 12 months after that (DoH 2000b). The legislation will give patients a right to independent advocacy.

Health benefits

There are four aspects of NHS provision that, though they are subsidised, are not necessarily free of charge: the supply of prescribed medicines (which are subject to a standard fixed charge per item); dental treatment and the provision of dentures (which may be provided on special terms by dentists practicing under an NHS contract); sight-testing and the supply of optical glasses; the supply of wigs and fabric supports. However, certain people are entitled to receive these free or subject to a reduced charge. Additionally, some people may also receive assistance with the cost of fares when they have to travel to hospital (for example, to attend out-patient appointments) and some expectant mothers and young children are entitled to receive free milk and vitamins. There are some rather complex variations in the rules pertaining to these different concessionary benefits (for exact details see, for example, CPAG's *Welfare Benefits Handbook*), but some or all of these entitlements extend, as may be appropriate, to:

- children and, in some instances, pregnant women (and women who have recently given birth) and pensioners;
- people in receipt of income support or income-based jobseeker's allowance and, in some instances, recipients of working families' tax credit and disabled person's tax credit or who may qualify for means-tested assistance under the low-income health benefits scheme.

Free prescriptions and sight-tests (and help towards the costs of glasses) are also available to people suffering from certain specified chronic illnesses or conditions and certain health care equipment or appliances – such as wheelchairs, hearing aids and incontinence pads – may be provided free of charge or on prescription.

Social care

Although the term social care is generally used to apply to social service provision for elderly and disabled people, I shall, as I have already announced, apply a wider concept of 'care' so as to encompass legislative arrangements intended to promote childcare, as well as discussing the rights of elderly and disable people to have their care needs assessed and to receive assistance with the costs of care.

Childcare

I have already indicated that there is a problem about defining the boundary between education and childcare. It also reflects a tension between children's rights to education and their parents' rights to work. In part it reflects the competing traditions and values associated with early years education on the one hand and nursery provision on the other. Finally, it reflects some deeper contradictions concerning our understanding of childhood: are children biological beings that must be dutifully tended and made ready for responsible adulthood and employment, or are they social beings and active agents in the very processes that construct the world they inhabit (see, for example, Moss 2000)? My purpose here, however, is to outline the framework within which childcare provision has developed, since the question of whose rights are served remains ambiguous.

Provision for children of pre-compulsory schooling age was not a high priority in Britain in the period following the Second World War. It consisted of nursery schools and nursery classes provided by a few local education authorities, a smattering of privately run day nurseries, and a number of local authority day nurseries provided 'to meet the special needs of children whose mothers are constrained by individual circumstances to go out to work or whose home circumstances are unsatisfactory from the health point of view or whose mothers are incapable for some good reason of undertaking the full care of their children' (1945 Ministry of Health Circular, quoted in Daniel and Ivatts 1998: 154). Legislation also provided that private childminders should be registered and subject to basic minimum standards. A declared commitment to the expansion of nursery education from the 1970s onwards had comparatively little effect, although there was a significant expansion in the admission of 'rising fives' into reception classes in primary schools. Also from the 1960s and into the 1970s a voluntary sector initiative, the pre-school playgroups movement, emerged. The 1989 Children Act extended the regulatory functions of local social services departments and the standards to be applied to private and voluntary sector daycare providers. However, the patchwork of provision that had emerged was geographically very uneven and heavily skewed towards low-cost private or voluntary sector providers – such as registered childminders and community playgroups – with, by international standards, comparatively little in the way of publicly funded services (Moss and Melhuish 1991).

The short-lived nursery voucher scheme introduced by a Conservative government before the 1997 General Election was destined to put additional funding into early years provision, but the evidence suggests that those re- sources were already being captured to fund the expansion of nursery and reception class provision in primary schools at the expense of other forms of provision (Daniel and Ivatts 1998: 163). The New Labour government moved swiftly to scrap the scheme and committed itself instead: to guaranteeing educational provision for all 4-year-olds whose parents want it, and to at least two-thirds of 3-year-olds by 2002; to the promotion of a National Childcare Strategy, involving local early years development and childcare partnerships; the regulation of early years education in both the private and voluntary sectors through the Office for Standards in Education (OFSTED) with speci- fied learning outcomes for pre-school children (Moss 2000).

This decisive shift towards education, rather than care, for pre-compulsory school age children has been accompanied, none the less, by a drive to fund additional childcare places in non-educational settings through the introduc- tion of childcare tax credits and to promote 'family-friendly' employment (see Chapter 6 above). While additional funds are being provided to promote out- of-school care for older children, there has been no attempt to legislate for a duty upon either education or social services authorities to provide these. Recent evidence indicates that the impact of this raft of policies to date has been modest: the number of children aged 0–8 per registered childcare place declined from 7.5 in 1999 to 6.9 in 2000 (Daycare Trust 2000). At the time of writing, further resources have been pledged for the expansion of childcare. What is less clear is whether there is any commitment in the longer term to establish a right to childcare, and whose interests that right should serve.

Needs assessment

Turning now to elderly people (should they be frail) and disabled people (including – for these purposes – people with learning difficulties or mental health problems should they require social care), the ambiguity of their right to care had, even in the post-Second World War period, been overshadowed by the institutional nature of state-provided care and its association with the tradi- tions of the Poor Law. The story of the transition from institutional care to pluralistic forms of care in the community is amply told elsewhere (e.g. Wistow et al. 1994). The manner in which that transition was driven during the 1980s and 1990s was characterised, on the one hand, by the new significance accorded to informal care and the desire that people requiring care should be enabled to live as far as possible in their own homes; and, on the other, by the emergence of managerialist approaches to service delivery and the insistence on separating the purchasing of care from its provision (see Chapter 1 above). While the New Labour government has sought to extend processes of quality control over com- munity care provision, it remains committed to the essential form of the system established by the Conservatives (Johnson 1999), which is best characterised as 'a needs-based yet cash-limited system' (Means and Smith 1998: 230).

During the 1980s a Conservative government had sought initially to expand provision within private sector residential care and nursing homes – at the expense of the public sector – by extending the entitlement of elderly and disabled people under the social security system. Means-tested IS could be used to meet the costs of care in private homes. However, the 1990 NHS and Community Care Act was intended to curtail such expenditure, by requiring local authority social services departments to undertake individual needs assessments and then purchase and manage 'packages' of care. Care was to be provided where possible in the service user's own home, and only otherwise in a residential setting. The clear intention was that local authorities should become primarily 'enablers' rather than providers. The greater part of the funding that was transferred from the social security budget to local authorities was to be spent in the private and/or voluntary sectors and local authorities were to be responsible for managing, funding and regulating provision.

The duties placed on local authorities imply that elderly and disabled people have a right to a needs assessment (although such a right in fact had already existed for people registered under the 1970 Chronically Sick and Disabled Persons Act). However, the value of that right may be questioned in at least four ways. First, as I have indicated, the system is cash-limited. If the old professionally dominated systems of provision had had a tendency to be service-led, there is little sense in which the new managerially dominated system is truly needs-led. A right to needs assessment does not give rise to a right to receive care, since local authorities are entitled to set their own eligibility criteria in the light of the resources at their disposal. There is no obligation on authorities to provide or commission services corresponding to the assessed level of need (Ellis 1993) and, in practice, the process of needs assessment rapidly became an exercise in reducing consumer expectations (Lewis and Glennerster 1996). Attempts to enforce an absolute right to have needs met have failed: the House of Lords has ruled that cash-strapped local authorities are entitled to revise their local eligibility criteria and withdraw care provision on financial grounds, even if a previous needs assessment had held such care to be necessary.

Second, needs assessment has been attacked from a user perspective for promoting 'pathology, inadequacy and inability as the basis of who has what services' (Jones, cited in Langan 1998: 170). As Langan (1998: 169) has put it: 'The position of users is that of quasi-customer, exercising sovereignty at second hand through the care manager'. A needs-based system is not necessarily consistent with a rights-based approach unless service users can have a say in what the *outcomes* should be (Balloch *et al.* 1999). Pressure from the user movement played a part in securing provision for direct payments by local authorities (see below), which can give service users a greater measure of independence over the management of their own care, but access to such payments is not a right.

Third, the needs of service users may conflict with the needs of informal carers. A needs assessment that results in a person being cared for in her own home can place unreasonable demands on a spouse or close relative who may be called upon to undertake a key role in providing care. It is possible, however, for informal carers to demand their own needs assessments and the Carers (Recognition and Services) Act of 1995 goes some way to ensuring that carers are supported as well as the people they care for. Conversely, there is a risk that care managers may on occasions privilege the demands of carers at the expense of service users (Balloch *et al.* 1999) and sometimes attention to the 'burdens' shouldered by carers distracts attention from the nature of the relations of power in which elderly and disabled people are enmeshed and the ways in which their rights are compromised (cf. Morris 1993).

Finally, as we shall see in a moment, needs assessments have to be carried out in conjunction with financial assessments or tests of means in order to determine the ability of the client to pay for care. This can stigmatise the process as a whole and deter people from seeking assessment (Davis *et al.* 1998).

Paying for care

While medical and nursing care is free to all and provided by or on behalf of the NHS, social care – including 'personal' care for elderly and disabled people – provided by or commissioned through local authority social services departments may be charged for, subject to means-testing (except in the case of certain aftercare and intermediate care packages that may be funded by the NHS). This is the situation (in England and Wales, but not Scotland) following the government's rejection of the recommendations of the Royal Commission on Long Term Care for the Elderly (1999, and see further discussion in Chapter 10 below). The government has accepted that all nursing care should be free, regardless of the setting in which it is provided, but at the time of writing it is in the process of making changes to the regime under which local authorities charge for social care. When account is taken of the various transitional arrangements that apply, the provisions are frighteningly complex and what follows is a very basic outline. For a detailed account, see, for example, CPAG's *Paying for Care Handbook*.

Elderly and disabled people may receive a variety of home care or domiciliary services; they may receive 'meals-on-wheels' in their own homes, or they may receive meals and other services in local day centres (for which transport may be provided); they may be provided with various aids or equipment for use at home. Home care provision may range from occasional help with housework and shopping to daily assistance with personal care (such as with getting in and out of bed, getting dressed, etc.). The basis on which users are charged for such services varies between local authority areas, but guidance from central government (that is likely to come into effect in 2002) will indicate that users' net income after they have met the authority's charges should not be reduced below basic income support level, with a 'buffer' of 25 per cent. In practice this means that local authorities may absorb in charges the full amount of any disability benefits that the user receives (see Chapter 5 above) and may additionally have regard when setting charges in an individual case to the extent of the user's savings and the resources available from other household members.

Provision also exists for the users of community care services to receive direct payments from a local authority so that they may purchase services themselves. Characteristically, payments are used to employ a carer or helper (although users are not allowed to employ their spouses or close relatives). Although the local authority must monitor any arrangements that are entered into, direct payments give service users a degree of independence and control over the planning and delivery of the services they receive. However, local authorities will not normally make direct payments that exceed the cost they would incur in providing services themselves and, at the time of writing, only some local authorities operate direct payment schemes. The government has taken powers to make provision for direct payments mandatory, but has not at the time of writing exercised that power. In any event, the decision to make direct payments in any particular case is discretionary.

An additional source of discretionary assistance with the costs of care is the Independent Living Fund (ILF). The original ILF, which was discontinued in 1993, was established in 1988 to provide discretionary payments that would enable disabled people to continue living in their own homes. The present ILF, which was set up to replace the original scheme, is similarly a discretionary fund, but is subject to more restrictive guidance. Though provided with a fixed budget by central government, the ILF is independently managed by a Board of Trustees who, working in partnership with local authority social services departments, may make payments towards the care needs of people who are severely disabled but can be cared for at home.

At the time of writing, services charges for the care, support or supervision of 'vulnerable' people in certain kinds of sheltered housing or hostel accommodation can be met from HB (see Chapter 7), but this arrangement will cease in 2003 when funding for this kind of support is to be transferred to local authority housing and social services departments.

People who cannot be cared for at home may be placed by local authorities in nursing homes or, more usually, residential care homes (most of which are now privately run but are subject to registration and inspection by local authorities). There are circumstances in which the care of people placed in nursing homes will be fully funded by the NHS (e.g. patients undergoing rehabilitation or palliative care), but generally, the costs of the social care element of residential home charges (including charges in homes that are still provided by local authorities themselves) will be met by the local authority and may be recovered in whole or in part from the service user.

The extent to which a service user is exempt from charges – or, conversely, of her liability to pay – is determined by way of a financial assessment. The assessment entails a means-test according to a national scheme, elements of which are similar to IS (see Chapter 5). Applicants with capital and savings above a certain limit do not qualify for any assistance and must meet the full amount of the charges (or make private arrangements). The capital limits are slightly higher than for IS but, within three months of being admitted on a permanent basis to a care home, the value of any home that the applicant owns in the community (unless it is still occupied by a spouse or close relative) will be included in the assessment. However, it is possible for service users who do not wish to sell their homes to defer payment of charges and for the local authority to recover payment at a later date. The assessment of income, unlike the IS means-test, takes full account of income from disability benefits like disabled living allowance or attendance allowance which are effectively, therefore, called upon to pay for the service user's care. However, there is provision that, following the assessment and the payment of charges, the service user should retain from her income a small allowance for personal expenses to meet the costs of clothing, toiletries, stationery, gifts, etc. Some local authorities operate a savings account system to help users administer their personal expenses allowances.

Service users have a right to choose the care home to which they are admitted, though the right is in practice limited since the accommodation must be adjudged suitable, and accommodation in the home must be available at a cost that the local authority is prepared to pay. If a service user wishes to enter a home that is more expensive than the local authority would normally pay for, it is possible for a third party (such as a relative) to make top-up payments to meet the additional cost.

At the time of writing, users on IS who have been in residential care since before 1993 can still have their charges met through IS and those who entered residential care subsequently receive an IS residential allowance towards the costs of their care. From 2003, however, virtually all funding for social care will be channelled through local authorities in the hope that they will be able in time to help more people remain in their own homes.

Summary/conclusion

This chapter has examined the ambiguous status of the rights of citizens in Britain within our education, health and social care services. While education and health services are sometimes referred to as the 'bedrock' of the welfare state, not least because they tend to enjoy near universal popular approval (Taylor-Gooby 1995), social care (childcare provision and the personal social services for elderly and disabled people) has often been referred to as the Cinderella of the welfare state since it attracts proportionately less popular support and fewer resources. We have observed, however, that the boundaries between education and health provision on the one hand and social care on the other can be contested and uncertain. We have also observed that substantive social rights across all three services are, perhaps surprisingly, tenuous.

Education is not so much a right for either children or their parents as an obligation, and it is not at all clear that the education system has ever existed to serve the interests of children or their parents. Though parents may enjoy certain limited rights in relation to the choice of schools for their children and to information about schools, they have few, if any, rights in relation to the content of the education their children will receive. Children with special educational needs have a right to have their needs assessed, but not necessarily to command the resources necessary to satisfy those needs. Children whose parents are on low incomes may have access to means-tested forms of financial assistance and to free school meals.

The NHS does guarantee a right of access to health services for all citizens, but not necessarily to any particular treatment. Once again, patients may enjoy certain limited rights in relation to the choice of doctors or hospitals and to information about health facilities, but they have few, if any, rights over the substantive nature of their treatment. Patients with mental health problems enjoy certain specific rights intended to guard their civil liberties. Patients on low incomes may be exempt from certain health service charges or be entitled to means-tested financial assistance in connection with their use of health service facilities.

Childcare provision in Britain is relatively poorly developed and, once again, it is not at all clear in whose interests it is being developed. While a right for older pre-compulsory school-age children to receive early years educational provision is emerging, a right to childcare is not. While low-income parents have a right to means-tested assistance towards the costs of childcare, there is no right of access to such care. Elderly and disabled people now have a right to have their need for personal social services assessed but, once again, they cannot assert a right to any particular level of service. Access to social care provision for elderly and disabled people is means-tested in so far that clients on low incomes may be exempted from direct charges.

Universal rights to education, health and social care are seldom what they seem. We may have rights to have our needs assessed, but not to say how those needs should be met. We may have limited rights to choose from whom we receive a service, but not to determine the nature and extent of that service. What is more, some of our rights may in effect be conditional upon a means-test. We may rely upon the state to educate us, to look after our health and attend to our social care needs, but we cannot in fact assume that we have unequivocal rights to such things.

Chapter 9

Rights of redress

Rights that remain unfulfilled or that are dishonoured do not necessarily cease to *be* in the formal sense, but to exist in a meaningful way rights must be effective. They must either be specifically enforceable, or else it must be possible for people who have been denied their rights to seek some form of redress. This applies as much to welfare rights as to any other kind. We have already seen that welfare or social rights are not the same as legal or civil rights, yet they depend for their definition upon the law-making process. The administrative machinery of a democratic-welfare-capitalist state will generally provide the individual with at least some means of redress if she cannot obtain or enforce those rights. This chapter is concerned with the enforceability of welfare rights and with individual rights of redress, but it will begin by addressing the relationship between welfare and law and the issues that are raised by the legalisation or 'juridification' of welfare. In so far that the legal basis of rights to welfare and the process by which redress may be sought can be highly technical, the chapter will also discuss the means by which people may obtain the expert assistance that may be required in order to exercise a right of redress. Finally, the chapter will address the comparatively limited role the courts may play in the enforcement of welfare rights and the very substantial array of procedures for administrative redress that exist beyond the courts.

The juridification of welfare

For the kinds of discretionary 'relief' that had once been administered to the poor to become welfare 'rights' it was necessary to insinuate a juridical element. The process, which Jowell once called 'legalisation', meant 'subjecting official decisions to the governance of predetermined rules' (1975: 2). This legalisation or 'juridification' or welfare presents what Teubner (1987) has called a 'regulatory trilemma'. His argument is that the law and social administration represent separate 'autopoietic systems', each with its own fundamental integrity and distinctive internal self-regulatory logic. When the law is applied instrumentally to serve social policy, three things can happen: the two systems may prove mutually incongruent; social policy may become over-legalised, so that its fundamental purposes are frustrated; or else the law may become over-socialised, so that its formal integrity is undermined.

Incongruity

The idea that social policy and the law are incongruous is hardly new. Opposition to the idea that the courts should meddle in matters of social administration can be traced back to Chadwick, one of the architects of the 1834 Poor Law. Chadwick was concerned that courts hearing individual pleas out of context would not take account of those 'large classes of cases and general and often remote effects, which cannot be brought to the knowledge of judges' (cited in Cranston 1985: 287). Similarly, throughout the twentieth century the incursion of the courts into the everyday administration of the welfare state was resisted by politicians as diverse as Winston Churchill and Aneurin Bevan. In 1911, Churchill, then a Liberal Home Secretary, expressed doubts about the capacity of the judiciary to handle public policy matters of concern to working-class people, since 'where class issues are involved, it is impossible to pretend that the courts command the same degree of general confidence [as in ordinary criminal and civil matters]' (cited in Cranston 1985: 288). In 1946, Bevan, as Labour's Minister of Health, was equally explicit that social policy reforms should, as far as possible, be insulated from 'judicial sabotage' (*ibid.*: 288–9).

Where they have been afforded a specific jurisdiction the courts have not always coped well. The inability of the county courts to deal with a flood of disputed claims under the Workmen's Compensation Act of 1897 was a factor that contributed to the view that specialist tribunals would provide a more suitable forum for handling the claims of working people (Abel-Smith and Stevens 1967). Not only were alternative adjudicative arrangements devised when unemployment insurance was first introduced in 1911, but also the workmen's compensation scheme was in time removed from the courts with the introduction of the industrial injuries scheme in 1946. At about the same time, the rent control functions of the county courts were entrusted to new tribunals and later, in the 1970s, the creation of the Industrial Tribunal (now the Employment Tribunal – see Chapter 6) also removed from the civil courts the bulk of litigation relating to the interpretation and enforcement of employment protection provisions and the law governing individual contracts of employment. Finally, whereas the lower courts had had a role in securing income maintenance for children, in the 1990s this jurisdiction was largely removed to the Child Support Agency (see Chapter 5), with rights of appeal to a specialised tribunal.

However, the political scepticism that has sought to distance welfare administration from the courts has in no way succeeded in keeping the law out of social policy. We shall see later in this chapter the extent to which alternative fora of redress have often become almost as formal and certainly no less technical in the legal sense. With or without the supervision of the courts, welfare rights are created in law.

Over-legalisation

The development of welfare rights has allowed the law to penetrate the social arena in a quite fundamental sense. Habermas regards juridification as part of the process by which technical welfare systems colonise the 'life world' of the individual subject (see discussion in Tweedie and Hunt 1994). A part of the argument here is that the law is simply an unsuitable instrument for the regulation of social welfare: its formality and rationality may undermine the ordinary patterns of social life and customary processes of social negotiation (e.g. Teubner 1987: 311). The argument can be interpreted in ways that support some of the critiques of welfare rights that are examined in Chapter 4 above. Conservatives may be critical of legally regulated welfare since it undermines the welfare functions of traditionally constituted families and the paternalistic responsibilities of the ruling order, while Fabians may be critical because it constrains the creative expertise of state welfare professionals.

The argument may be taken further than this, however, in so far that legalisation not only bears upon welfare administrators, but upon the objects of their decision making. The individual subject is constituted as an object of decision making, as a juridical entity, a bearer of rights and an observer of rules (see Dean 1991). Entitlements may be calculable rather than arbitrary, but they are also – as we have seen throughout Part II of this book – largely conditional and dependent upon a variety of predetermined factors. The legally arbitrated rules and conditions of the system appear as the correlative duties to the social rights of citizenship. The relationship between the state and the individual becomes, in Garland's words, 'fundamentally depoliticised – referenced in terms of welfare instead of power' (1981: 43). Law is the instrument by which this is achieved.

Habermas's answer to the problem of juridification is to argue for an ideal concept of law as the 'external constitution' or framework within which the uncoerced negotiation of our social relations and welfare needs may take place. Tuebner suggests a similar concept, 'reflexive law', as a medium for the self-regulation of welfare systems. A less idealised version of such arguments is that legal regulation should apply only to procedural matters and not to substantive welfare rights, which are the proper concern of social policy. The latter in essence is the case advanced by contemporary administrative reformers and will be critically discussed in Chapter 11 below.

Over-socialisation

Implicit in many lawyers' concerns about the juridification of welfare is the extent to which it is social policy that is corrupting the purity of the law: the law has been reduced to an overstrained political instrument (Luhmann 1987). Dicey's (1885) classical nineteenth-century legal theory – which still represents the orthodoxy of the legal establishment (see Harden and Lewis 1986) – would reject the very idea that the courts should be beholden to policy, rather than to the law. The guarantee that has supposedly underpinned the British (or English) constitution since the late seventeenth century is 'the rule of law' or, more precisely, 'government under the law'. It is a two-fold guarantee to ensure the protection of the people from any exercise by government of arbitrary power: first, that sovereignty should reside in a representative parliament; second, that the role of the courts should be the preservation of the common law. By this means, governments must, in theory, account to Parliament for the policies they pursue and to the courts for the legality of their actions.

In practice, as some constitutional authorities have long realised and many textbooks on government and politics will argue (e.g. Kingdom 1999), government under the law has become a fiction. The nature of modern party politics and the sheer complexity of modern government are such that, in most circumstances, a prime minister and the cabinet with an electoral mandate can so control the policy making agenda and the processes of administration as to wield almost absolute power. The checks and balances to be provided by Parliament on the one hand and the courts on the other are of strictly limited effect. Much of the machinery of the welfare state has been generated with decision making powers which are far beyond any routine scrutiny or intimate knowledge on the part of either Parliament or, still less, the courts. In fact the problem for all democratic-welfare-capitalist societies is that of how the law, as an autonomous system, could ever develop a constructive role in matters of social policy. Luhmann has argued that:

> law, particularly in its conceptual structures, has not yet adapted to the exigencies of a highly differentiated society. Legal doctrine is still bound to the classical model of law as a body of rules enforceable through adjudication. The legal order lacks a conceptual apparatus adequate for the planning and social policy requirements that arise in the interrelations among specialised social subsystems. (quoted in Harden and Lewis 1986: 34)

The problem is especially acute for the English common law tradition, which has remained 'stuck in a constitutional time warp' (*ibid.*). The argument of constitutionalists and systems theorists is that the development of legal rights in relation to matters in the public sphere of policy and administration has lagged behind the development of legal rights in relation to matters in the private sphere of property and contract. Therefore, while the substantive body of statute law has been harnessed to serve policy objectives, prevailing legal doctrine (not to mention the judiciary), it is argued, are not equipped with any of the principles that might be appropriate to a role in the oversight of social policy.

Access to legal expertise

In the context of these wider issues, how can individual subjects seek to enforce their welfare rights or to secure redress? The individual's right of access to redress and to the advice, assistance and advocacy this might require is itself an issue. Is this a legal right, a social right or, as the National Consumer Council (1977) once claimed, a 'fourth right of citizenship'? The technical character of welfare rights is such that the capacity to seek redress is for many citizens dependent upon the availability of expert help. The rule of law requires that we should all have equal access to redress: mechanisms to ensure this are part and parcel of our legal rights. To the extent that poor or disadvantaged people may have particular kinds of legal problems, it may be argued that they are, or ought to be, entitled to receive publicly provided legal services (see, for example, Royal Commission on Legal Services 1979). At another level, the meeting of legal needs, like the meeting of health needs, is fundamentally necessary to our capacity to function as full citizens: access to legal aid is therefore a social right (T.H. Marshall 1950). There is, however, a further sense in which *all* our rights of citizenship require that we should have information about our entitlements and, if needed, the assistance of experts in order to pursue our remedies. Access to legal expertise has been provided in the past partly through a system of state funded but privately provided legal aid, and partly through the development of independent advice and law centres within a wider welfare rights movement. More recently, these have – after a fashion – been brought together with the creation of the Community Legal Service (CLS).

Legal aid

Prior to the Legal Aid and Advice Act of 1949 such limited concessionary provision as had been made available to poor people by the legal profession had been essentially charitable in nature. Ancient traditions relating to the prosecution of civil proceedings and the 'dock brief' system for the defence of criminal proceedings allowed persons without means to have counsel assigned from among any willing to take on their cases free of charge (Zander 1978). The introduction of a publicly funded legal aid scheme was based on the Rushcliffe Report of 1944 and implemented by the reforming post-war Labour government. In such circumstances, it might be supposed that the scheme would have followed the Beveridgian principle of universal provision. It did not. There was to be no National Legal Service. Though public funding was to be made available, it was to be channelled through a privately organised and self-regulating legal profession and eligibility was to be based on a means-test. It amounted to a system of 'judicare', analogous to 'medicare' in the USA.

The original legal aid scheme was restricted to civil proceedings, but developed over the years that followed until by the 1970s it had incorporated a formal system of criminal legal aid (that is required in any event to comply with human rights obligations) and a scheme for the provision of legal advice and assistance (that came to be known as the 'green form scheme'). Legal aid was not available for all types of court proceedings and civil legal aid was subject not only to a means-test, but also to a merits-test. The merits-test applied both to the legal merits (does the applicant have a good case in law?) and the wider merits of an applicant's case (would a solicitor advise a paying client of modest but sufficient means to run the risk of the litigation contemplated?). Intended to prevent the abuse of public funds, these additional hurdles placed poorer citizens with uncertain or unusual cases, or cases involving small rewards but important principles, at a disadvantage compared with more affluent litigants. The green form scheme enabled lawyers to recover fees up to a modest set limit to advise and assist clients on low incomes on a wide range of matters, including welfare rights. However, the scheme did not allow lawyers to represent clients before tribunals or at administrative hearings.

During the 1980s and 1990s Conservative governments had sought to curtail the spiralling costs of legal aid by reducing the financial eligibility limits, thus reducing the number of people who could qualify for assistance; they began to reduce the scope of civil legal aid, by providing that certain classes of action – such as personal injuries cases – should in future be undertaken by lawyers on a conditional fee basis (i.e. 'no win-no fee'), underwritten where necessary by private insurance arrangements; and they began to change the system by which individual legal firms could be remunerated for work carried out under the scheme by introducing a system of 'franchising' (Blake 2000).

The right to legal aid has always been a qualified right. Cranston has suggested that it is as a consequence of the charitable origins of legal aid that the right to it had been so slow to develop (1985: 89). It is perhaps ironic that the other ways in which attempts have been made to advance the achievement of the 'fourth right of citizenship' should have involved new forms of charitable endeavour. Charitable status is the common thread that has underpinned the development of independent advice and law centres and of the major pressure groups that comprise the 'poverty lobby'.

The welfare rights movement

The 1960s and 1970s in Britain witnessed the birth of a radical new enthusiasm for 'rights'. This was fuelled to an extent by the civil rights movement in the USA, by the popularisation of new ideas about community action (exemplified in the works of Alinsky 1969 and Friere 1972) and the pioneering approach of American neighbourhood law firms first sponsored under the US Economic Opportunity Act of 1964.

New proactively oriented grant-aided advice centres sprang up in inner-city areas as part of a wider growth in community development initiatives. The British law centre movement was founded with a mission to use the law to tackle the structural causes of poor people's disadvantage (see Cooper 1983). A new breed of national charities, including Child Poverty Action Group, Shelter, Low Pay Unit, Disablement Income Group, National Council for One Parent Families, emerged not with a traditional emphasis upon fund-raising and voluntary service, but with a view to campaigning on policy issues and for the rights of disadvantaged groups (Whiteley and Winyard 1983). Local authorities sometimes sought to develop welfare, housing and consumer advice centres of their own, but the nature and scope of these has always been variable and, in so far that local government has its own responsibilities as a welfare provider, such agencies can never be regarded as independent.

The defining character of the new movement was its independence. It was their independent status that enabled advice and law centres (most of which were registered as charities) and the charitable national pressure groups to work for or on behalf of whole groups of clients as well as individuals and, for example, to take up or support individual test-cases in the area of welfare rights. The 'test-case strategy' (see Prosser 1983) became a major weapon in the armoury of welfare lawyers and the poverty lobby. The cases of individual social security claimants, homeless people or council tenants were taken before the higher courts with a view to establishing more general points of principle by which to clarify or develop the law or to force changes in policy. I shall return to discuss the role of rights-based reformism in Chapter 11. However, the contribution that independent advice and law centres could make in terms of helping individuals to achieve their welfare rights was always limited.

Citizens Advice Bureaux (CABx) had provided a national network of advice bureaux since the Second World War (and therefore pre-dated the movement of the 1960s and 1970s), but these were staffed almost entirely by volunteer advisers and were able to fulfil a quite restricted information-giving role. They have since become a part of the wider welfare rights movement, and in certain locations they now employ full-time staff (including lawyers) and provide expert assistance and advocacy services, but most of the 2,000 or so bureaux are still primarily staffed by volunteers. The new generation of independent advice centres, whose numbers have fluctuated over time (there are at the time of writing just over 900 in membership of the Federation of Independent Advice Centres) are often very small, few (about 80) employ lawyers, and they tend to be concentrated in particular urban locations. The number of law centres – whose impact is acknowledged to have been 'out of all proportion to their size' (Royal Commission on Legal Services 1979) – is even smaller: at the height of their development there were only 62 such centres, but at the time of writing this has declined to just 51. The independent advice and law centre movement has been dependent on a patchwork of funding arrangements entailing a precarious mixture of local authority and charitable grants, legal aid funding and, more recently, National Lottery funds. However, where people do have access to independent advice and law centres, there is evidence to suggest that they find them more approachable and effective than private legal firms (McAteer 2000).

The Community Legal Service

A major reform introduced in 2000 by the New Labour government has, on the one hand, qualified the scope of legal aid and, on the other, formally recast key elements of the welfare rights movement as not-for-profit legal service providers.

Responsibility for legal aid passed from the Legal Aid Board to the Legal Services Commission under whose aegis the Criminal Defence Service has assumed responsibility for criminal legal aid and the CLS, through its Regional Legal Service Committees, administers a reformed version of civil legal aid and the 'legal help' scheme (a revised version of the 'green form' scheme). It has been argued that the overriding purpose of the reforms was to contain legal aid expenditure rather than to harness the potential of community-based legal services to New Labour's social inclusion agenda (Stein 2001). While criminal legal aid expenditure is still demand led, because there is an overriding obligation to guarantee legal representation for citizens charged with serious crimes, the overall legal aid budget is now capped, so that expenditure on civil legal aid is constrained. Most civil legal aid and 'legal help' work is now undertaken under block contracts by a mixture of specially franchised private law firms and not-for-profit legal services providers (including law centres and some of the more specialised advice centres). CLS providers are required to achieve a 'quality mark', by demonstrating that they meet certain minimum standards, and they contract to undertake a fixed volume of work, usually within clearly defined legal specialisms. Lower levels of quality mark (but not funding) are also awarded by the CLS to basic information points (in libraries and hospitals, for example) and general help agencies that may together provide co-ordinated local referral networks to complement the specialist legal providers. Specialist providers can now obtain funding for certain kinds of public interest and high-cost cases and, for example, for immigration appeals, but most money-based claims are now excluded (and must be pursued on a conditional fee basis), while other cases are still subject to a discretionary merits-test (see above). In addition to these rationing devices, access to funded legal services continues to be subject to a means-test.

The CLS is 'decidedly not a national legal service' (Blake 2000: 221). None the less, in an attempt to ensure that it is responsive to local needs, local CLS partnerships – involving CLS providers, local authorities and community representatives – have been given a role in the planning of provision. The government claims that by 2002 at least 90 per cent of people in England and Wales will have the benefits of a CLS partnership in their area (LCD 2000). Even if this were achieved, it would not ensure universal availability. Participation by private legal firms is now restricted to a smaller number of practitioners than under the old legal aid scheme. Local authorities, which have played a major role in funding not-for-profit advice and law centres in the past and who now participate in CLS partnerships, are under no obligation to contribute to the funding of independent advice and law centres: constraints on local government spending mean it is difficult for them to do so and many have recently cut back their funding (Stein 2001). The right to civil legal aid is now more restricted and, because of budget limits, less certain than in the past. At the same time, as parts of the welfare rights movement are drawn in to contractual arrangements and subject to quality controls by the CLS, there is a danger that the independence that has characterised the movement may be compromised and that its proactive potential will be diluted (see, for example, Patterson 2001).

The role of the courts

I have already indicated that policy makers have often sought to deny or to minimise the role of the courts in relation to welfare rights. In so far that the courts do none the less have a role to play, it is important to understand the basis of the court system, the distinctive nature of the English legal tradition, and the different circumstances in which the courts have either refrained from intervention or else have actively sought it.

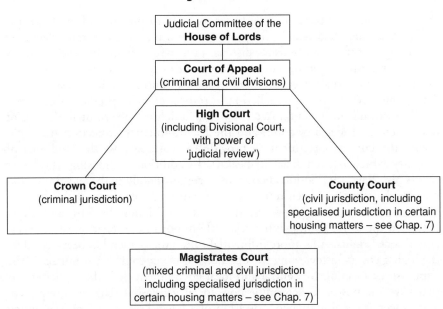

Figure 9.1   Court hierarchy of the English legal system

The system

There are, broadly speaking, three ways in which the courts may be drawn into the arena of welfare rights. First, in a general sense, the courts have a constitutional responsibility as the final arbiters of how social legislation should be interpreted. Second, the courts are responsible for ensuring the 'legality' of the executive's administrative actions. The inherent prerogative or supervisory jurisdiction of the *higher* courts therefore enables them to intervene to review the decisions or actions of government ministers or welfare administrators. More recently, the courts have also been able under the Human Rights Act of 1998 to consider whether legislation is consistent with the provisions of the European Convention on Human Rights, although – unlike courts in the USA – they do not have power to strike down primary legislation. Third, certain of the *lower* courts may have a specific jurisdiction conferred upon them by legislation that gives them either a direct or an incidental function in relation to welfare rights.

The hierarchical nature of the court system – see Figure 9.1 – is such that lower courts are bound by precedents decided in higher courts, and appeals against decisions in lower courts are heard in the higher courts. For a fuller account readers are referred to one of the many textbooks on the English legal system (e.g. Slapper and Kelly 1999).

In spite of the tendency in the field of social welfare to create specialised tribunals to deal with justiciable issues where these arise, the ordinary courts cannot avoid the affairs of poor and working-class people in such areas as landlord and tenant law, which has been a concern of social policy. County courts are routinely concerned with claims by both private and public sector landlords against their tenants for possession, but may also entertain claims by tenants against their landlords for disrepair, unlawful eviction or other breaches of covenant. Since 1996 the county court has also dealt with appeals on points of law against internal review decisions by local authorities in homelessness cases. The magistrates court has jurisdiction in respect of such specific legislation as the Protection from Eviction Act 1977 (which defines the criminal offences of harassment and illegal eviction) and the Environmental Protection Act 1990 (being the current enactment to provide remedies against the landlords of property which is prejudicial to health). In addition to housing, the lower courts also have specific jurisdiction over certain family and child protection matters that have not been touched upon within the confines of this book.

It remains the case, however, that social legislation has, by and large, entrusted the lower courts with a relatively minor role in relation to the exercise of social rights. A far more influential role is that which has been seized by the higher courts in reviewing the decisions of lower courts or tribunals or the administrative actions of central and local government. It is the higher courts that have the power to determine how social legislation shall be interpreted. The power arises either when a decision of a lower judicial forum is appealed against or upon an application for judicial review. Judicial review is the legal remedy by which judges may ensure that the powers exercised by public authorities are kept within legal bounds.

The English tradition

The court systems of modern welfare states have generally developed as part of a process by which state power has grown and become centralised. In place of the ad hoc assemblies of mediaeval times, at which disputes were resolved in accordance with local custom by the sovereign or his local representative, there have emerged uniform and centrally regulated institutions for the dispensation of justice. The precise manner in which this has occurred has differed between countries but we are concerned here with the role of the English (and Welsh) courts. However, there is an important preliminary point to be made about what distinguishes the basic tenets of English law (which have been adopted in other English-speaking countries of the world) from that of Roman or 'Continental' law (characteristic of other Western European nations). The classical sociologist Max Weber remained puzzled by the inherent irrationality of English law, compared with its Continental counterpart. For Weber, the adherence of English law to adversarial procedures and a common law tradition (rather than inquisitorial procedures and codification) was inconsistent with the degree of predictability required to underpin the economic calculus of free-market capitalism (see, for example, Hunt 1978).

The adversarial procedure that characterises English law is descended from the ancient practice of trial by combat. Though combat now takes place by way of formalised verbal argument, the judge is not required to enter the contest between the disputing parties, merely to enforce the rules of combat and determine who has won. It is a procedure that, without substantial safe-guards, will tend inevitably to disadvantage weaker parties at the expense of the powerful. Adversarial procedure constrains the nature of judicial interven-tion in procedural matters. On the other hand, the common law tradition affords great flexibility to judges in matters of legal interpretation and gives them power in effect to create law. The common law is so called because it imposed itself in place of a variety of local customs: it is none the less a form of law determined not by any code or statute, but which is built up over time by *judicial* custom. Judges are required to make decisions not by following any central logical precepts, but on the basis of precedents established in earlier judgments. The effect of this, it has been argued, is that it enables the courts 'to hide behind a screen of verbal formulae of apparent logically formal rationality, those considerations of substantive rationality, that is, of social policy, by which the decision has been actually motivated but which judges are reluct-ant to reveal to the public and, often enough, to themselves' (Rheinstein, cited in Hunt 1978: 124).

Under the English legal tradition, the courts have lacked procedural power to protect the weak, while simultaneously possessing the legal power to advance a very particular social policy agenda. Griffiths (1991) has argued that the English judiciary is influenced by its own perception of what constitutes 'the public interest'. According to Griffiths, the supposed neutrality of the judiciary is not only put into question by the outcome of certain celebrated 'political' cases, but has never been anything more than a myth. His assertion is:

> that judges in the United Kingdom cannot be politically neutral because they are placed in positions where they are required to make political choices which are sometimes presented to them, and often presented by them, as determinations of where the public interest lies; that their interpretation of what is in the public interest and therefore politically desirable is determined by the kind of people they are and the position they hold in our society; that this position is a part of estab-lished authority and so is necessarily conservative and illiberal. From all this flows the view of the public interest which is shown in judicial attitudes such as tender-ness towards private property and dislike of trade unions, strong adherence to the maintenance of order, distaste for minority opinions, demonstrations and protests, indifference to the promotion of race relations, support of governmental secrecy, concern for the preservation of the moral and social behaviour to which it is accustomed . . . (1991: 319)

The social background of judges (predominantly white, male and upper or upper-middle class), their education (predominantly independent school and Oxford or Cambridge University), their training (based conventionally on a long and successful career as a barrister) and the method of their appointment (effected upon the advice or recommendation of the Lord Chancellor) inclines them towards 'a strikingly homogeneous collection of attitudes, beliefs and principles, which to them represents the public interest' (*ibid.*: 275). Recent attempts have been made to broaden the social spectrum from which judges are drawn, but this by itself does little to blunt Griffiths's underlying point which is that senior judges, in particular, are part of a small establishment elite that represents authority within, he claims, an essentially and increasingly authoritarian society. Historically their role has been to defend property rights and the stability of the existing order. To the extent that they are also charged with the defence of the individual against the power of the state, it is only exceptionally and in quite particular circumstances that they have been prepared to challenge the authority of the government of the day.

In drawing attention to the inherently conservative nature of the judges, Griffiths does not imply that the judiciary as an institution is in any way passive. On the contrary, judicial creativity is essential to the political function of the courts in the maintenance of social order. In charting the application of such creativity in a number of controversial cases – especially in the spheres of industrial relations, public order, property rights and 'race' and immigration – Griffiths bolsters his case that, while the neutrality of the courts is a myth, their power is real.

Judicial intervention

The essence of judicial power is that judges have discretion either to intervene or to refrain from intervention. In the case of the social security system, not only had the administration of social security been effectively insulated from the interference of the courts, but the courts were for many years largely insulated from all acquaintance with social security. However, the emergence of the welfare rights movement in the 1970s resulted in a number of cases being forced before the courts (see Prosser 1983). The resulting decisions were inconsistent, but tended to fall into one of two categories: those by which the courts sought to avoid involvement and to leave matters to the 'common sense' of tribunals and administrators; and those in which the courts felt obliged to displace policy-directed decision making with the individualistic logic of liberal jurisprudence. The clearest examples of the former approach related to cases involving litigants such as students and young unemployed people, while perhaps the clearest examples of the latter related to cases involving elderly and disabled people. Arguably, the courts were prepared to give closer attention to 'deserving' than to the 'undeserving' poor. In one case the court went so far as to say that, because the social assistance scheme of the day was supposed to be administered with as little technicality as possible, the court should hesitate to interfere with a tribunal's decision even if it was legally erroneous. When, in contrast, the court elected to intervene, it sought to apply the principle of administrative law that requires that discretion must be exercised with regard to the merits of an individual case and not fettered by the adoption of a rigid policy.

Where decisions in favour of claimants were made, this generally resulted in hasty legislative changes to nullify the effect. Eventually, a wholesale reform of the social assistance scheme translated established administrative practices into statute and a mass of detailed regulations (Walker 1993), the implementation of which would be less vulnerable to judicial criticism. The courts unwittingly helped pressure the government into having Parliament squeeze nearly all elements of discretion out of the scheme (so setting the scene for the introduction of even greater rigidity at a later stage – see Chapters 5 and 6 above). Since the 1970s a right of appeal in respect of decisions affecting social security benefits has lain from the Social Security Commissioners directly to the Court of Appeal, though the volume of litigation has been small and the Court of Appeal has remained, by and large, content to bow to the expertise of the Commissioners. There have been exceptional cases in which the court has ruled that regulations made by the Secretary of State are *ultra vires* (i.e. that the Secretary of State had exceeded the powers conferred by Parliament), but they have been few. Above the Court of Appeal, the House of Lords has generally proved itself 'unwilling to probe deeply into the subtleties of social security law' (Ogus and Barendt 1988: 587).

A more direct influence on British social security policy has been the European Court of Justice (ECJ). There have been two instances in which rulings of the ECJ have forced Britain to make legislative changes. Both have arisen as a result of EU equal treatment directives (see Baldwin-Edwards and Gough 1991). The first was in 1985 when a case was successfully brought against the British government, claiming that the British invalid care allowance (ICA) scheme unlawfully discriminated against married women since it excluded them from benefit upon the assumption that they would in any event have been available to care for a disabled spouse in a way which men would not. As a result, ICA was subsequently extended to working-age married women. The second instance relates to ECJ judgements which compelled Britain to amend the state regulation of occupational pension schemes so as to ensure that men and women retiring or being made redundant at any given age shall receive parity of treatment; and which more recently resulted in moves to equalise the state pension age for men and women.

In the field of housing policy, involving as it does matters of property, the domestic courts have had a rather more substantial role. In some instances, legislation has necessarily impinged upon the rights of property owners and landlords. This has applied, first, in the case of public health and regulatory planning legislation by which local authorities may require the improvement or even the wholesale clearance of property and, second, in the case of legislation that creates rights for tenants against their landlords in respect of security of tenure, rent levels and repairs. Both kinds of legislation have generated conflicts to be resolved in the courts. There are other instances in which social legislation has imposed duties on public authorities with regard to the provision of housing; duties which individuals have attempted to enforce through the courts. A thorough exposition of the history of judicial intervention in such matters is beyond the scope of this chapter. However, the overall tendency in judicial decision making has been to side with property owners against local authorities and tenants, but with the local authorities against, for example, the 'undeserving homeless' (see Cranston 1985; Griffiths 1991). This is not to say that there have not been some important judicial rulings whose effects have served to advance welfare rights, but that the net impact of the courts' role has inclined towards the restraint rather than the development of housing policy.

The courts' insistence upon strict interpretation and enforcement of procedural safeguards for property owners has on occasions inhibited the implementation of local planning decisions, although in eviction proceedings, for example, the courts could at times be quite permissive in overlooking procedural safeguards for those homeless people who had resorted to squatting. The courts were often sympathetic to the legal manoeuvres by which private landlords sought to evade the Rent Acts, but they have generally been unsympathetic towards litigants who have sought to force local authorities to incur public expenditure upon the maintenance of public infrastructure. The courts have on occasions been critical of capricious decision making by local authorities, but they have, by and large, been supportive of local authorities seeking to resist the demands of homeless people upon the public housing stock and have failed to use their power to support a fundamental right to shelter.

Similarly, in the arena of health and social care we have seen in Chapter 8 that the courts have ruled that, although citizens may have rights of access to medical treatment and the assessment of their needs, they do not have an automatic claim upon the resources of health and social services authorities in order to obtain particular forms of treatment or care. Critics have claimed that where the judges have had the opportunity to review the substance of policy they have, for the most part, 'treated the idea of policy in the most crude fashion' (Harden and Lewis 1986: 207). They have failed to make some fundamental distinctions, for example, between the values which inform policy, the specific objectives to be served by a policy, and the measures required to implement that policy. More optimistic advocates of public interest law and of policy advocacy before the courts, such as Harlow and Rawlings (1992), suggest that lately there have none the less been significant shifts in judicial thinking. Additionally, some would argue that the Human Rights Act now provides an opportunity for the judiciary to have an enhanced role in advancing social, and not just legal, justice (Stein 2001).

Administrative redress

More important than the courts – certainly in terms of their day-to-day impact – is the bewildering array of 'administrative' mechanisms or procedures by which welfare rights are, or might potentially be, protected or advanced. By convention the mechanisms in question are distinguished from the 'legal' or 'judicial' procedures that are provided by the courts. They include *tribunals* that can be clearly 'quasi-judicial' in character; *ombudspersons* who, like the courts, are constitutionally independent; *complaints* procedures that are constituted as adjuncts to the administrative machinery; and *reviews* that are in fact internal to the administrative process. It would not here be possible to outline in detail the jurisdiction and function of every forum that exists for the redress of grievances in relation to state-governed welfare provision, but Table 9.1 provides a simple summary.

In classifying the jurisdictions of the various fora in Table 9.1, it may be noted that – except in the case of bodies having a more general statutory

Table 9.1   Principal statutory fora for administrative redress

Forum	Jurisdiction
Social Security	
The Appeals Service (TAS) tribunal (there is a further right of appeal from a TAS tribunal to the Social Security Commissioner)	appeals from decisions relating to most social security benefits (including housing benefit and council tax benefit and *mandatory* social fund payments) and determinations by the Child Support Agency
Tax Appeal Commissioner	appeals from decisions relating to the payment of national insurance contributions
Social Fund Inspector	reviews of decisions relating to the *discretionary* social fund
Parliamentary Commissioner for Administration	petitionary complaints about maladministration by a central government department or agency
Local Commissioner for Administration	petitionary complaints about maladministration by a local authority
Department of Work and Pensions and Inland Revenue complaints procedures	personal complaints about standards of conduct or administration
Employment	
Employment Tribunal	statutory jurisdiction in relation to disputes between employees and employers
Tax Appeal Commissioner	appeals from decisions relating to statutory sick pay and statutory maternity pay
Housing	
Rent Assessment Committee	statutory jurisdiction in relation to private sector rents
Local authority internal homelessness reviews	reviews of decisions relating to applications by homeless persons
Local Commissioner for Administration	petitionary complaints about maladministration by a local authority
Education	
Governing body and/or local education authority complaints procedures	personal complaints in relation to curriculum matters
Admission Appeal Panels	appeals from decisions by governing bodies or local education authorities in relation to school admissions
Exclusion Appeal Panels	appeals from decisions by governing bodies in relation to the exclusion of a pupil from school
Special Educational Needs Tribunal (SENT)	appeals from decisions relating to statements of special educational need
Local Commissioner for Administration	petitionary complaints about maladministration by a local authority

Table 9.1   *(continued)*

Forum	Jurisdiction
Health	
NHS complaints procedure (a two-stage procedure culminating in an independent review panel)	personal complaints in relation to health care treatment and/or conduct of NHS staff Note: there is also a special procedure for the review of decisions in relation to the discharge of patients from hospital
Mental Health Tribunal	statutory jurisdiction in relation to the use of compulsory powers to treat or detain people with mental health problems
Health Service Commissioner	petitionary complaints about maladministration by health authorities and/or NHS providers
Social care	
Social services complaints procedure (a three-stage procedure culminating in an independent review panel)	personal complaints in relation to the provision made or commissioned by local authority social services departments
Local Commissioner for Administration	petitionary complaints about maladministration by a local authority

Notes: This excludes (1) voluntary or extra-statutory complaints or review procedures such as those provided by many local authorities; (2) instances where a right of appeal may lie directly to the relevant Secretary of State; and (3) mechanisms of judicial redress available through the courts.

jurisdiction – I distinguish between 'appeals', 'petitionary complaints', 'personal complaints' and 'reviews'. Very broadly speaking, these are the kinds of jurisdiction that are appropriate respectively to tribunals, ombudspersons, complaints procedures and internal reviews, but – as will emerge shortly – these classifications do not always fit with the titles and official descriptions of the fora concerned. To make sense of the different forms of administrative redress it is necessary to go behind the way these various fora are described and address the assumptions upon which they are based. In Chapter 1 I drew a distinction between the doctrinal and the claims-based conceptions of rights. Redress within the doctrinal conception of rights may take different forms, depending on the focus. If the focus of redress is upon the obligations of the state then redress will take on the form of an appeal and the appellant is constituted as a juridical subject exercising rights against the welfare state; but if the focus is upon the demands of the individual then redress will take on the form of a personal complaint and the complainant is constituted as a 'heroic consumer' (cf. Warde 1994; Bauman 1998) demanding effective welfare services. Similarly, redress within the claims-based conception of rights may take different forms. If the focus of redress is upon the obligations of the state then redress will take on the form of a petitionary complaint and the complainant is constituted as an angry

Table 9.2 Forms of redress: a model

Conception of rights	Focus of redress	Form of redress	Implied status of the individual
doctrinal	the state's obligation	appeal	juridical subject
	the individual's demands	personal complaint	heroic consumer
claims based	the state's obligation	petitionary complaint	angry (active participating) citizen
	the individual's demands	review	passive client

citizen who actively seeks to expose the shortcomings of the welfare state; but if the focus is upon the demands of the individual then redress will take on the form of a review and the supplicant is constituted as a passive client beseeching that her case be looked at again. This model, which is represented diagram-matically in Table 9.2, will help to guide us through the account that follows.

Tribunals

Tribunals provide the classic forum for appeals. Bodies that function as tribunals, such as the Tax Commissioners, had existed since before the modern welfare state. Although many tribunals have nothing to do with social policy, the development of the welfare state has represented the biggest single factor in the emergence of tribunals (Wraith and Hutchinson 1973). The first tribunal with a welfare rights jurisdiction was established in 1911 with the creation of the Court of Referees: a three-member independent tribunal, chaired by a lawyer, which dealt with disputes arising under the unemployment benefit scheme. The arrangement was a concession to offset the possibility of working-class resistance to the idea of compulsory national insurance contributions (see Dean 1991: ch. 5). A similar political motive was evident in the creation in 1934 of a rather different tribunal, the Unemployment Appeal Tribunal, whose existence ministers hoped might deflect popular resentment against an unpopular means-test (Lynes 1975). This tribunal did not have lawyers as chairpersons and one of its members was a direct nominee of the government agency whose decisions the tribunal was supposed 'independently' to review: in effect, therefore, it was a review body, rather than an appeal tribunal. These two tribunals evolved over time, one dealing with insurance-based benefits, the other with social assistance benefits. Eventually, they merged to become the Social Security Appeal Tribunal and more recently they have been ab-sorbed into The Appeals Service (TAS), a streamlined appeals process that has also absorbed such fora as the Medical Appeal Tribunal, the Child Support Tribunal and Housing Benefit Review Panels. (It should, incidentally, be noted that a process of internal review will usually precede an appeal to TAS.)

It has been observed that 'once an administrative tribunal is set up, it appears to give such satisfaction that it is never replaced by the ordinary courts' (Street 1975: 10). Certainly, policy makers, especially after the Second World War, began to see tribunals as a satisfactory way of handling disputes in many areas of public administration. Tribunals were created under the Rent Acts (though, following deregulation of the private rented sector, the Rent Assessment Committee is the only surviving vestige of that system). As we have seen, tribunals were instituted to handle employment disputes, and specialist tribunals have been created with jurisdiction relating to such matters as mental health and special educational needs. Certain 'panels', such as those that deal with appeals against decisions in relation to school admission or exclusion decisions, are sometimes regarded as tribunals, although once again these are in some respects more like review bodies.

When tribunals first began to proliferate, concern that politicians and officials might be relying on them too much led to the commissioning of the Franks Report (1957). Franks endorsed the role of tribunals, and made clear that they were to be regarded as 'the machinery provided by parliament for adjudication rather than as part of the machinery of administration'. Franks none the less expressed the advantages of tribunals over courts, namely their greater 'cheapness, accessibility, freedom from technicality, expedition and expert knowledge' (1957: para. 38). In his recommendations he laid down three fundamental principles for tribunals: 'openness, fairness and impartiality' (*ibid.*: para. 41).

The Franks Report marked not only the acceptance of tribunals as *adjudicative* fora, but also the beginning of a process by which tribunals became increasingly judicial in character (Dean 1991: ch. 5). Properly constituted tribunals are characteristically chaired by qualified lawyers and other lay members are selected for their independence of any relevant administrative authority and will characteristically have some appropriately specialised expertise or experience. Tribunals specialise in areas of law which are policy-relevant and may therefore be more 'policy conscious' than the judiciary, but the idea that tribunals administer policy while only courts administer law is, according to Abel-Smith and Stevens, a myth: 'Properly understood, tribunals are a more modern form of court' (1968: 228).

The ideal implied by the Franks principles is that tribunals provide a form of justice that is more informal and accessible but no less rigorous than other courts. But does this render tribunals a more appropriate forum for the realisation of welfare rights, which may reflect collective as much as individual objectives? Large numbers of social security or school admissions appeals, for example,

> may be good for individual justice but they may have the consequence of promoting individualistic values to get a larger share of what is being provided at public expense. They encourage selfishness. The consequence may be an overall reduction in what is being provided collectively, a diminution in efficiency and no means to ensure that the same problems are not repeated. (Lewis and Birkinshaw 1993: 90)

A judicial approach, even when adopted by a specialist tribunal, can as easily undermine social rights as advance them, a point to which I shall return in Chapter 11. Though no less judicial in their approach to decision making, tribunals are less formal than courts, if only in matters of procedure. Research commissioned by the Lord Chancellor's office (Genn and Genn 1989) has demonstrated that the varying degrees of informality that tribunals exhibit (as to seating arrangements, forms of address, order of proceedings, rules of evidence, etc.) may be quite superficial. In every case, the complexity of the law that the various tribunals had to apply proved such as to necessitate the injection of a considerable degree of technicality and formality into the conduct of hearings. Genn and Genn point to a fundamental conflict between the requirements of openness, fairness and impartiality on the one hand, and the desire for cheapness, expedition, informality and freedom from technicality on the other.

The model that tribunals tend to adopt is that of the English legal system and, though some claim to subscribe to an inquisitorial rather than an adversarial style, this is not necessarily reflected in the perceptions of the participants. Tribunals such as the Employment Tribunal, because they resolve disputes between employees and employers, are *explicitly* adversarial. Other tribunals resolve disputes between citizens and state administrators and, though some of these publicly proclaim their inquisitorial nature, there is perhaps a danger that instead of tribunals presiding over an unequal adversarial contest between a trained departmental official and an unrepresented social security claimant there will be substituted an accusatorial inquisition by the tribunal itself (cf. Ganz 1974). This author's own research (see Dean 1991: ch. 6) has suggested that there is an unresolved tension between the adversarial tradition and the inquisitorial aspirations of the tribunals. The tribunal is seldom 'informal' but tends to adapt its formal nature, depending on the circumstances, so as to 'manage' the appellant and her appeal.

If tribunals therefore offer little advantage over the ordinary courts by way of informality, what of their supposed advantages in terms of cheapness and speed? From the appellant's point of view, tribunals may be cheap because, usually, no fees are charged upon the issue of proceedings and, generally, unsuccessful litigants cannot be held liable for costs (there are exceptions). None the less, if an appellant requires representation then, as we have seen, legal aid is seldom available. Unless an appellant has access to an advice agency, law centre or trade union able to represent free of charge, the cost of representation may be prohibitive. From the government's point of view, the cheapness of the tribunal system lies partly in the use that is made of tribunal members who are, for the most part, part-time unpaid volunteers, but more particularly because of the absence of legal aid. This is in spite of a considerable body of evidence that demonstrates that representation undoubtedly increases an appellant's chances of success. As for speed, largely because tribunal proceedings have become so complex, they have been hardly better than other courts in combating delay (see Genn and Genn 1989).

Ombudspersons

Ombudspersons provide the classic forum for the petitionary complaint. The 'ombudsman' concept has its origins in Scandinavia and dates back some two centuries (see, for example, Stacey 1978). The Scandinavian states differ in several respects from Britain (see Chapter 3). In particular, their traditions of government were, and are, less dependent upon the concentration of administrative power that characterises the Westminster model. The distinctive idea of an independent and universally accessible citizen's champion has spread around the world and been adapted to provide mechanisms of redress within a variety of quite different jurisdictions. Britain's interest in the idea dates from the 1960s.

Three main statutory ombudsperson schemes have been established: the Parliamentary Commissioner for Administration (PCA); the Commissioners for Local Administration (CLA) or local ombudspersons (consisting of a body of commissioners for England and Wales and a separate commissioner for Scotland); and the Health Service Commissioner (HSC). There is a separate Commissioner for Complaints for Northern Ireland. There is also a number of private or voluntary ombudsperson or arbitration schemes – for example, the Insurance Ombudsman and an experimental Independent Housing Ombudsman for private landlords – and some local authorities have established a voluntary ombudsperson (or complaints executive officer) scheme as part of their internal complaints procedures, but these non-statutory schemes will not be considered here. (Nor are we concerned with the role of the Parliamentary Commissioner for Standards who, though she is called an 'ombudsman', is not to be confused with the PCA).

Classical ombudspersons enjoy independent investigatory powers and, in theory, may 'dig where the courts and tribunals cannot trespass' (Lewis and Birkinshaw 1993: 78). While the proceedings of courts and tribunals are primarily adversarial, those of an ombudsperson are truly inquisitorial. In the Nordic tradition, ombudspersons are allowed to point up systemic weaknesses in policy and administration and to propose improvements. However, the statutory ombudsperson schemes introduced in Britain are significantly compromised versions of the Nordic ideal. The PCA is empowered to investigate complaints where personal injustice is alleged to have been suffered by an individual as a result of 'maladministration' on the part of a central government department. The jurisdiction of the PCA has been extended to include the government's executive agencies and certain 'quangos'. Complaints against health authorities and NHS Trusts are dealt with separately by the HSC. Since 1994 the PCA (and the HSC) have also had power to consider complaints under the Code of Practice on Access to Government Information (provisions which are soon to be superseded by new Freedom of Information legislation). The power of the PCA, when compared with that of ombudspersons in several other countries, is fettered in two ways: first, by the way the PCA has been made an adjunct to Parliament; second, by the restrictive notion of 'maladministration'.

Citizens may not complain directly to the PCA but must first complain to their Member of Parliament who may, at her discretion, refer the complaint for investigation by the PCA. This 'sifting mechanism' is defended on the basis that 'In effect, every individual MP is himself an Ombudsman and deals in his elected capacity with many complaints without having to seek recourse to the PCA' (Select Committee on the PCA 1987–8: para. 9). The PCA is thus portrayed as a way of assisting MPs who may lack the time and resources to pursue enquiries on behalf of their constituents. The inability of citizens to approach the PCA directly is widely perceived as a 'weakness' (Stacey 1978: 170). The PCA reports on individual investigations to the sponsoring MP and the department or agency investigated. Where maladministration leading to injustice is found to have occurred, the PCA may recommend a remedy, including *ex gratia* compensation to the person aggrieved and/or changes in administrative procedures. Where such recommendations are not acted upon, the PCA may lay specific reports before Parliament. The PCA also makes general periodical reports to Parliament and is supported in her work by the Select Committee on the PCA. There is no legal sanction by which government departments or agencies may be compelled to respond in compliance with the PCA's findings. Ultimately, the only sanction is beyond the control of the PCA and lies within the vagaries of the political process.

The other related weakness of Britain's PCA is that her brief has been restricted so as to exclude matters of policy (which are for Parliament) and law (which are for courts and tribunals) and to concentrate on 'maladministration'. Maladministration has no statutory definition and the only definition to be offered during the passage of the relevant legislation came from the minister responsible who cited the examples of 'bias, neglect, inattention, delay, incompetence, ineptitude, perversity, turpitude, arbitrariness' (*Hansard*, vol. 734, col. 51, 18 October 1966). Any of such failings might seriously obstruct the exercise of social rights, but they are failings of procedure, not policy.

In the 1970s the ombudsperson concept was extended from central to local government with the creation of the LCAs. The local commissioners' terms of reference were modelled directly on those of the PCA. They were restricted to investigating allegations of personal injustice occasioned by maladministration on the part of local authorities and, initially, such complaints could only be referred by elected members of the local authorities concerned. Since 1988, however, citizens have been able to complain directly to local commissioners. LCAs have gone further than the PCA in publicising their existence and promoting their function. They have also been quite imaginative in their approach by, for example, investigating group complaints; in one instance, by parents aggrieved by their local authority's schools admission procedures and, in another, by a group of local advice agencies who advanced a complaint based on their clients' shared experiences of their local authority's homeless persons' unit. LCAs have been able, for example, to draw attention to deficient administrative standards and practices in local authority Housing Benefit offices. Though LCAs have arguably done rather more than the PCA to interpret their brief, they have also experienced more difficulty in enforcing their recommendations. LCAs report the findings of their investigations directly to the local authorities concerned and, if they have found that an injustice arising from maladministration has occurred, the local authority must respond to the report. Should the LCA be dissatisfied with any response, she must make a further report with recommendations and, if this is not acted upon by the local authority, that authority may be directed to publish a statement giving details of the local commissioner's findings and recommendations and its reasons (if any) for failing to comply. Though local authorities do, by and large, comply with LCA recommendations, such compliance is not assured and may sometimes be only partial or tokenistic. As with the PCA, there are no legal sanctions to ensure compliance.

Finally, the PCA also acts under a separately created jurisdiction as the Health Service Commissioner (HSC), a responsibility conferred in 1973. The HSC has since become a final 'court of appeal' in respect of complaints under the NHS complaints procedure (see below). The HSC is free to investigate not only complaints of maladministration, but also complaints about treatment, care and service standards. She may not, however, investigate issues where other remedies (such as for medical negligence) may exist, or in the case of complaints concerning the substantive merits of clinical or administrative decisions.

British ombudspersons do not enjoy the more free-ranging powers available to ombudspersons in other countries, such as the Scandinavian countries, but also to varying degrees New Zealand, Australia, Canada, France and Austria. They cannot conduct investigations without first receiving an explicit complaint, they are prevented from investigating complaints where a complainant has alternative means of redress, and they must not investigate matters encroaching on organisational, personnel or contractual matters. What is more, the peculiarly British notion of 'maladministration' has had several implications. First, it tends to assume the applicability of narrow but generic principles of administration and therefore to preclude a broad and informed view in specialist policy areas. Second, a preoccupation with administration without regard to the purposes of social policy may provoke defensive blame-avoidance behaviour on the part of welfare administrators, so stunting initiative and flexibility in service provision. Third, the term may come to be so restrictively interpreted as to preclude any challenge to policy or to the level of resources available for welfare provision (Harlow and Rawlings 1984). In the British context, it is difficult to tell whether the ombudspersons' function is to remedy individual injustices or merely to promote good administration. Certainly, they do not function as unfettered champions of the people.

There are, however, other potential fora for petitionary complaints. Some years before the trend towards individualised complaints procedures, which I shall discuss below, local government had been enjoined to combat their monolithic corporate tendencies through the development of participative fora, such as extra-statutory neighbourhood councils and complaints committees. Comprehensive complaints procedures could allow citizen participation by way of representations made directly to a special committee of locally elected councillors (Redcliffe-Maud 1969). Some 'progressive' local authorities responded to these suggestions and, although many of these voluntarily established complaints procedures have since been adapted for the disposal of *personal* complaints, there had been at least a few that actively sought to promote the hearing of complaints as an exercise in responsive governance (McCarthy *et al.*

1992). There is a sense in which these democratically oriented complaints committees fulfilled a function very similar to that of an ombudsperson. Indeed, the CLA (1978 and 1992) has provided guidelines to local authorities on setting up authority-wide complaints procedures with an emphasis on complaints monitoring as a means to detect trends that may require changes in policy or procedure.

Critics have dismissed such initiatives for providing little more than a 'ritual of participation', since they orchestrated public criticism only as a means to control it (Mathieson 1980). However, McCarthy *et al.*'s observations of such committees suggested that they did provide opportunities for *vox pop* to be heard. Commenting on an instance in which a chief local government officer had received an 'uncomfortable grilling' before one such committee, they observed, 'Cynics may dismiss this as little more than a bureaucratic *tableau vivant* staged for the benefit of an angry citizen, but the fact that it took place at all is in many ways significant' (1992: 94–5). Petitionary complaints are ends in themselves and are not necessarily instrumental or goal-directed. They may represent an attempt to elicit an appropriate 'social response' from a welfare authority (cf. Mulcahy and Lloyd-Bostock 1992) or an assurance that what the complainant has experienced will not happen to anybody else (Genn 1995; Dean *et al.* 1996).

Complaints procedures

Contemporary formal complaints procedures, including the statutory procedures operated by local authority social services departments and the NHS, though they may sometimes have to field complaints received from petitionary complainants, are primarily constituted to receive personal complaints.

The ethos for the new generation of complaints procedures was provided in the 1990s by the *Citizen's Charter* (see Chapter 1, and Dean 1996). The specially created Citizen's Charter Complaints Task Force defined redress in terms of 'the whole range of responses which organisations can offer to the user who has suffered sub-standard service. Redress heals the breach with the user that poor service has caused' (CCCTF 1994: para. 1.1). The managerialist orientation is clear. The provision of welfare is regarded as a business like any other in which customer grievances must be turned into complaints and the information they generate must be regarded as a management tool (Pfeffer and Coote 1991). Staff must share the mission of the organisation for which they work, they must be trained to deal proactively and expeditiously with complaints, to disarm aggrieved customers and ensure the organisation's mission is achieved. The aim is to ensure that heroic consumers of welfare, by their complaints, and motivated providers, by their responses, will drive up the quality of services. The ideological fiction on which this depends assumes not only parity of status between consumers and providers, but also that the 'customer' and her wishes are sovereign. In reality, of course, those who consume, for example, health and social care services may be especially powerless and vulnerable, while unemployed people who claim social security benefits or homeless people who seek assistance from a local authority are unlikely to be 'customers' through choice.

Local authorities were first required to establish further statutory complaints procedures under the Children Act 1989 and under the community care provisions of the NHS and Community Care Act 1990. The first procedure is for children aggrieved by matters relating to their care; the second is for service users and carers aggrieved by matters relating to services or, for example, the discretionary needs assessments and associated assessment of means which local authorities conduct (Gordon 1993). The model for both procedures is a process in three stages: first, an informal problem-solving stage, at which attempts are made to mediate and resolve the complaint; second, a formal 'registration' stage, at which an unresolved complaint is formally recorded and investigated by specially designated staff who may make recommendations for the resolution of the complaint; third, a review stage, at which unresolved complaints are referred to an independently chaired review panel.

Following the recommendations of the Wilson Report (1994) a broadly similar two-stage complaints procedure was adopted within the NHS in place of the confusing array of procedures that had applied before, though the operation of the new system is currently under review. The procedure, which relates to complaints about health authorities and all NHS trusts and other providers (including private sector providers where they are treating NHS patients), is operated at local level and provides: first, an investigation stage, during which the relevant chief executive or complaints manager should investigate the complaint and must respond within 28 days; second, a review stage at which unresolved complaints may be referred to an independent review panel.

Complainants who remain dissatisfied after the review stage may refer the matter to the HSC (see above). The government has proposed (DoH 2000a) that to assist patients with complaints there should be a patient advocacy and liaison service (PALS) based in all NHS and primary care trusts and local independent statutory patients' fora. However, there has been considerable opposition to the proposed abolition of Community Health Councils (see *The Guardian*, 15 February 2001), which had previously fulfilled a general role as the patients' advocate, and, at the time of writing, alternative arrangements for supporting complainants are being considered.

In practice, complaints procedures may not always conform to the model prescribed by policy makers and, in particular, independent review panels may often attempt to function in ways more reminiscent of other fora for redress (Dean *et al.* 1996). None the less, Charter oriented complaints resolution implies a different kind of service ethos to that implied by the application of appeals procedures or ombudspersons. The emphasis is less upon the standards of decision making, more on compliance with performance targets; less on interpreting citizens' rights, more on achieving customer satisfaction. As Gray and Jenkins have put it, when commenting in more general terms upon the impact of new public management upon the welfare state: 'A stress on honesty, fairness and equity leads to a different administrative structure than one on speed of response and cost minimization. It is therefore essential to determine what values administrative structures are attempting to serve' (1993: 22). According to the original defenders of the Charter approach to complaints, redress and standard setting in the public sector, it is competition or the fear of it, and not judicial or administrative authority, that will make providers take complaints seriously (Pirie 1991). As 'customers' citizens have a right to complain, but this is a right founded upon a notional contract: it has the form of a civil not a social right.

Reviews

Internal review represents, in one sense, the oldest means by which administrative redress may be sought. Like the eponymous hero of Charles Dickens's novel, *Oliver Twist*, the clients of welfare services could always try to ask for more – or to have their cases looked at again. There is a long tradition of welfare providers of various kinds holding case conferences to review the treatment they are meting out to any particular individual. In the past bodies supposedly constituted as tribunals – such as the old National Assistance Tribunal – had been criticised for functioning not as adjudicators, but more in the manner of 'an assessment or case committee, taking a further look at the facts and in some cases arriving at a fresh decision' (Franks 1957: para. 182). More recently, however, certain *statutory* internal review procedures have been introduced.

In 1982, when the housing benefit (HB) scheme was first introduced, challenges to determinations of entitlement by local authorities were made subject to a two-stage internal review procedure: the first stage involved a re-examination by local authority officers; the second a review by a Housing Benefit Review Panel composed of elected members of the local authority concerned. The Review Panels did not have any independent element and research into their functioning (Eardley and Sainsbury 1991) had recommended that their role would be better entrusted to the Social Security Appeal Tribunal. In the event, in 2000, adjudication in disputed HB cases was passed to TAS (see above) and is now carried out by tribunals.

The discretionary social fund, which was established in 1988 (see Chapter 5 above), replaced certain social assistance provisions that had been subject to a right of appeal to a tribunal. A more limited right was provided for claimants wishing to challenge decisions by social fund officers, which enabled them to have their case examined again by a social fund inspector. More recently, local authorities have been required to institute internal review procedures in relation to decisions in homelessness cases (see Chapter 7) though the Court of Appeal has recently ruled that the lack of an independent element in such reviews amounts to a breach of human rights (*The Guardian*, 15 December 2001).

These procedures represent an alternative to independently constituted tribunals and a model to which policy makers have occasionally turned. It is possible for internal review mechanisms to exhibit some of the hallmarks of a 'tribunal-like' adjudicative approach. For example, the social fund internal review procedure has been able to achieve standards of procedural fairness and efficiency that even critics of the social fund and its discretionary nature have acknowledged to be 'impressive' (Lewis and Birkinshaw 1993: 96). In some local authorities, in contrast, the standards of decision making by Housing Benefit Review Panels – before they were abolished – were subject to widespread inconsistencies (Eardley and Sainsbury 1991). Internal administrative review, however, is best understood as a form or style of redress that is the polar opposite of judicial review and may be formally or informally adopted in response to the supplications of a powerless client.

Summary/conclusion

In addressing the ways in which people may seek redress in relation to their welfare rights this chapter has raised a number of questions concerning the relationship between legal rights and social rights.

First of all, the relationship between the legal system and the welfare state is in some ways inherently problematic. The law – and especially the English common law tradition – is not necessarily well suited to the protection of welfare rights. Second, although welfare rights find expression in statutory legal form, rights to legal advice and assistance have not been developed on the same footing as other social rights. Third, although the administration of welfare has been developed largely beyond their gaze, the courts do potentially possess considerable power either to create or frustrate social policy. Finally, the welfare state has developed its own mechanisms of redress. The different forms of redress that have emerged reflect different conceptions of welfare rights and can constitute the welfare subject as the bearer of those rights in different ways. In the next chapter the ways in which the welfare subject is constituted will be examined in greater detail.

Part III

Rethinking welfare rights

Chapter 10

Discourses of citizenship, rights and responsibility

Having explored the practical realities of welfare rights – of the rights we obtain through social policy – I propose in this chapter to re-open the various theoretical controversies that I touched upon in Part I concerning different approaches to welfare and citizenship and different understandings of rights and redress.

One of the fundamental premises of this book has been that rights and citizenship are creatures of ideological discourse. The distinction has been drawn between civil rights (the legal framework upon which capitalism depends), political rights (upon which 'liberal' democracy is founded) and social rights (which found expression in the creation of the welfare state). T.H. Marshall has argued that such rights developed as reflections of competing values, but that the existence and continuing equilibrium between these three kinds of rights were functionally necessary to the survival of 'modern' capitalism. Social or welfare rights are ambiguous, however. They are bestowed in legal form, but as a consequence of processes that are political. It is also possible that the goods and services to which social rights allow access, though to varying degrees detached from the processes of the market economy, may none the less assume the form of quasi-commodities.

Upon the premise that poverty is inimical to full citizenship, the supposed function of social rights is to guarantee the satisfaction of human need. The problem is that definitions of poverty and human need are contested and that the relevance of social rights to citizenship is not clear. The relief of poverty may be a necessary condition for the achievement of human emancipation, but the prescription of rights and responsibilities may militate against the achievement of a form of citizenship from which nobody may be excluded. Certainly, there is no universal formula for human emancipation. The organisation of human welfare differs around the globe and there is little evidence that any one form of social rights will attain ascendancy. What is clear is that social rights in Western-style welfare states are ineluctably associated as much with controlling human behaviour as with meeting human need. It may be argued that, not only do social rights co-exist uneasily with other kinds of rights, they also have the propensity to be exploitative, disciplinary and/or divisive.

Though Britain is by no means a typical case, this book has considered the manner in which rights to subsistence, to work, to housing and (more briefly) to education, health and social care are currently guaranteed. In so far that

185

the highly complex British social security system guarantees the subsistence needs of its citizens, it does so selectively, treating different social groups in different ways; it functions so as to enforce particular patterns of family dependency and social exclusion. British social legislation does not guarantee a right to work; it provides limited protection to employees and subsidies to support the incomes of some low-paid employees; it imposes stringent conditions upon those who are unemployed or who are incapable of work. Similarly, British social legislation does not guarantee a right to a home; it provides increasingly selective subsidies to enable people to meet housing costs and a diminishing level of control over excessive housing costs; it gives powers to local government to remedy deficient housing stock, but only a limited duty to secure accommodation for homeless persons. Finally, British social legislation does provide a right to education and basic health care and a more conditional form of right to social care, but most pupils/students have limited control over their education, much publicly provided health care is rationed and the only enforceable right in relation to social care is a right to be assessed and not a right to substantive services.

To be of value rights must be enforceable. Within liberal democracies, this means they must be legally enforceable. The British courts have shown themselves to be capable both of advancing and obstructing the exercise of social rights; of tempering or colluding with the administrative power of the welfare state. By and large, however, the enforceability of social rights has been entrusted to administrative forms of redress: to tribunals, ombudspersons and complaints and review procedures. Such remedies have shown themselves capable of providing for citizens a strictly technical or procedural form of justice, but also of catering to the needs of welfare administrators and providers.

This leaves unanswered two major questions. First, can social rights be constituted as a meaningful and necessary component of citizenship? Second, can social rights provide more dependable guarantees of human welfare than is currently the case in Britain? The second of these questions I shall address in the next chapter, but in this chapter I address the first. The chapter will discuss the different discursive traditions that are embodied in the concept of citizenship and the ways these have been conflated in more recent debates; the conflicting ways in which welfare subjects, welfare principles and welfare regimes may be constituted through the various discourses of rights; and the way in which the discourse of social rights is currently being displaced by a discourse of individual responsibility.

Traditions of citizenship

The late twentieth century witnessed a renaissance of interest in the concept of citizenship that has succeeded in pushing debate about rights and welfare beyond the bounds of the seminal theory of citizenship first espoused by T.H. Marshall (e.g. Turner 1986; Jordan 1989; Oldfield 1990; Roche 1992; Twine 1994; Bulmer and Rees 1996; Lister 1997; Dean with Melrose 1999). Though this is not the place to recount a detailed history of citizenship as a concept, it is worth recalling that the term originally denoted residence of a city or, more precisely, the status of the free men of that city. Citizenship was concerned with freedom, whether it was the freedom of a self-governing patrician elite in the cities of ancient Greece or Rome, or the freedom from feudal servitude that had been won by the burghers of the late mediaeval cities of Western Europe. In neither case did women, slaves or servants count as citizens. Although citizenship was specific to a territory, it was not defined in relation to the city, the nation, the culture or the people so much as by the political practices of free men and the state that they had created (Habermas 1994).

The emergence of modern citizenship, though it was fashioned by the outcome of wars, migrations, political struggles and social movements, was intimately associated with the ideological upheavals of the Enlightenment and the social and economic upheavals wrought by the transition from feudalism to industrial capitalism (Turner 1986). What was entailed was the renegotiation of sovereignty, or as Dahrendorf has put it 'the domestication of power' (1996: 41). In this respect the Enlightenment principles encapsulated in the French revolutionary slogan – *liberté, egalité, fraternité* – represented mutually inimical demands that could not be accommodated in conjunction with each other (cf. Hobsbawm 1962). One solution, the liberal or contractarian citizenship tradition, privileged the demand for *liberté* or individual freedom and sought a compromise that entails a notional social contract by which sovereign power is negotiated between the individual and the state. The other, the republican or solidaristic tradition, privileged *fraternité* or social solidarity and subordinated the sovereignty of the individual to the need for mutual support and social cohesion.

Neither of these traditions was *necessarily* concerned to accommodate the demand for *egalité* or social equality. To the extent that either of them has done so, they have tended to interpret equality quite differently: the logic of liberal/contractarian citizenship may admit a concern with *formal* equality or the universality of individual opportunity; republican/solidaristic citizenship a concern with *substantive* equality or a universality of social outcomes. Contemporary Anglophone welfare states might be taken to represent differing versions of a contractarian citizenship model that are to varying degrees tolerant of social inequality while promoting procedural equality. The classic Nordic welfare state might be taken to represent egalitarian interpretations of a solidaristic citizenship model, while the classic Bismarkian welfare state represents a less egalitarian version. (See the discussion of welfare regimes in Chapter 3 above.)

I have sought elsewhere (Dean with Melrose 1999) both to develop this theoretical dichotomy between liberal and republican models of citizenship and to locate it within both popular and political discourse. The distinction I draw between contractarian and solidaristic approaches relates more concretely to people's expectations of a political community than the distinctions that may be drawn, for example, between the abstract ideological theories of liberalism and communitarianism (cf. Dwyer 2000). I have argued that the inherent ambiguity of public opinion towards the British welfare state stems from the way in which people draw on conflicting discursive repertoires about the nature of citizenship. At the heart of the dichotomy between contractarian and solid-aristic notions of citizenship lie fundamentally different ideas about the nature of the human condition. At one extreme lies an essentially Hobbesian view that society is composed of self-interested and inherently competitive indi-viduals whose mutually destructive propensities require a contractual arrange-ment by which certain individual freedoms must be 'traded' in return for social order achieved through state regulation. At the other extreme lies a view that the human subject is endemically vulnerable and to survive requires collectively organised mechanisms for mutual co-operation and support: what matters, as Richard Rorty has put it, 'is our loyalty to other human beings clinging together against the dark' (cited in Doyal and Gough 1991: 19).

My own qualitative research on popular discourses of citizenship has illus-trated that although people in Britain are seldom able to engage coherently with the concept of 'citizenship' they usually can and do convey what they understand with regard to rights and responsibilities and the nature of their and other people's relationships as individuals to society. In their attitudes to redistributive state welfare, people tend to exhibit an ostensibly contradictory mixture of guarded altruism and pragmatic instrumentalism (cf. Rentoul 1989; Brook *et al.* 1996; Dwyer 2000). The participants in our study were, by and large, predisposed to ideological principles that would underpin more contractarian or individualistic self-sufficiency, but they none the less valued key elements of the solidaristic or collectivist principles on which the welfare state was originally founded. Judged in terms of their explicit opinions, our sample was, on balance, more individualist than collectivist in outlook. The way they answered questions conformed, by and large, to the assumptions about popular opinion upon which New Labour policy has been constructed. However, close examination of the participants' underlying discourses revealed a subtler reality. Our findings suggested that people are capable of both selfishness *and* altruism, but that what most aspire to above all is ontological security. By implication, their preference was for a form of citizenship that protects against poverty before it secures the opportunity to pursue wealth. There remains a fundamental tension within pop-ular discourse between contractarian and solidaristic expectations of citizenship.

Citizenship remains an ambiguous concept in political as well as popular discourse. I observed in Chapter 1 how the Conservative government in the 1980s sought to appeal to an ostensibly solidaristic but distinctly inegalitarian concept of 'active citizenship' and the idea that comfortably-off citizens should assist their less fortunate neighbours on a voluntary basis. But in the 1990s the Conservative government promoted the 'Citizen's Charter' in which the citizen was envisaged in quintessentially contractarian terms as a consumer of welfare services. Similar confusions applied on the left of the political spectrum. Labour Party policy documents (1988, 1989 and see Plant 1988) began to promote the concept of citizenship, while the left-of-centre weekly magazine *New Stateman and Society* launched the 'Charter 88' Campaign, demanding a new political settlement, based on citizenship principles. Citizenship was regarded simultan-eously as a solidaristic antidote to unbridled market individualism *and* as an essentially contractarian organising principle for postmodernity or 'New Times' (see Hall and Held 1989). In the event, prior to the 1992 General Election, Britain's main political parties were all vying with each other to establish different visions of a 'citizen's charter' (Dean 1994: 103–4).

Significantly, such rhetoric did not feature so explicitly in either the 1997 or 2001 election campaigns. None the less, the language of citizenship lies at the heart of New Labour's project and, in particular, its proposals for welfare reform. The policy documents that began to emerge from New Labour (e.g. Labour Party 1996) began to speak of 'Labour's contract for a new Britain', of building both a 'stakeholder economy' and a 'one nation society'. The Labour manifesto (Labour Party 1997) to which the electorate subsequently gave its endorsement perpetuated this mixture of discourses, drawing on contradictory notions of citizenship. In his introduction to the manifesto, Blair drew on solidaristic discourse when he spoke of wanting 'a Britain that is one nation, with shared values and purpose'. However, he also drew very explicitly on contractarian discourse, not least in his final flourish, which claims 'This is our contract with the people'. The 'bond of trust' which Labour seeks to forge is with 'the broad majority of people who work hard, play by the rules [and] pay their dues'. By implication, it would seem, the contract is conditional on behaviour and there will be those who are not included. The welfare reform agenda outlined in the manifesto (to which I shall return later in this chapter) is 'based on rights and duties going together'. This is not the unconditional language of the 'old' Labour Party which had presided over the creation of the modern welfare state, but a discourse that flows from the party's qualified acceptance of key recommendations of the Commission for Social Justice, originally established by the late John Smith, Blair's predecessor as Labour leader. This had called for an 'investors' strategy' which would 'combine the ethics of community with the dynamics of a market economy' (CSJ 1994: 95). Here we have the makings of a regime that draws on the contractarian discourse of economic liberalism *and* the solidaristic discourse of social conservatism.

In Labour's 2001 manifesto Blair reiterated his government's central aim – 'to refashion the welfare state on the basis of rights and responsibilities, with people helped to help themselves, not just given handouts' (Labour Party 2001: 3). However, the section of the manifesto dealing with 'A modern welfare state' was concerned more with employment than with citizenship. Explicit references to citizenship only really appeared in the section of the manifesto that was devoted to 'Strong and safe communities', in which the declared aim was 'a new social contract where everyone has a stake based on equal rights, where they pay their dues by exercising responsibility in return' (*ibid.*: 31). A curious chain of association is constructed in the manifesto between crime, social order, personal responsibility and community regeneration. The language is contractarian, but the substance is redolent of an essentially authoritarian solidaristic tradition.

Interpreting rights

The underpinning tensions and contradictions between contractarian and solidaristic traditions of citizenship are reflected in diverse interpretations of rights and it is to rights rather than citizenship that I wish now to return. In Chapters 1, 2 and 3 I drew out a number of broadly inter-related distinctions between doctrinal and claims-based conceptions of rights, between distributive and relational approaches to human need and between constitutionalist and absolutist forms of political settlement. What I now want to explore is the way in which each of these distinctions intersect with the distinction between the contractarian and solidaristic citizenship traditions in ways that imply quite different interpretations of welfare rights.

A diagrammatic representation of the argument that follows is provided in Figure 10.1. The horizontal axis in the diagram represents a continuum between contractarian approaches to citizenship on the one hand and solidaristic approaches on the other. The vertical axis represents a continuum that draws

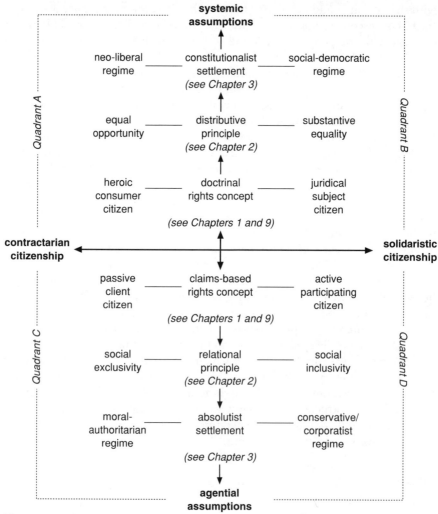

Figure 10.1 Interpreting rights

upon the distinction I introduced in Chapter 2 between *systemic* assumptions that privilege the role of social and political structures on the one hand and *agential* assumptions that privilege the role of either individual or collective human action on the other. We are concerned here with assumptions about the nature of governance within the confines of democratic-welfare-capitalism. Hindess has observed that 'the community of autonomous persons' envisaged by liberal democracy is an inherently ambiguous construction: it appears both as '. . . the basis of government in some contexts and as artefact of government practices in others' (1996: 73). Systemic assumptions are those that regard welfare rights in terms of the means by which inherent needs should be met. Agential assumptions are those that regard welfare rights as the outcome of struggle or negotiation over interpreted needs.

The model is of course no more than a general heuristic or explanatory device that relates strictly to dominant interpretations within welfare state capitalism. It does not account for specifically situated interpretations by any particular thinker or movement, not does it accommodate the critical interpretations that might be offered by, for example, feminists, socialists or ecologists.

The construction of the welfare subject

My starting point is the distinction between doctrinal and claims-based notions of rights. The former are inherently systemic in the sense that they are premised on some overarching rationality or set of immanent principles. The latter are inherently agential in the sense that they are premised on the demands or expectations of living human actors. In Chapter 9 I discussed the different ways in which rights of redress in relation to welfare provision can constitute the welfare subject: I wish to suggest that the various forms of rights of redress reflect different underlying approaches to rights themselves and that it is these that account for the various ways in which we may be constituted as the bearers of rights.

The contractarian version of doctrinal rights (see Quadrant A in Figure 10.1) is founded on an instrumental rationality and a deontological concept of correlative rights and duties. The individual subject is constrained by negative duties to her fellow subjects, but is otherwise free to exercise her rights as a consumer in the market place; to demand welfare goods and services upon the most advantageous terms; to withhold her custom when the terms are not right; to complain when things go wrong. The good citizen is a heroic consumer. The solidaristic version of doctrinal rights (see Quadrant B in Figure 10.1) is founded on an ethical rationality and a universalistic concept of consequential rights and duties. The individual subject is constrained by a positive duty to ensure the welfare of her fellow subjects (through an obligation to pay taxes) and a right to collectively provided or financed welfare goods and services; to insist upon her entitlements; to appeal when things go wrong. The good citizen is a responsible juridical subject.

In contrast, the contractarian version of agential rights (see Quadrant C in Figure 10.1) is founded upon ontological fears and expectations; the hope that the market will provide and that the Leviathan state may mitigate its predations. The individual subject has the right to demand the satisfaction of her wants, but is constrained by the vagaries of the market place and the authority of state administrators. The good citizen may be self-seeking, but is obedient; a passive client. The solidaristic version of agential rights (see Quadrant D in Figure 10.1) is founded on particularistic allegiances; the idea that rights embody collective goals. The individual subject has the right to the satisfaction of her needs by virtue of her birth into a particular society or her membership of a particular class or group within that society, but is constrained by her duties towards that society, class or group. The good citizen is a loyal champion of the collective cause and the rights it espouses; an active participating citizen.

The construction of welfare principles

In Chapter 2 (see Figure 2.1) I suggested a certain correlation between doctrinal approaches to rights and distributive approaches to need and a similar association between claims-based approaches to rights and relational approaches to need. I intend now to turn from the discussion of the ways in which the welfare subject may be variously constituted depending on the way in which rights are conceptualised to a discussion of the various ways in which welfare principles are constituted depending on the way in which needs are conceptualised.

The contractarian version of the distributive approach to needs satisfaction (see Quadrant A in Figure 10.1) is founded upon a notion of equity. Equity in its strict sense does not imply substantive equality, but equivalence of rewards based on merit or desert. From this perspective the unequal distribution of rewards that results from the operation of market forces is equitable provided there are rules that ensure a 'level playing field'; provided the market system allows every subject or 'player' to compete on free and equal terms; provided the competition is procedurally fair. Welfare intervention is required to guarantee equality of individual opportunity and to ensure that everyone has a chance of satisfying her own needs. The solidaristic version of the distributive approach to needs satisfaction (see Quadrant B in Figure 10.1) is founded upon a notion of social justice. Social justice is not concerned with equivalence of reward so much as the universal moral worth of all members of society. From this perspective it is important to correct the unfair outcomes that will foreseeably result from the operation of market forces; to ensure that the basic needs of all may be met, regardless of their circumstances; to ensure that procedural equality does not obscure the exploitation of the weak by the strong. Welfare intervention is required to ensure a measure of substantive equality.

In contrast, the contractarian version of the relational approach to needs satisfaction (see Quadrant C in Figure 10.1) is founded upon a kind of social Darwinism: the idea that only the fittest in society should be allowed to survive or, at least, that only compliant subjects should be allowed to participate. From this perspective the social and economic milieu that we inhabit is inherently hostile and competitive; our participation in that milieu is a matter of fate rather than choice, and an obligation rather than a right. Therefore, those who disrupt or offend the given norms that guarantee survival should be sanctioned or excluded. State intervention may be required to ensure the social exclusion of those – the criminal, the insane and the undeserving – who are unfit to participate. The solidaristic version of the relational approach to needs satisfaction (see Quadrant D in Figure 10.1) is founded on the right to social participation or membership. From this perspective those in society who are disadvantaged by economic exploitation or by personal circumstances are entitled none the less to belong; to benefit from mechanisms that do not necessarily ensure equality, but inclusion. State intervention is required to promote social inclusion, to underwrite the cohesiveness of society, to contain or ameliorate social divisions and/or to integrate or re-insert those who are excluded.

The construction of welfare regimes

Just as principles of welfare tend to be fashioned or constructed from concepts of need, so different kinds of welfare regime – affording different kinds of welfare rights – tend in turn to be fashioned or constructed from different kinds of welfare principle. In earlier works of mine (Dean with Melrose 1999; Dean 1999 and 2001) I have sought to demonstrate the relationship between different ideal-typical welfare regimes and the different discursive moral repertoires upon which they are premised. My task here, however, is slightly different, in so far that I am concerned not with the differing kinds and degrees of egalitarianism that are exhibited in different welfare regimes, as the fundamentally different notions or rights and needs that underpin them. In Chapter 3 above I drew on Mann's work to make the distinction between constitutionalist and absolutist (or, more precisely, post-absolutist) forms of political settlement. The distinction, though it helpfully enables us to differentiate Anglophone and continental European historical traditions, has been criticised by Turner (1990) because it overemphasises the significance of class relationships and underemphasises the significance of rights. None the less, I would regard the distinction as conceptually significant since it resonates with the continuum in the vertical axis of Figure 10.1. The principles of a constitutionalist settlement are inherently systemic: they are predicated on rule-bound resolutions and determinate structures. The principles of an absolutist settlement are inherently agential: they are predicated on pragmatic resolutions and negotiable structures.

The contractarian version of a constitutionalist political settlement (see Quadrant A in Figure 10.1) is best exemplified (using Esping-Andersen's schema – see Chapter 3 above) by a neo-liberal welfare regime in which the constitutional role of the state is that of 'enabler'. The welfare state provides a constitutional framework in which market forces can function; in which a skilled labour force can be reproduced; in which citizens can provide so far as possible for their own welfare. The solidaristic version of a constitutionalist political settlement (see Quadrant B in Figure 10.1) is best exemplified by a social-democratic welfare regime in which the state furnishes the constitutional means for the regulation of markets; the protection of labour; the provision of welfare services.

By contrast, the contractarian version of an absolutist political settlement (see Quadrant C in Figure 10.1) is perhaps a counterfactual construct (or, at least, it is not exemplified by any of the conventional regimes in Esping-Andersen's schema), though it might be characterised as a moral-authoritarian regime in which sovereign state power remains absolute; sovereign power is not bargained away but attains a degree of popular legitimacy in relation to the regulation and control of human conduct; a legitimacy based in tradition, pragmatism or 'common-sense'. Arguably, this might represent a description of the paternalistic, so-called 'Confucian' welfare state emerging in East Asia. As a heuristic construct, however, it may just as easily be applied to certain *aspects* of the Benthamite utilitarianism and the Fabian welfarism that had informed the early development of the British welfare state: distinctly illiberal tendencies that, though premised on conflicting ideological doctrines, could cater in rather similar ways to populist authoritarian demands by offering distinctly non-constitutionalist means for the exercise of state power in the interests of the (imagined) greater good. Finally, the solidaristic version of an absolutist political settlement (see Quadrant D in Figure 10.1) is best exemplified by a conservative or corporatist welfare regime in which absolute sovereign power has struck compromises with the representatives of society's principal classes or communities of interest; in which provision for social welfare is brokered on behalf of society's members; in which welfare concessions cement the social order.

Just as concepts of citizenship draw upon contradictory traditions, so associated concepts of social or welfare rights are capable of conflating disparate interpretations of rights. No given welfare regime or set of welfare principles or individual welfare subject is constituted by a single set of forces or a single set of ideological concepts. I am not necessarily seeking to develop the kind of typological thinking promoted by Esping-Andersen, so much as contribute to debate about the nature of the discourses that inform current processes of welfare reform. A better understanding of welfare rights depends on a deeper understanding of the complex and conflicting array of interpretations that may underpin them. Ruth Levitas (1998), for example, has developed a taxonomy that distinguishes redistributionist discourse ('RED'), which would be broadly consistent with Quadrant B in Figure 10.1; social integrationist discourse ('SID'), which to my mind embraces two distinctive strands – one entrepreneurial and the other communitarian – and in fact straddles Quadrants A and D in Figure 10.1; and moral underclass discourse ('MUD'), which would be consistent with Quadrant C in Figure 10.1.

In the British case, it would seem, the New Labour government, in spite of its social democratic heritage, seldom draws on interpretations drawn from Quadrant B (equating with Levitas's RED). Instead, the interpretations that explicitly drive the development of welfare rights are drawn primarily from quadrants A and D of Figure 10.1 (or Levitas's SID), though often the substantive effects of policy intervention imply a logic drawn from quadrant C (Levitas's MUD). The citizen is sometimes looked to as a heroic consumer and sometimes as an active participating citizen, but in practice she is often *treated* as a passive client. Distributive principles of welfare are sometimes premised on equality of opportunity, sometimes on the goal of social inclusion, but in practice the effect is often to *underline* the exclusion of the non-compliant citizen. The emergent welfare regime is predominantly neo-liberal, but with certain conservative tendencies, though such tendencies are informed by American-style communitarianism (see below) rather than European-style corporatism, and in practice the style of *intervention* is sometimes best characterised as moral-authoritarian. The key to understanding the ambiguity of welfare rights in British policy discourse probably lies in emergent discourses of responsibility.

Rights and responsibility

We have already observed that the language of rights within New Labour's discourse has been coupled to a language of responsibility. The clearest manifestation of this is to be found in the change made in 1995 to Clause IV of the Labour Party constitution: a commitment to social equality was replaced with a commitment to a society in which 'the rights we enjoy reflect the duties we owe'. Rights were in effect made conditional on the fulfilment of responsibilities. Here I shall explore the implications of conditionality and rights in relation to New Labour, before opening up a wider discussion of responsibility and welfare.

The conditionality of rights

The increased emphasis on the conditionality of welfare rights was given shape in the British government's 1998 welfare reform Green Paper (DSS 1998). Explicitly or by implication this accepted as inevitable the end of the protectionist welfare state. It insisted on social inclusion through 'work for those who can' and, through a preoccupation with benefit fraud, it tempered a commitment to security for those who cannot work by reinforcing a culture of suspicion around the receipt of welfare benefits (see Dean 1999). As we saw in Chapter 5, the government's welfare-to-work programme has encompassed the 'New Deal' intended to assist a wide range of working-age target groups – including unemployed people, lone parents and disabled people – into the labour market (e.g. Millar 2000). The very expression, 'New Deal', it has been suggested, articulates a populist interpretation of contractarianism; a trade-off between the government and the people (Fairclough 2000: 39). The New Deal has now been extended through the creation of a single agency – JobCentre Plus – that administers the full range of social security benefits for claimants of working age and, through compulsory 'work-focused' interviews, provides them with guidance and support in relation to employment opportunities.

New Labour's political discourse frequently elides references to rights in favour of the language of opportunities. As is consistent with a neo-liberal discourse it subordinates equality of outcome to equality of opportunity, though it sometimes obscures this by appealing to a superficially solidaristic notion of 'equal worth'. For example, in a recent speech by the Prime Minister, he declared:

> ... the belief in the equal worth of all [is] the central belief that drives my
> politics ... Note: it is equal worth, not equality of income or outcome; or, simply,
> equality of opportunity ... So: let us start applying this principle to modern
> Government ... We do so on the basis of building a community where citizens are
> of equal worth. Opportunity to all; responsibility from all ... I don't think you
> can make the case for Government, for spending tax payers' money on public services
> or social exclusion ... without this covenant of opportunities and responsibilities.
> (Blair 2000)

This might be interpreted as meaning that social rights are being reduced to
labour market opportunities and those who abjure the responsibility to rise to
such opportunities are unworthy and, by implication, justifiably less equal. In
so far that rights to social protection are acknowledged, it would appear that
they are seen as conditional on the acceptance of responsibilities. The citizen
is offered the opportunity to access certain institutionally embodied entitlements, but must accept the responsibility that comes with such opportunity.
The 'worth' of the citizen is measured by a social contract or 'covenant' in
which she surrenders irresponsible freedoms in return not directly for rights,
but for 'opportunities'.

Turning to recent developments in social care policy, as we have seen in
Chapter 8, these would seem to reflect a similar, if more ambiguous, preference
for contractarian as opposed to solidaristic conceptions of citizenship rights.
While the emerging political consensus may accept the proposition that individuals should so far as possible assume responsibility for their own welfare,
public opinion has been resistant to the idea that this should extend to the
provision of long-term care during extreme dependency in old age (Parker and
Clarke 1998). The New Labour government established a Royal Commission
on Long-term Care for the Elderly (1999) in the ostensible hope that it could
generate proposals that would carry popular consensus. Though the majority
report urged that all forms of care should be provided free and without a
means-test, it none the less perpetuated a conceptual distinction between
'nursing care' and 'personal care' and so failed to transcend the medical model
of disability in order fully to adopt a more holistic social model (e.g. Parker
2000). In its subsequent plans for the NHS (DoH 2000a) the government did
not adopt the specific recommendation of the majority report, but proposed
that while nursing care would be provided as an unconditional right, personal
care would still be conditional upon a means-test. However, the lives of frail
elderly and disabled people are hazardous. What might be called 'personal
care' ensures their physical and ontological security and, as such, would be
regarded as a fundamental right to safety or 'asylum' (in the original meaning
of the term) within a solidaristic citizenship framework.

At the same time that the British government claimed to be 'bringing rights
home' through the enactment of the Human Rights Act 1998 (that incorporates
into domestic law the provisions of the European Convention of Human Rights
– see Chapter 1 above), it was attempting specifically to displace the language
of rights in relation to the provision of social protection. Collective provision
is giving way to an emphasis on social responsibility and self-provisioning.

While the Human Rights Act does provide a right to life (which does not necessarily but might imply a right to basic health and nursing care) and a right to education, it does not provide a universal right to adequate subsistence, shelter or 'personal' social care. The Human Rights Act may well contribute to a shift in domestic political discourse and a changing context for the development of social policy.

The ground for this latest re-interpretation of rights was laid in part during the 1980s by the New Right, but it was fuelled by a variety of cultural and intellectual influences. Roche (1992), for example, has contended that since the crisis of the welfare state in the 1970s the 'dominant paradigm' of social citizenship has come under attack from across the political spectrum as a 'discourse of duty', as well as rights, emerged. This discourse has taken several forms, ranging from New Right and neo-conservative claims that welfare rights undermine the 'traditional' obligations that people have to sustain themselves through work and to provide for each other through the family, through to claims by new social movements that a *dirigiste* welfare state denies oppressed people any real autonomy. Though Roche opposes the New Right's rejection of social rights, he accepts the case for rethinking the absolute priority that he believes has been given to social rights and urges a need 'to reconsider the moral and ideological claims of personal responsibility, of parental and ecological obligations, of corporate and inter-generational obligations, and so on.' (1992: 246).

Such arguments prefigured those that occurred within the British Labour Party in the late 1980s and 1990s and the principles eventually advanced by the New Labour government that I have already outlined above. Prominent academics who have been close to the Labour Party have endorsed, and even nourished, the trend: Raymond Plant, who has done much to defend the idea that social rights are equal in importance to civil and political rights, none the less argued in a seminal Fabian Society pamphlet 'that welfare rights should depend on performing corresponding obligations of a workfare or learnfare sort' (Plant 1988: 14); and Tony Giddens, who has done much to characterise the challenges that late modernity poses for welfare citizenship, has none the less concluded that 'a prime motto for the new politics [is] *no rights without responsibilities*' (Giddens 1998: 65).

In common with the New Democrats in the USA during the Clinton era, New Labour was also strongly influenced by an emergent strand of communitarian thinking emanating particularly from American political scientists like Etzionni (1995). Jordan (1998) has argued that the appeal of this form of communitarianism to the present politics of welfare stems from the connections it makes between individual choice and collective responsibility. It offers an almost nostalgic appeal to the rural village or the close-knit working-class neighbourhood; it speaks to the moral intuitions of small-town America or traditional English values; and it seeks to translate the principles of reciprocity appropriate to membership of a small association to the realisation of the common good within a national community. This, Jordan suggests, lies at the heart of a newly emerging and increasingly hegemonic orthodoxy in an age when all prescriptions for welfare reform are informed by a perceived need to limit public spending and sustain labour market flexibility. There is a role for governmental intervention, especially in stimulating the supply side of the economy, but it is necessary that the rights of citizens should strictly reflect their observance of duties and obligations to and within the community. More persuasive communitarian theorists, such as Putnam (1993), have sought to demonstrate the efficacy of a vigorous civil society in which associational networks facilitate democratic self-government and actively promote welfare – either independently of the state or by facilitating the development of services (cf. Hirst 1994). But as Foweraker and Landman point out, 'rights do not enter [Putnam's] definition of "civicness"' (1997: 240). Welfare appears almost as a by-product of 'civicness'. It is guaranteed neither by the top-down prescription of experts, nor through political struggle from the bottom up.

Communitarianism, it has been suggested, 'offers Labour modernizers a political vocabulary which eschews market individualism, but not capitalism; and which embraces collective action, but not class or the state' (Driver and Martell 1997: 33). New Labour's brand of communitarianism reflects some features of European-style Christian democracy, but in other respects it is quite different. Driver and Martell acknowledge that New Labour is essentially conservative rather than progressive, in so far that it is profamilial and more authoritarian than permissive; it is prescriptive rather than voluntaristic in so far that it will countenance compulsion in the interests of social cohesion; it is moralistic in so far that it has eschewed increased socio-economic redistribution in favour of policies to promote opportunity. In spite of a certain commitment to pluralism, constitutional reform and the devolution of power, New Labour has a tendency to be conformist in that it seeks to retain power centrally in certain key policy areas and, on occasions, appears rhetorically to conflate the powers and responsibilities of 'the community' with its own powers and responsibilities as a government. In two important respects, however, New Labour's communitarianism is more distinctively American.

First, it is a strictly conditional communitarianism and, I would contend, it lapses into an essentially contractarian form of moral authoritarianism. As we have seen, the reciprocal and proportionate nature of rights and responsibilities are determined with reference to a narrow calculus. In spite of New Labour's insistence that vulnerable people will always be protected, the overwhelming implication is that social rights can be conceded only if they are earned or, exceptionally, deserved. There are no unconditional rights of citizenship. Though it has been claimed that Labour's new direction reflects a move away from socialist dogma and towards substantive social justice (Plant 1995; Blair 1996), Blair himself insists that 'the most meaningful stake anyone can have in society is the ability to earn a living and support a family' (*ibid.*). Such a 'stake' becomes in effect the *sine qua non* of social justice. Jordan (1998) has argued that the prevailing orthodoxy may be seen, in the name of social justice, to be extending the surveillance and control of 'deviant' minorities; to be expanding processes for counselling and compelling unemployed people, lone parents and disabled people towards the labour market. In this, Jordan suggests,

New Labour is observing regulatory principles espoused in the nineteenth century by the utilitarian philosopher Jeremy Bentham. Here I think Jordan is correct, not because Bentham was a communitarian, but in the sense that the disciplinary techniques associated with the development of administrative power are continuously available to be refined and applied (Foucault 1977; Dean 1991); and because utilitarianism approved of coercion in the cause of the greater good. New Labour thinking here chimes with that of Mead, who had argued that the goal of social policy should be to promote 'equal citizenship', a process which

> does not require that the disadvantaged 'succeed', something not everyone can do. It requires only that everyone discharge the common obligations, including social ones like work. All competent adults are supposed to work or display English literacy, just as everyone is supposed to pay taxes or obey the law. (1986: 12)

Second, according to Driver and Martell (1997), New Labour's communitarianism is more individualistic than corporatist. Once again, I would argue, this makes New Labour's approach contractarian rather than solidaristic. By this they mean that New Labour's concept of 'stakeholding' is less about the corporate economic responsibilities of companies and organisations (as advocated, for example, by Hutton 1996) as about the personal moral duties of individuals.

It is in this context that New Labour's welfare reform Green Paper sought to define 'a new contract between the citizen and the Government, based on responsibilities and rights', a contract which it illustrates using a table that defines the respective *duties* of the Government and the individual (DSS 1998: 80). By sleight of hand, therefore, the broad concept of responsibility is recast in terms of a narrower notion of duty and the citizen is recast as an individual. The Government's essential duty is to provide a supportive framework in which individual subjects are obliged, if they are able, to seek training or work, to take up the opportunity to be independent, to support their children and other family members, to save for their retirement and not to defraud the taxpayer.

Interpreting responsibility

Current discourses of responsibility tend, as we have seen, to embrace a variety of specific responsibil*ities* and to conflate a number of concepts to do with duties, obligations and obedience (see Dean and Doheny 2001). I wish to return to the conceptual framework I developed earlier in relation to the interpretation of rights in order to discuss the interpretation of responsibility. A diagrammatic representation of the argument that follows is provided in Figure 10.2. Once again the horizontal axis in the diagram represents a continuum between contractarian approaches to citizenship on the one hand and solidaristic approaches on the other. The vertical axis represents a continuum that draws upon the distinction between systemic assumptions about the nature or responsibility on the one hand and agential assumptions on the other.

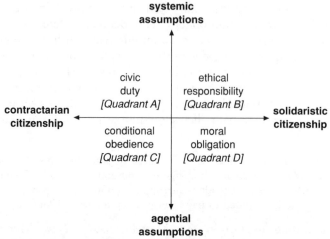

Figure 10.2 Interpreting responsibility

Responsibility, when it is socially constructed from within a contractarian understanding of citizenship, but from a systemic perspective (Quadrant A in Figure 10.2), takes the form of civic duty. The citizen's freedom as a consumer is premised upon such duties as she owes to other citizens that may be necessary to ensure that their freedoms are not infringed. Each person's duty to fulfil or refrain from certain actions thus flows from a system of expectations that are reciprocal and symmetrical, but duties themselves are individualised. In so far that rights are constructed in terms of individual interests, one's duties arise from the need to ensure, as far as can reasonably be expected, that one's interests can be met without unfairly prejudicing the interests of other individuals. The observance or performance of duties becomes, ideally, a self-regulating process.

However, when a solidaristic notion of responsibility is constructed from within a systemic perspective (Quadrant B in Figure 10.2), responsibility assumes a more strictly ethical and universalistic form. It is important to remember that what is being presented is a heuristic model and, arguably, an ethical notion of responsibility, such as might fully be realised only within an unfettered global communication community (Apel 1980 and 1991; and see Chapter 11 below) has never in reality been applied. The rational ethic that has informed even the most collective strands of state welfare capitalism has arguably been premised upon an essentially Kantian notion of responsibility: a notion that regards responsibility as innate to an individual having free will, rather than as constructed through the nature of social relationships. None the less, this notion of responsibility is essentially rational, reflexive and democratic. It recognises that responsibilities are shared, as much as individual; that they may have to be asymmetrically distributed, rather than reciprocal; that they depend none the less on general assent.

In contrast, when it is constructed from within a contractarian notion of responsibility, but from an agential perspective (Quadrant C in Figure 10.2), responsibility takes the form of conditional obedience. Self-interested behaviour in the absence of systemic self-regulating duties is likely to result in irresponsibility and, in this context, the function of the state relates not to the promotion of responsibility, but the governance of irresponsibility (cf. Lund 1999; Dwyer 2000). This entails the imposition of penalties and sanctions on the one hand and the identification and stigmatising of irresponsibilities on the other. We have seen already that certain approaches to social exclusion may be criticised because the remedy for exclusion would seem to have more to do with social *integration* than with social inclusion. In the same way, a contractarian approach to the governance of irresponsibility is likely to have as much to do with eliciting *obedience* as with promoting responsibility. Rights that are conditional upon behaviour do not necessarily promote responsibility, since this also depends on trust (see Dean 2000).

When a solidaristic approach to responsibility is constructed from within an agential perspective (Quadrant D in Figure 10.2), it assumes the form of moral obligation. Responsibility is constructed with reference to collective loyalties and traditions; to moral norms and shared values; to the necessary and incontestable expectations that arise from membership of a particular community. Fulfilment of obligations gives rise to pride and a strengthening of social inclusion, failure to do so in shame and a risk of social exclusion.

As with the model I present in Figure 10.1, I would not wish to make overinflated claims for that which I present in Figure 10.2. It by no means exhausts the possibilities for discussion. There are notions of ethics that sit beyond this framework. Bauman (1993) has argued that the postmodern epoch creates a space for entirely new and authentically ethical discourses. Foucault, in rejecting the Kantian orthodoxy that informs the ethic of universal welfare, argues that what counts is individual ethical obligation to the self-governing self (e.g. Hunter 1996). Rose (1996) contends that in a 'post-social' era, governments seek to promote not only personal human capital and individual prudentialism, but the ethical skills necessary to self-management.

My own argument, however, is that what distinguishes ethics from morality is its systemic nature and that what distinguishes responsibility from mere duty or obedience is that it is a solidaristic imperative. The device that I am presenting here helps to illustrate the competing interpretations upon which New Labour draws. When New Labour insists that rights and responsibilities go together, the meaning of 'responsibility' conflates the duties that flow from a civic/social contract and the obligations that are endemic to an ordered community. At the same time, it seems to me, New Labour is promoting a project for the governance of irresponsibilities – for eliciting obedience rather than self-responsibility. The dominant assumption is that in so far that the human condition gives rise to 'rights', these are to be met by guaranteeing individual opportunity, before collective protection. Personal responsibility – construed in terms of duties and obligations – is in practice preferred to a reflexively constructed ethic of responsibility. New Labour does not, in my contention, embrace ethical responsibility.

Summary/conclusion

Whether welfare rights can be constituted as a meaningful and necessary component of citizenship therefore depends, first, on how citizenship itself is understood; second, on how rights are interpreted; third, on how rights are conceived in relation to responsibility.

This chapter has argued that we may discern two principal traditions of citizenship. The first is contractarian. Though strongly associated with liberalism, the essence of the contractarian tradition lies in the expectation that the individual citizen has a notional contract with the state; a contract that civilises the self-interested conduct of others while guaranteeing the freedom of the self. The second tradition is solidaristic. Though strongly associated with civic republicanism and/or communitarianism, the essence of the solidaristic tradition lies in the expectation that the individual citizen is a protected member of a particular society; that the interests of the self are bound up with the interests of others.

From different understandings of citizenship flow different interpretations of rights, depending in turn upon whether rights are seen as part of a system of governance or as a part of a 'life-world' inhabited by social actors. Rights may constitute the welfare subject as a heroic consumer, entitled to equality of opportunity within a neo-liberal regime; as a juridical subject, entitled to substantive equality within a social-democratic regime; as a passive client, entitled to the benefits of state controls within an essentially moral-authoritarian regime; as an active participating citizen, entitled to social inclusion within a conservative regime.

Current approaches to welfare rights and welfare reform draw in ostensibly contradictory ways upon several of these interpretations of rights. The central thread of the current orthodoxy is an emphasis upon responsibility and an insistence that rights should be conditional upon responsibilities. However, this discourse of responsibility conflates concepts of civic duty, moral obligation and conditional obedience and fails, I have argued, to establish a clear ethical basis for responsibility.

My contention would be that rights remain conditional, subordinate and inadequate within current concepts of citizenship. Welfare rights are caught up in a fundamental but poorly articulated conflict between, on the one hand, a contractarian calculus that assumes that rights are conditional upon and must equate with responsibilities and, on the other, a solidaristic guarantee that assumes that membership of society gives rise unconditionally to rights and responsibilities alike. The question to which I must return in the next chapter is – can welfare rights provide more dependable guarantees of human welfare than is currently the case in Britain? What are the chances of a more reflexive approach to welfare rights? Will this depend upon reform or resistance?

Chapter 11

Welfare reform or social resistance?

In this final chapter I shall discuss alternative strategies for the future development of welfare rights. I want to suggest that there are two broad kinds of
strategy available, though each is susceptible to widely differing interpretations
and neither by itself contains a sufficient answer to the question of whether
welfare rights may yet provide more dependable guarantees of human welfare.
The first kind of strategy is premised on reformism and the second on resistance.
What distinguishes reformism from resistance is that the former seeks to compromise with or improve upon the existing social order, while the latter seeks
to subvert or supersede it. Reformism is likely to look upon the advancement
of rights as an end in itself. Resistance is likely to regard rights as a means to
an end. The distinction drawn earlier in this book between systemic and agential
assumptions comes into play. Reformism focuses on the modification or creation
of systems. Resistance focuses on the harnessing or the promotion of different
kinds of agency. However, as with the models that are presented in Chapter
10, this distinction intersects with another – that between contractarian
expectations of the relationship between citizen and state on the one hand
and solidaristic expectations on the other. The analysis in the next part of this
chapter is therefore summarised in Figure 11.1, which illustrates two kinds of

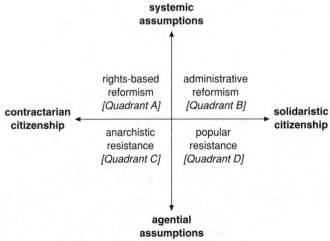

Figure 11.1 Strategies of reform and resistance

reformism – rights-based reformism and administrative reformism; and two kinds of resistance – anarchistic resistance and popular resistance.

Because reformism and resistance represent different kinds of opposition to the status quo, Figure 11.1 does not map straightforwardly, for example, on to the Figures 10.1 and 10.2, which I presented in the last chapter. The reformism that flows from systemic interpretations of rights and principles demands more of the same (i.e. more effective welfare rights or better welfare administration), whereas the resistance that flows from agential interpretations of rights and principles demands something different (i.e. the end of the state or the victory of the people). Accordingly, the types of reform and resistance that I shall discuss are not necessarily peculiar or appropriate to any particular kind of welfare regime, though they are all framed as responses to democratic-welfare-capitalism. In the final part of the chapter I shall explore the possibility that we might learn from the pitfalls of reformism and resistance in order to transcend them both.

Welfare reformism

The distinction I seek to draw between rights-based and administrative reformism is, of course, conceptually driven. Reformism has many camps and there are several bridges between those camps. By highlighting axiomatic differences, however, we may better understand, on the one hand, the scope for alliances between reformers and, on the other, the inherent limitations of welfare rights as a vehicle or focus for reform.

Rights–based reformism

Rights-based reformism (see Quadrant A in Figure 11.1) is the creed that characteristically motivates welfare rights workers and welfare lawyers. It is a systemic creed in so far that it is premised upon a critical acceptance of a framework of rights. It is contractarian in so far that those rights are construed as a feature of a formal relationship between the individual subject and the state. It arises out of a concern to empower the disadvantaged and oppressed through rights to individual redress. It is potentially a radical creed that can exploit the contradictions of a legal system that is constructed to ensure the freedom of the property-owning individual and equity between participants in market exchanges. Equally, however, it may become a conservative creed, since it may end up perpetuating a status quo based on property ownership and market forces.

Rights strategies have been a significant feature of certain kinds of campaign against poverty (see, for example, Alcock 1993/1997: ch. 15). In the USA in the 1960s, President Johnson's 'War on Poverty' sought the empowerment of impoverished communities through the introduction of community action and legal services programmes, organised through an Office of Economic Opportunity. The first OEO director referred to legal services as the 'heavy artillery' in the war against poverty: poverty was thought to result as much from people's failure to exercise their rights as from any deficiency in those rights. In Britain in the 1970s, the Home Office sponsored Community Development Projects in twelve inner-city areas, generating a variety of self-help initiatives and welfare rights services. As has been seen in Chapter 9, the 1970s also witnessed the emergence of the British law centre movement, a major expansion of the Citizens Advice Bureaux and other independent advice centres, and attempts by national charities like Child Poverty Action Group to employ new forms of 'test-case strategy'.

A debate about the uses of law in the struggle for rights has continued among 'radical' or 'critical' lawyers (see Travers 1994). While some critical legal scholars maintain that law is necessarily subordinate to a dominant power in society, others are prepared to argue about the possibilities of counter-hegemonic rights strategies (Hunt 1990) and of law as a mode of resistance to law itself (Fitzpatrick 1992). However, the relationship between critical legal theory and progressive legal practice has been said to be 'at best problematical and at worst non-existent . . . Most practising lawyers are too busy getting on with their work to notice, let alone worry about, the relationship between their activities and legal theory' (Economides and Hansen 1992).

In spite of this, rights strategies founded in progressive legal practice or in advice and community work clearly can succeed in securing social security benefits for people who are entitled to them, in curbing bad employment practices, in improving local housing conditions and in securing access to education, health and social services for those who have been excluded. However, the improvements they can bring to the living conditions of poor people are often marginal and there are several reasons why this is so.

First, such strategies cannot by themselves improve the levels at which social security benefits are set, they cannot create new jobs or homes and they cannot secure increased resources for education, health and social care. Second, the advantages obtained even from ground-breaking test cases may be short lived given the capacity of the legislature to nullify each victory (Prosser 1983). Third, when resources are rationed, those who exercise their 'rights' successfully may do so at the expense of others: for example, successful social fund applicants may, by using up the local office budget, deprive other applicants of assistance; local authority tenants who successfully exercise their rights under the Environmental Protection Act to obtain improvements to their homes may, by using up the local authority's investment allocation, prevent their neighbours from having essential works carried out (see, for example, Reidy 1980). In this way, the exercise of rights may even be inimical to social justice.

Fourth, the technical legal process on which rights strategies depend can individuate, frustrate and disempower the poor. It can isolate them and deliver them to the ministrations of experts and professionals. Alternatively, it may offer them knowledge and skills that are of little or no practical use. Reference was made in Chapter 4 to neo-Marxist critiques of rights strategies. Writers like Bankowski and Mungham have long since dismissed as 'a waste of time' any attempt at social or political change through the pursuit of rights and legal remedies. Even they, however, concede that there are occasions 'when people are caught up in the coils of the law, when they have to fight on the stage provided by it' (1976: 112). Drawing on the experiences of campaigns fought in the Rio squatter settlements, de Sousa Santos (1979) argues for a strategy that subverts or enlarges litigation and adjudicative processes so as to encompass 'real' social issues, not narrow 'legal' definitions. Such a possibility is not without precedent in Britain. In the 1970s, more radical welfare rights activists and claimants' unions often adopted a 'carnival-style' approach to tribunal appeals that, as Hilary Rose describes, insinuated a 'slice of real life' to the artificiality of the proceedings.

> The bumpy spring-broken mattress, the worn out sheets, the children and their too small vests are brought to the appeal as evidence to challenge the social security decisions. The individuated humiliation of the home visit is turned into an offensive weapon to expose and ridicule the meanness of the social security system. The representative becomes compere and produces exhibit after exhibit while the witnesses – whose role is audience as well as evidence givers – switch mood from laughter, to anger, to pain as the charade is played out . . . As when the silent speak, these sorts of appeals enter into the mythology as occasions when 'we showed them'. (1982: 151)

Such tactics were undoubtedly memorable, but by themselves they were seldom effective. Twelve years' experience as a welfare rights worker taught this writer that what counts for most people when they are 'caught up in the coils of law' is to win substantive rather than merely moral victories. The implication of my argument in Chapter 10 is that at a time when late modernity casts the poor as 'flawed consumers' (Bauman 1998), the ultimate object of reform based on a systemic/contractarian rights-based strategy is to equip or re-motivate even the most disadvantaged welfare subject as a 'heroic consumer'. However, the successful consumer requires more than competence to empower her. In the absence of social redistribution the danger in the longer term is that this strategy will demoralise rather than empower. Especially for those for whom meaningful labour market opportunities do not exist, enhancing their competence as welfare consumers will emphasise rather than ameliorate their experience of poverty.

The fifth and final reason for the limited scope of rights-based reformism is that the activists upon whom such strategies depend can all too easily be co-opted or diverted. Claimants' unions, like the Welfare Rights Organisations that had preceded them in the USA (Piven and Cloward 1977), proved to be transient organisations and have failed to sustain themselves as an integral movement. Their activities remained outside the mainstream of the democratic political process, and their grass-roots leaders were often co-opted into more conventional forms of pressure group activity. Claimants' unions and welfare rights organisations never in themselves became a vehicle for political mobilisation to secure social rights. We have seen in Chapter 9 that the autonomy of welfare rights advisers in Britain is increasingly compromised – most recently, for example, by a pervading 'contract culture', imposed forms of 'partnership' involving other agencies, processes of 'Best Value' review, and/or the restrictive regime and 'Quality Marking' mechanisms associated with the new Community

Legal Service. Piven and Cloward have concluded that a rights strategy focusing upon individual 'grievance work' is of limited organisational value and they echo a view expressed by Schiengold (1974), that recourse to litigation and individual rights can only be one tactic in any plan for a broad mobilisation for change. Schiengold himself has dismissed as a 'myth' (*ibid.*: 5) the very idea that the definition and realisation of social rights can be achieved through the pursuit of enforcement action.

This is not necessarily to say that such action is without its own significance. There is a case for 'rights without illusions' (Hunt 1990: 326); for exploiting a discourse of rights as a tactic within a *political* strategy. Such a strategy would seek to broaden a discourse based on individualised or 'legal' rights so as to encompass 'social' rights. This must contend, however, with a 'blocking' tendency that arises precisely because of the association within dominant hegemonic discourse between 'liberty' and 'rights' (*ibid.*: 315); an assumption, in other words, that rights cannot be 'social' in a collective sense, but are protections that must function within the limits of individually guaranteed civil and political freedoms.

Rights-based reformism, I would argue, has three principal roles to play:

1. I have already – in Chapters 1, 3 and 10 – touched upon the potential significance for Britain of the Human Rights Act of 1998. It is a reform that will probably, for the reasons already discussed, have relatively few direct applications so far as welfare rights advisers and welfare lawyers are concerned, but more generally it will introduce into our judicial and political culture a new way of thinking about rights. Potentially there is scope to capture the idea of a right to security, safety or 'asylum' as a basic human right; to develop the language of rights in ways that embrace and even celebrate human interdependency. Social security provision offers asylum from the risks of an exploitative labour market and social housing offers asylum from the risks of homelessness, just as social care offers asylum from the risks accompanying the impairment and isolation that can be associated with disability or old age. If 'social inclusion' means anything, it means being dependent upon those around us. Rights-based reformism – if it is willing – can play a part in counteracting the tendency of neo-liberal political discourse to obscure this interpretation of human rights.

2. The casework experiences of welfare rights workers and welfare lawyers can be used to impress upon policy makers that the increasingly conditional framework within which welfare rights are being provided can as easily disempower people as empower them. This has been a traditional role for the advice and legal services movement, but it is important that the new terms of engagement that are affecting so many welfare rights advisers should not diminish their capacity to speak out against the contradictions and perverse effects of policy when these are observed at first hand. Britain's New Labour government places great rhetorical store on the principles of 'evidence based policy making' (see, for example, Performance and Innovation Unit 2000) and the adage that 'what counts is what works' (Labour Party 1997: 4).

Rights-based reformism can play a part in making a reality out of such rhetoric by demonstrating which rights work and which do not, and what the implications are when rights are curtailed.

3. The implication of my argument in Chapter 10 is that a strategy based on systemic/contractarian rights-based reformism will be locked in to a notion of responsibility based on civic duty rather than collective responsibilities. None the less, rights-based reformism can have things to say about the extent of the duties of government as well as the duties of the individual subject. There are limits to the extent to which welfare rights groups and federations of advice agencies can engage directly in political debate: there are constraints that arise from their charitable status and/or the codes of professional conduct to which legally qualified staff may be subject. However, it is precisely because welfare rights advisers can legitimately claim a degree of professional autonomy that they may be able to lend their support to claims for the broadening of the duties of government in relation to the provision of welfare.

Administrative reformism

Administrative reformism (see Quadrant B in Figure 11.1) is the creed shared by social democratic politicians and by a great many social policy academics. It is a systemic creed in so far that it is premised on the idea that human welfare can be ensured through administrative intervention. It is solidaristic in so far that such intervention is construed to be in the collective interest. It arises out of a concern to mitigate structural disadvantage through the deployment of administrative power and the provision of welfare. It is, in essence, the orthodoxy of social administration: the discipline that gave rise to modern social policy. In Chapter 1 I focused on the seminal definition of social rights provided by T.H. Marshall (1950). Marshall's argument was that the emergence of social rights – rights to health and social care, education, housing and income maintenance – represented the fulfilment of modern citizenship. However, this conception of rights provided the supports for a 'big tent', capable of accommodating different strands of thought (Lund 2000: 24). Administrative reformism – especially in the British context – has consistently fallen short of social democratic ideals and has in practice been shaped by two strands: social liberalism on the one hand and Fabianism on the other. Social liberals and Fabians agree that citizenship entails responsibilities as well as rights, but there are differences of emphasis with regard to questions of enforceability.

Marshall himself was primarily a social liberal who subscribed, implicitly at least, to the 'organic' theory of society espoused by liberal thinkers like Hobhouse and Hobson (see Lund 2000), who assumed that human society was akin to an organism that evolved, not in a Darwinian sense by virtue of natural selection, but by virtue of ethical reasoning. The social liberal strand of reasoning has been perpetuated in more recent times by Raymond Plant. Plant argues that social rights (and 'economic' rights, by which he refers to rights to income and to work that are here encompassed within the term social rights) 'are not in fact categorically different from civil and political rights' (Plant 1992: 17). In response to neo-liberal critiques (which I have discussed in Chapter 4), Plant asserts that positive social rights cannot be dismissed as mere desires, interests or claims, unless one is prepared similarly to dismiss the 'negative' rights associated with civil and political freedoms. Social rights may make claim to the allocation of scarce resources, but this is no different to such rights as the right to physical security, the enforcement of which may entail the allocation of considerable resources upon the apparatuses of law and order. Social rights are invariably predicated upon contestable conceptions of need, but this is no different to such rights as the right to privacy, the definition of which is no less problematic and no less susceptible to changing social expectations and technological contexts. It is difficult to achieve consensus about the extent of social rights, but this is no different from other kinds of rights, which depend upon achieving a measure of political consensus as to what is just. The defenders of 'negative' freedoms insist that free markets cannot be blamed for unjust outcomes provided such markets have been constituted with just intentions, but Plant argues that the injustices which demonstrably flow from the free play of market forces, though they may not be intended, are foreseeable. Measures to ensure social justice are therefore as logically and morally necessary as any civil or political freedoms.

The essence of Plant's argument is 'that the freedoms and immunities which are guaranteed [by] civil and political rights remain wholly abstract if people do not have the social and economic resources to be independent citizens' (*ibid.*: 21). Our liberties and our abilities are in no way categorically different. We cannot be free to do that which we are not able to do. The freedom to own one's home is not a freedom if one cannot afford and is not enabled to pay the mortgage. The freedom to compete for a high-paid job is not a freedom if one does not have the necessary ability – whether in terms of training or, for example, access to childcare. The 'progress' of industrial capitalism has been based upon an expansion in the range of some people's abilities and this has been associated with a necessary growth in certain constraints upon human conduct in the organisation of productive processes: the expanding range of human abilities has none the less increased rather than diminished the scope of human freedoms. After all, 'what makes freedom valuable to us is what we are able to do with it' (*ibid.*: 25). Abilities underwritten by social rights are no less constitutive of citizenship than freedom underwritten by civil and political rights.

Having argued that social rights are equal in status and importance to civil and political rights, Plant becomes more hesitant when he approaches the question of the enforceability of social rights. He acknowledges that because social rights do involve rights to scarce resources, this often involves rationing and the exercise of administrative or professional power. Here he links the concept of social rights with the notion of citizen empowerment and the idea that it is through rights that citizens may enforce their claims against welfare administrators and professionals. But how? Coote (1992) has taken Plant's argument as the basis upon which to endorse a strategy that would entail the enactment of a British Social Charter. This would specify certain rights and provide a framework within which to interpret and develop social legislation, but, unlike a Bill of Rights (or the Human Rights Act that has now reached the statute book), it would not be directly enforceable by individuals. Rather, it would provide a 'supportive environment' for the promotion of procedural rights to welfare, based on consistent principles of fairness in relation to all welfare services. Coote's argument is that:

> if all individuals in a society were comfortably housed and enjoyed reasonable stand-
> ards of health care, education and social insurance, but had no civil rights, that society
> would offer them no constitutional means of winning the rights they lacked. By con-
> trast, a society in which individuals enjoyed the right to vote, and freedoms of speech,
> assembly, movement and so forth, would hold out the possibility of winning social
> rights through the democratic process. Civil rights can thus be seen as a means of
> achieving social rights. Social rights may be necessary for the just enforcement of
> existing civil rights (since abilities make liberties worthwhile), but on their own they
> cannot be a means of achieving civil rights. And indeed, without civil rights, social
> rights are almost certainly unenforceable and therefore meaningless. (1992: 8)

Coote is right to point out that social rights are dependent for their enforce-ability upon civil rights and for their development upon political rights, but it is surely neither necessary nor consistent to accept that social rights ought therefore to remain subordinate to civil and political rights. In practice, the social liberal champions of social rights are equivocal about asserting them on an equal footing with civil and political rights.

The Fabian strand of administrative reformism is different. It is best associated with Richard Titmuss (1958), the 'father' of social administration, who believed like Marshall that the function of the welfare state was to compensate for the diswelfares of capitalism; that it provided a means to counteract the destructive reign of market forces. However, he also believed – unlike Plant and Coote whom we have just discussed – that social rights did not require the legalistic proportionate justice appropriate to civil rights, so much as a creative indi-vidualised justice to be administered by enlightened officials and professionals (Titmuss 1971). In this Titmuss was heir to an older Fabian tradition: that of the Webbs. The ultimate vision of a fully comprehensive and highly specialised interventionist welfare state was embodied in the dissenting Minority Report of the Royal Commission on the Poor Laws of 1905–1909, a report written by Beatrice and Sidney Webb (1909). The authoritarian, if benign, purpose of that vision is perhaps best encapsulated in a Soviet slogan which, years later, the Webbs were to note and quote with approval: this spoke of 'mending the human race on scientific principles' (Webb and Webb 1935: 805). Fabians character-istically favour extensive social spending, but *dirigiste* methods of administration.

The most recent standard bearer of the Fabian strand has arguably been Frank Field, veteran anti-poverty campaigner and Labour MP who was briefly appointed as New Labour's Minister for Welfare Reform following the 1997 election. The proposals that Field had endorsed before New Labour's election victory had been based on a wholesale onslaught against means-tested provision (1995). To this end he advocated individualised stakeholder pensions on the one hand and an extended but 'mutualised' form of national insurance provision on the other; but he coupled this with a 'proactive' approach to income support in order to compel those who are able to work to do so and to eliminate fraud. It is only the latter, moral-authoritarian elements of Field's approach that have found their way into New Labour's legislative programme.

New Labour's approach combines the social liberals' diffidence about the enforceability of social rights with Fabian enthusiasm for the enforcement of social responsibility. The result is at best a poor example of administrative reformism. And arguably New Labour does not represent administrative reformism at all since some of its primary influences are drawn from outside the administrative reformers' tent. Administrative reformism remains an inherently ambiguous if not a counterfactual type of strategy.

None the less, administrative reformism has been the principal motor and creator of social rights and can continue to advance their cause and effectiveness, provided:

1. It can take seriously the contention that welfare rights created by social policy can be rendered equivalent to civil and political rights and need not be subordinate to them. The implication of this is that a welfare right becomes an unequivocal claim upon resources, not a juridical fiction. The challenge of this for social policy making is that welfare rights would become democratically demand led. This would mean either unrestricted social spending, or the emergence through democratically accountable mechanisms of more detailed and explicit codes for the distribution of welfare goods and services.
2. It can avoid lapses into the contradictory logic of moral authoritarianism. In a sense, this means taking both the solidaristic tradition of citizenship and a systemic approach to reform more seriously. Once again, this would entail a greater democratisation of welfare and the development of more effective means of professional and administrative accountability.
3. A major shift could be achieved towards a more reflexively ethical notion of responsibility. This is a key issue to which I shall return in the conclusion to this chapter.

Social resistance

Once again, I must caution that the distinction I am drawing between anarchistic and popular resistance is conceptually driven and framed by the context of democratic-welfare-capitalism. There are social movements, including feminism and ecologism, which straddle or arguably transcend the distinction. The purpose of the analysis, however, is to help situate our understanding of welfare rights in relation to the potential for resistance.

Anarchistic resistance

Anarchistic resistance (see Quadrant C in Figure 11.1) embraces an impulse that has a romantic appeal to certain political activists and an intellectual attraction to many contemporary social scientists. Anarchistic resistance is agential in so far that it is premised on the freedom and integrity of the individual subject. It is contractarian in a paradoxical sense because it can only conceptualise that freedom in relation to 'unfreedom': as the *absence* of the constraints imposed by the contract between the individual and the state. The central purpose of anarchistic resistance is to defy or discard that contract. It arises on the one hand out of a deeply conservative strand of individualism and, on the other, out of a profoundly radical opposition to the intellectual premises of the existing order. Its essence lies in the negation of systemic rights. Anarchistic resistance has two distinct strands. The first I would characterise as essentially nihilist, the second as quixotic.

The nihilist strand of anarchistic resistance has been powerfully influenced by Nietzschean ideas. The Nietzschean legacy, founded in the individually self-affirming conception of 'the will to power', represents an element that is held in common by certain nineteenth-century anarchists and by certain late twentieth-century post-structuralists alike. Nietzsche's reputation as a founder of Fascism is in fact quite erroneous, but he remains none the less the most misanthropic of individualists. He sought to distinguish between the Apollonian tendency of the state to curtail human creativity and the Dionysian potential of the self-fulfilling individual or 'Superman'. What matters is the creative realisation of self. As a consequence his own thinking was characterised by extreme elitism and indifference to human suffering.

The point about the nihilistic strand of anarchistic resistance is that it rejects the very concept of rights. This is most clearly represented in the writings of nineteenth-century anarchist thinkers like Bakunin and Stirner. Thus, for Bakunin, the state is predicated on violence and oppression, the 'democratic' state is a myth, and the concept of a legal or politically created 'right' is 'nothing but the consecration of fact created by force' (cited in Marshall 1993: 296). While Bakunin argued that 'democratic' rights were the contradiction or negation of human rights, Stirner went further in rejecting the existence of any natural, moral or social rights: for him right is only might and '[w]hat you have the *power* to be you have the *right* to . . . [T]here is no right *outside* me' (cited in Marshall 1993: 226). There is a resonance between this kind of rejection of rights and that found in contemporary post-structuralist critiques of law. Peter Fitzpatrick (1992), for example, presents modern law as a mythology; an inherently racist mythology, what is more, predicated as it is upon imagined distinctions between civilisation and regulation on the one hand, and barbarism and disorder on the other.

But if this strand of thinking rejects the existence of rights, how can it constitute a strategy? There is an anarchic rights strategy that self-consciously exploits rights without accepting the authority of those who administer them. Harking back for a moment to the claimants' union movement of the 1970s, Jordan (1973) has identified within it two quite different approaches. Drawing on the distinction made by E.P. Thompson (1968) between the English and the Irish working-class traditions, he observed that unions in the English tradition were organised as mutual aid societies, while those in the Irish tradition pursued a 'claims maximisation' approach. The former collectively cultivated allotments to grow vegetables, organised the bulk purchasing of food, and conducted relations with the social security authorities in an orderly and responsible manner. The latter ruthlessly wrung from the social security system every advantage obtainable for their members, adopting a combative and abrasive relationship with the authorities. The claims maximisation approach owes its coherence, like that of immigrant Irish workers in nineteenth-century England, to a rejection of Puritan values, a contempt for authority, but an acute knowledge of legal procedure. Elements of the approach are also adopted by those welfare rights activists who see their task as that of manipulating the welfare state to maximum advantage while minimising its controlling effects.

The second, quixotic, strand of anarchistic resistance is altogether gentler. It has something in common with what Nick Deakin has mischievously characterised as 'hobbit socialism' (1994: 227), after the diminutive creatures who, in J.R. Tolkein's novels, triumphantly collaborate against a nasty and brutish world. Deakin refers to a vision in which the distinction between client and professional, civil society and the state is dissolved and people are allowed to relate to each other on the basis of genuine equality. He charges the unnamed proponents of this model with naivety. In the event, it is a depiction that calls to mind the anarchist Emma Goldman's vision of 'a society based on voluntary co-operation of productive groups, communities and societies loosely federated . . . [and] . . . actuated by solidarity of interests' (cited in Marshall 1993: 403). Here Goldman was giving expression to the thinking of a group of nineteenth-century anarchist thinkers, such as Godwin and Kropotkin, who were very different from Bakunin and Stirner. Godwin was prepared to acknowledge the existence of rights, albeit just two kinds of right: the right (or rather the freedom) to exercise private judgement, but also the right to the assistance of one's neighbour (and the correlative duty to render assistance to a neighbour in need) (see Marshall 1993: 204–5). Similarly, Kropotkin, rejecting the egoism of Neitzsche, gave a central place to the need for altruism: his vision was of a society based on mutual aid and voluntary co-operation.

In the event, such a vision resonates with a range of more contemporary arguments by so-called civil-society socialists and radical democrats, such as Keane (1988) and Waltzer (1983), whom I have already mentioned in Chapter 4. It also resonates with Colin Ward's observation that 'an anarchist society, which organises itself without [state] authority, is always in existence, like a seed beneath the snow' (1973: 11). This is more anarchistic than socialist. What is offered is the alluring prospect of provision for human welfare without the necessity for the overbearing might of a welfare state. It remains quixotic because first we must contend with the state as we find it. While the nihilists leave us with no strategy or hope of resistance (or at best a tactical device), the quixotic anarchists would seem to inhabit a world that is accessible only by a leap of the imagination.

The possibilities that anarchistic resistance provides may yet make a contribution to the advancement of an emancipatory form of welfare rights:

1. The libertarian impulse that inspires anarchistic resistance tends to obscure both the defining nature of human interdependency and the role that rights can play in mitigating power. The Nietzschean legacy is inimical to the recognition of human interdependency, while the more quixotic forms of anarchistic resistance fail adequately to account for relations of power. None the less, anarchistic resistance contains a necessary insight concerning the risk that rights may merely reflect the exploitative might of those who bestow them.
2. The intrinsic elitism of the Nietzschean legacy would never aspire to self-realisation for all, while the quixotic resistor's preoccupation would seem to be with the road to self-realisation, rather than its actual achievement or the means to guarantee it. None the less, the ideal of creative self-realisation remains a valid aspiration, and it represents something that the rights of citizenship could protect, rather than destroy.
3. Anarchistic thinking contains some important ethical elements that bear upon the nature of responsibility, as opposed to mere obedience. Most strands of anarchistic resistance are bound together by an ideal of self-responsibility (a feature of anarchistic thought that is little understood). Anarchistic resistance need not be preoccupied with disobedience or the avoidance of obedience to authority; it can also challenge the irresponsibility of authority.

Popular resistance

Popular resistance (see Quadrant D in Figure 11.1) embraces an impulse that is opposed to the power of capital and the state. However, it is distinguishable from anarchistic resistance because it is pragmatic, rather than romantic, in its vision; populist, rather than intellectual, in its appeal. Popular resistance is agential in so far that it is premised upon the possibility of human action. It is solidaristic in so far that such action is construed in relation to the people as a collective entity. The central purpose of popular resistance is to defy imposed solidarities and to remake authentic ones. Its essence lies in the possibility of resistance through everyday practices and discourse, though it may be more grandly conceived in terms of cultural strategies of power (cf. Gramsci 1971).

Though popular resistance is no doubt a timeless phenomenon our understanding of it is aided by recent post-structuralist critiques of administrative state power. The key thinker here is Foucault (1979). To Foucault resistance is integral to power: 'Where there is power, there is resistance' (*ibid.*: 95). Power is relational, he argues. It is vested in the entire network of human relationships and depends not upon a single oppositional relationship between ruler and ruled, but upon a multiplicity of points of resistance. The power of the state rests on the institutional integration of power relationships, but similarly it is the 'strategic codification' of resistances that would make revolution possible.

However, when it comes to the creation and the exercise of rights, it must be remembered that popular rights and popular justice are potentially inimical to state-administered systems. Foucault (1980: ch. 1) has questioned whether any form of popular justice is achievable through the medium of even the most accountable form of adjudicative apparatus. A court, tribunal or adjudicator – even a lay arbitrator – represents a 'third element' who must necessarily claim independence from, rather than allegiance to, the parties; who must adhere to some ideal of justice that is not 'popular' but claims absolute or universal validity over the people; who has the power to enforce decisions and must therefore remain alien to the people. Popular justice would not necessarily guarantee social justice. It is difficult to see how popular demands could be framed in terms of welfare rights; still less how they might be enforced. Popular resistance may occasionally impact upon policy – as it did in Britain when there was intense popular opposition to the Poll Tax in the 1980s (Bagguley 1994) and as has been achieved by campaigns organised on behalf of particular social groups, enjoying widespread popular support, such as pensioners. It has been suggested that 'dual power' situations during revolutionary crises may enable the emergence of popular forms of rights and justice that function in parallel if not in opposition to conventional or bourgeois forms (de Sousa Santos 1979), but there are few if any instances in history in which rights have been specifically formulated through genuine popular resistance as opposed to demands that may have been manufactured and 'popularised' through the intervention of political elites.

Bill Jordan has argued that in practice most popular resistance against oppression occurs not through autonomously elaborated counter-discourses or alternative theories of justice, but through such substantive practices as petty fraud, pilfering, go-slows and sabotage (Jordan 1993); that particular 'communities of fate' entrapped by poverty in a world of narrowing mutualities may develop a retaliatory 'culture of resistance' and survival strategies based on informal economic activity or even organised crime (Jordan 1996). On the one hand Jordan draws perceptively on the work of Scott (1985) to argue that the way that disadvantaged people frame their claims is often through the artful manipulation of dominant discourse: 'they choose not to challenge the dominant order, but seek a measure of autonomy and opportunistic gain within it' (Jordan 1993: 215). On the other hand, Jordan (1996) also suggests that there are marginalised social groups which, to circumvent their exclusion, behave in accordance with distinctive strategies (which can none the less be counterproductive since they invite further repression).

Jordan at least implies that some potential for popular resistance lies 'out there' waiting perhaps to be harnessed to some project that would humanise the welfare state, that would articulate welfare rights in popular form. As it happens, my own research over a ten-year period tends to suggest otherwise. I shall refer very briefly to key findings from three research projects. The first was a study of the so-called 'Dependency Culture' to which long-term social security recipients are alleged to fall prey (see Dean and Taylor-Gooby 1992). The findings from this study indicated that long-term social security recipients are very much a part of mainstream culture and belong to neither a culture of dependency, nor a culture of resistance. Though many of the respondents in that study did feel that they were trapped by the benefits system, they none the less exhibited the same sorts of aspirations, expectations and prejudices as the rest of the community. The second study explored the attitudes of fraudulent social security recipients; people who were, for the most part, illegally engaged in the informal economy (see Dean and Melrose 1997). The findings suggested that, to the extent that respondents were engaged in acts of resistance, it was a very conservative form of resistance: many did feel that their legitimate expectations of the welfare state had been betrayed and believed this justified their dishonesty, but they aspired not to challenge the state, but to get a 'proper' job and achieve a decent but modest living standard. Finally, the most recent study has been an investigation of popular discourses around the themes of poverty, wealth and welfare (see Dean with Melrose 1999, and Chapter 10 above). The findings indicate that popular discourse is chaotic and contradictory, but that it draws upon a range of largely conventional moral repertoires. Popular attitudes may best be characterised as a complex mixture of guarded altruism and pragmatic instrumentalism. This is reasonably encouraging for the cause of administrative reformism, but it offers little hope that any systematic basis exists for popular resistance. Reformism is to some extent latent within popular discourse, but resistance is not.

In so far that it at present exists at all, popular resistance – as opposed to more intellectually predisposed notions of anarchistic resistance or intellectually orchestrated notions of a politics of discourse (e.g. Laclau and Mouffe 1985) – is highly fragmentary and deeply conservative. None the less, popular resistance may yet have a role:

1. It is possible, for example, that the growing preoccupation both in Britain and elsewhere with increasingly coercive work-welfare regimes coupled with increasingly intrusive anti-fraud measures may eventually – especially in the event of an economic downturn – exceed the level of popular support that such measures currently enjoy. In neighbourhoods or locations in which there are no formal labour market opportunities engagement with alternative survival strategies may cease to represent isolated acts of resistance and become the norm (Sullivan and Potter 1998; Turok and Webster 1998), while the resentment experienced by increasing numbers of working-age social security claimants may provoke a backlash and authentically popular (though not necessarily coherent) demands for enhanced welfare rights.
2. It is possible that social groups who are excluded or marginalised from mainstream welfare provision may – if they cannot organise alternative provision – become more cohesive and vocal. To an extent, British Muslims represent an example of a marginalised community that is becoming increasingly militant, though there are dangers that this process may reinforce potentially conservative and internally repressive aspects of the community's culture rather than promote popular demands for the recognition of their rights to welfare (Dean and Khan 1997 and 1998). It cannot be assumed that popular forms of power, once mobilised, will necessarily be inclusive or democratic.

3. The view of popular resistance that has been advanced by Gramsci is premised on such notions as the 'war of position'; the idea that social groups may struggle to achieve hegemony for their own ideology or view of the world. This may be achieved in quite non-reflexive ways, through the 'hidden transcripts' of a popular vernacular (J. Scott 1990). However, to promote rights through popular resistance does require a reflexive ethic: 'only the social group that poses the end of the state and its own end as the target to be achieved can create an ethical state, one which tends to put an end to the internal divisions of the ruled, etc., and to create a technically and morally unitary social organism' (Gramsci 1988: 234). It is to such a possibility that my concluding section now turns.

The autonomous subject and the ethical state

The challenge, therefore, is to conceive of welfare rights as rights that are created for autonomous subjects within an ethical state. The ethical state is necessarily an object of both resistance and reform. Welfare rights have been problematised in current political discourse because it is assumed that dependency and responsibility are incompatible. My argument is that they are not and that resistance is required in order to assert the autonomous subject's right to dependency, while reform is required in order to create an ethical framework through which to realise social responsibility.

Rights and autonomy

Turner, drawing on philosophical anthropology, has argued that 'it is from a collectively held recognition of individual frailty that rights as a system of mutual protection gain their emotive force' (1993: 507). It is the frailty of the human subject that both requires her to be in various ways dependent and exposes her to the risk of exploitation. Dependency and exploitation are intimately related. The human species' exploitation of the planet's natural resources has been a consequence of our physical dependency on such resources. Class exploitation and, most particularly, capital's exploitation of labour, arises because our social existence is also dependent on the application of human labour power. Men's exploitation of women initially arose out of the interdependency that is required for the reproduction of such labour power. Dependency in each instance is inevitable. Exploitation is not. Rights have the propensity to protect the dependent from the consequences of exploitation.

Sociologists from Durkheim to Marx have demonstrated that the more advanced a society is, the more interdependent its members become. However, the nature of that interdependency is generally obscured or 'fetishised' (see Dean and Taylor-Gooby 1992: ch. 6). The social democratic justification for the welfare state had been that the vicissitudes of the market generate unnatural 'states of dependency' that should be ameliorated (Titmuss 1958). The New Right's critique of the welfare state was based on the denigration of the 'sullen apathy of dependence' and the assertion that human happiness is to be found in the pursuit of 'independence' (Moore 1989). Neither view embraced the reality that frailty and interdependency remain an enduring and defining feature of the human condition. In fairness, New Labour does sometimes acknowledge human interdependence and recognises that ours 'is a world with a paradox at the heart of it: greater individual freedom; yet greater interdependence' (Blair 2000). However, the resolution that Blair offers to this paradox is a 'community' constructed not around rights, but upon notions of opportunity and responsibility. Yet individual freedom implies risk; and communities generally demand protection against risk. Interdependence represents the basis for personal security; and communities can properly demand that such security be underwritten or guaranteed. Such demands represent the essence of our welfare rights.

Relationships of dependency are also relationships of power (see, for example, Walker 1987). And power can entail exploitation – within households and communities; in employment; in market transactions; in the processes of state administration. While we may accept with Doyal and Gough (1991) that personal autonomy is a basic human need, it would be a mistake to presume that dependency precludes autonomy. It is power that threatens autonomy, and exploitation that negates it.

An alternative to Marshall's classification of citizenship rights is to be found in the work of David Held (1994) whose analysis hinges not on an antagonism of principles between the market and the state, but upon relations of power and the various sites of power in society. While the state and the market are each sources of power, they do not by themselves encompass 'the range of conditions necessary for the possibility of a common structure of action' (Held 1994: 51). The basis for the 'common structure of action', which Held equates with citizenship, is that of 'equal autonomy'; what a democratic community requires is 'a framework which is, in principle, equally constraining and enabling for all its members' (*ibid.*: 48). What Held calls 'nautonomy' (i.e. the negation of autonomy) occurs when relations of power in society are such as systematically to generate asymmetries of life-chances. Such asymmetries in life-chances may correlate with geography, class, gender or 'race'. Deprivation and ill-health, for example, are to be found clustered

> among countries of the South, among non-whites, among the poor and working classes and among women. These correlations and clusters are not, however, restricted to countries of the South, and can be found widely in the North as well. The patterns of social closure and opportunity among men and women, working, middle and upper classes, blacks and whites and various ethnic communities profoundly affect their well-being across all categories of health in both Europe and the United States. (*ibid.*: 52–3)

While Marshall spoke of three kinds of rights, Held differentiates seven sites of power and seven related categories of rights. Held's sites of power are the body, welfare, culture, civic associations, the economy, regulatory and legal institutions, and organised violence and coercive relations. In relation to each site of power there are conditions which must be fulfilled in order to have

Table 11.1 Categories of rights

Held's 'sites of power'	Corresponding categories of rights	Marshall's categories of rights
Body	**Health** (right to physical and emotional well-being, including control over fertility)	Social
Welfare	**Social** (right to social security, childcare and education provision)	
Economy	**Economic** (right to guaranteed minimum income – and to work)	
Coercive relations and organised violence	**Pacific** (right to due process, physical security, peaceful co-existence)	Civil
Culture	**Cultural** (freedom of thought and expression)	
Civic associations	**Civil** (freedom of association)	
Regulatory and legal institutions	**Political** (right to vote and to participate in debate/electoral politics, etc.)	Political

autonomy: physical and psychological well-being, the means of subsistence, security of personhood and cultural identity, the ability to participate in the economy, in community life, in political processes and to act without becoming vulnerable to physical force or violence. Rather like Marshall, Held asserts:

> Bundles of rights which are pertinent to each of the spheres of power must be regarded as integral to the democratic process. If any one of these bundles is absent, the democratic process will be one-sided, incomplete and distorted. If any one of these categories of rights and obligations is missing or unenforced, people's equal interest in the principle of autonomy will not be fully protected. (*ibid.*: 54)

Held's categories of rights can loosely be equated with Marshall's categories (see Table 11.1). Clearly, Held introduces a greater degree of specificity, but the difference between the two taxonomies goes deeper than this. In the concept of nautonomy we have a sense of the vulnerability of the citizen to the power of others in society: not only the vulnerability of the working class to the capitalist class or the vulnerability of the individual to the state, but the vulnerability of women to patriarchy, of minority ethnic groups to racism, and of the citizens of poor countries to the interests of rich countries.

The point to be drawn from this is that welfare rights that are conditional – that seek to elicit responsible behaviour – may undermine rather than enhance autonomy. Social security and social care regimes that encourage or coerce citizens into the acceptance of low-paid or exploitative employment and unsatisfactory or abusive care relationships are not so much promoting responsibility as undermining autonomy. Similarly, one might say that regeneration grants that are conditional on partnership arrangements and overseas aid packages that are conditional upon fiscal restraint may not so much empower the urban communities or developing countries involved as circumscribe their autonomy.

The relevance here of resistance strategies is that they will tend to oppose or frustrate the imposition of conditions that undermine autonomy. Conversely, the relevance of reform strategies is that they can work for rights that will promote autonomy because they are unconditional. An important example has been provided by Janet Finch who has demonstrated how, since the days of the Victorian Poor Law:

> On each occasion when government was attempting to impose a version of family responsibilities which people regarded as unreasonable, many responded by developing avoidance strategies; moving to another household, losing touch with relatives, cheating the system. If anything it has been the state's assuming responsibility for individuals – such as the granting of old age pensions – which has freed people to develop closer and more supportive relationships with their kin. (Finch 1989: 243)

The example is apt because it demonstrates how an understanding of the kind of rights that will promote autonomy may be drawn from everyday human experiences of the kinds of obligations and expectations that are socially negotiated over time, within relationships and between the generations (cf. Finch and Mason 1993). Such rights and responsibilities are more concrete and immediate than those that arise through the legal fiction of a social contract. They provide a sounder basis for conceptualising citizenship and for envisaging ways of achieving a just and sustainable distribution of resources. The argument resonates with feminist notions of an ethic of care (see Sevenhuijsen 1998 and 2000; and see discussion in Chapter 4 above) which contend that inclusive relationships cannot be imposed by ascribing rights and responsibilities to citizens: what is required is a set of values premised upon a recognition that vulnerability is endemic to the human condition.

The demand for autonomy, if it is to be framed in terms of welfare rights, must embrace the nature of human dependency, while resisting the threat of exploitation.

Towards an ethical state

We are left with the problem of the state: both in the sense that it is an extant reality (and therefore a part of the problem), and in the sense that regardless of whether we should like the state to 'wither away', it will remain necessary for the foreseeable future if we are to sustain any meaningful form of welfare rights. In so far that the demise of the welfare state is widely predicted, there is an abundance of speculation as to what might lie beyond it (e.g. Pierson 1998), or of what indeed a postmodern 'welfare society' might look like (Rodger 2000). While I have at several points above conceded the possibility of welfare without the state, Rodger's assertion is that 'self-organised welfare in a civil society in which state control is at "arms length" may come to pass through sheer necessity' (*ibid.*: 188). This notion of a 'welfare society' is altogether different from Gramsci's notion of an 'ethical state'. Gramsci equates the ethical state with a 'regulated society' in which coercion is superseded and law subsumed. The state is not some 'phantasmagorical entity', but a collective organism with a collective consciousness (Gramsci 1988: 244). Rights in a regulated society, as I understand it, would be no more and no less than human capacities that are consensually conferred and guaranteed (cf. Hirst 1980, and see discussion in Chapter 1 above).

What this entails is a view that transcends even the most developed forms of welfare rights to be found in social democratic welfare state regimes or, indeed, any of the 'conventional' models I have delineated in Chapter 10. To think about it we need to be able to conceptualise welfare rights in terms of global responsibilities on the one hand, and in terms of local needs on the other.

The question of global responsibilities has been addressed by the philosopher Karl Otto Apel. Apel (1980; 1991) argues that responsibility is the key normative feature in political discourse because by addressing any problem in argument we are implicitly acknowledging a responsibility – both at an individual and a collective level – for solving that problem. According to Apel, however, liberalism as the dominant ideological paradigm of modernity has effectively paralysed the possibility of an ethic of social responsibility because it separates the public sphere of scientific rationality from the private sphere of preferences and values. What is required is an ethical principle of 'co-responsibility'. This might become possible, upon three conditions.

First, it would have to be rational and transcend tradition. Second, it would require a global communication community, something made possible by cultural, technological and economic globalisation such that already 'we have become members of a real communication community' (1991: 269). This idea has obvious resonance with Habermas's (1987a) counterfactual notion of the 'ideal speech situation'. The ideal speech situation is an abstract political objective through which it would become possible for human beings to engage in undistorted and uncoerced kinds of negotiation, though Apel, for his part, is actually taking account of the concrete possibilities for collaborative scientific interpretation that are opened up, for example, by information and communication technologies. Third, says Apel, a principle of co-responsibility would require that scientific and ethical claims to truth be taken equally seriously. This idea has an obvious resonance with Beck's (1992) demand for the demonopolisation of science and a form of reflexivity based on negotiation between different epistemologies. The ethical fulcrum of such negotiation is human need:

> . . . the members of the communication community (and this implies all thinking beings) are also committed to considering all the potential claims of all the potential members – and this means all human 'needs' in as much as they could be

affected by norms and consequently make *claims* on their fellow human beings. As potential 'claims' that can be communicated interpersonally, all human needs are ethically *relevant*. They must be *acknowledged* if they can be justified interpersonally through arguments. (Apel 1980: 277)

Apel's concept of 'co-responsibility' implies the universalisability of human needs through a global form of rights. It is a riposte to postmodernity's claim that 'the foolproof – universal and unshakably founded – ethical code will never be found' (Bauman 1993: 10). It presupposes that there are certain basic human needs whose optimal satisfaction must precede the imposition of any social obligations (cf. Doyal and Gough 1991) and that it is possible to negotiate the empirical, ontological and normative consensus that is required to translate the particular demands of diverse social movements into universalisable human rights (cf. M. Hewitt 1993). The importance of this is that it implies a relationship between rights and responsibilities that goes far beyond the narrow contractarian calculus implied by the 'Third Way' motto – 'no rights without responsibilities' (Giddens 1998: 65) – because responsibility is by nature co-operative and negotiated, not an inherent obligation or *a priori* doctrine.

It is hard to articulate Apel's abstract reasoning about global responsibilities to concrete struggles over rights, but in some of the emerging 'anti-globalisation' literature, for example, we can see attempts to develop our understanding of human rights as a means to something other than the imposition of a global democratic-liberal orthodoxy; as something more than a kind of postmodern folklore that 'compresses' moral issues to the right of individuals to be left alone (cf. Bauman 1993: 243). De Sousa Santos (2001) has envisaged the possibility of a kind of counter-hegemonic globalisation process through which what he calls 'native languages of emancipation' may be re-interpreted to provide the basis for a 'bottom up', cosmopolitan and progressive form of multiculturalism driven from the local level by a wide range of indigenous peoples, groups or organisations and by movements from the periphery of established national and supranational systems. Though it is not necessarily a prototype, the paradox of the so-called anti-globalisation movement is that, through the power of the internet, it has established a counter-hegemonic global communication community of sorts (e.g. Yeates 2001).

This brings us to the question of local needs and back, I shall suggest, to Nancy Fraser's conception of a 'politics of needs interpretation' (1989) that I discussed in Chapter 2. It is precisely because we do not inhabit a 'welfare society' that a politics of needs interpretation is required in order to enlarge the scope and reach of welfare rights guaranteed by the state. A politics of needs interpretation would seek to define in specific contexts and for specific social groups what is required for personal autonomy; it would stretch beyond the essential or 'thin' definitions espoused by Doyal and Gough (1991) and Held (1994) to encompass enlarged or 'thick' definitions (see Drover and Kerans 1993). This would entail not only demands for redistribution, but for recognition (Fraser 1995): for rights that recognise specific needs stemming from social differences constituted by gender, ethnicity, age, disability and sexuality. It would entail not only demands for opportunities, but for safety or 'asylum' in its most basic sense (see above), including protection against exploitation and provision that ensures ontological as well as bare material security. What this implies in my view is struggles against conditionality (i.e. means-testing and work-testing) and against the commodification of essential services.

Summary/conclusion

This concluding chapter has sought to make the case for welfare rights. In doing so it has considered different kinds of reformist strategies, including the rights-based strategies of welfare rights professionals and the administrative strategies of mainstream social policy; and different kinds of resistance strategies, including the anarchistic strategies of intellectual radicals and the popular strategies of everyday protest. However, none of these by themselves hold the key to making welfare rights work.

The question that has been posed is – how is it possible to ensure the autonomy of the human subject through the medium of an ethical state? To this end I have advanced two essential arguments. First, the recognition of human dependency is not inimical to, indeed it requires, the promotion of social responsibility. Second, it is possible to envisage a regulated society that guarantees provision for human need.

The reader may accept neither argument. None the less, I hope she will accept a more general conclusion that flows from this book, namely that welfare rights matter. They matter because whether or not they succeed at present in preventing or containing poverty, they are critical to people's lives; and to some people more than others. They matter because they remain for the time being a constitutive component and are critical to maintaining the existence of what has been characterised as democratic-welfare-capitalism. They matter because in their present form they raise critical questions about the capacity of late modern societies to accommodate the needs of their members.

References

Abbott, E. and Bompas, K. (1943) 'The woman citizen and social security', reproduced in Clarke, J., Cochrane, A. and Smart, C. (eds) (1987) *Ideologies of Welfare*, London: Hutchinson.

Abel-Smith, B. and Stevens, R. (1967) *Lawyers and the Courts*, London: Heinemann.

Abel-Smith, B. and Stevens, R. (1968) *In Search of Justice*, Harmondsworth: Penguin.

Ainley, P. (1993) 'The legacy of the Manpower Services Commission: Training in the 1980s', in Taylor-Gooby, P. and Lawson, R. (eds) *Markets and Managers*, Buckingham: Open University Press.

Alcock, P. (1993/1997) *Understanding Poverty*, Basingstoke: Macmillan.

Alinsky, S. (1969) *Reveille for Radicals*, New York: Random House.

Amin, K. and Oppenheim, C. (1992) *Poverty in Black and White: Deprivation and ethnic minorities*, London: Child Poverty Action Group.

Anderson, D. (1991) Paper to 25th. Annual Conference of the Social Policy Association, *The Politics of Social Policy*, University of Nottingham, 11 July.

Apel, K. (1980) *Towards the Transformation of Philosophy*, London: Routledge.

Apel, K. (1991) 'A planetary macro-ethics for humankind', in Deutsch, E. (ed.) *Culture and Modernity: East–West philosophical perspectives*, Honolulu: University of Hawaii Press.

Association of Community Health Councils (ACHC) (1994) *Access to Health Records Act 1990: The concerns of CHCs*, London: ACHC.

Bacon, R. and Eltis, W. (1978) *Britain's Economic Problem: Too few producers*, London: Macmillan.

Baggott, R. (1998) *Health and Health Care in Britain*, second edition, Basingstoke: Macmillan.

Bagguley, P. (1994) 'Prisoners of the Beveridge dream? The political mobilisation of the poor against contemporary welfare regimes', in Burrows, R. and Loader, B. (eds) *Towards a Post-Fordist Welfare State*, London: Routledge.

Balchin, P. (1995) *Housing Policy: An introduction*, third edition, London: Routledge.

Baldwin, P. (1990) *The Politics of Social Solidarity*, Cambridge: Cambridge University Press.

Baldwin-Edwards, M. and Gough, I. (1991) 'EC social policy and the UK', in Manning, N. (ed.) *Social Policy Review 1990–91*, Harlow: Longman.

Ball, M. (1983) *Housing Policy and Economic Power*, London: Methuen.

Ball, S. (1998) 'Education policy', in Ellison, N. and Pierson, C. (eds) *Developments in British Social Policy*, Basingstoke: Macmillan.

Balloch, S., Butt, J., Fisher, M. and Lindow, V. (eds) (1999) *Rights, Needs and the User Perspective: A review of the NHS and Community Care Act 1990*, London: NISW/Joseph Rowntree Foundation.

Bankowski, Z. and Mungham, G. (1976) *Images of Law*, London: Routledge & Kegan Paul.

Barnes, H. and Baldwin, S. (1999) 'Social security, poverty and disability', in Ditch, J. (ed.) *Introduction to Social Security: Policies, benefits and poverty*, London: Routledge.

Barnes, M. (2000) 'Ending child poverty: Can New Labour succeed?' *Benefits*, Issue 29.

Barrientos, A. (2001) 'Welfare regimes in Latin America', paper presented at *Social Policy in Developing Contexts* workshop, University of Bath, 1–2 March.

Bauman, Z. (1987) *Legislators and Interpreters*, Cambridge: Polity.

Bauman, Z. (1993) *Postmodern Ethics*, Oxford: Blackwell.

Bauman, Z. (1998) *Work, Consumerism and the New Poor*, Buckingham: Open University Press.

Beck, U. (1992) *Risk Society: Towards a new modernity*, London: Sage.

Bentham, J. (1789) 'An introduction to the principles and morals of legislation', in Warnock, M. (ed.) (1962) *Utilitarianism*, Glasgow: Collins.

Beresford, P. and Croft, S. (1986) *Whose Welfare: Private Care or Public Services?* Brighton: Lewis Cohen Urban Studies Centre.

Berghman, J. (1991) '1992 and social security', in Room, G. (ed.) *Towards a European Welfare State?* Bristol: SAUS.

Berlin, I. (1967) 'Two Concepts of Liberty', in Quinton, A. (ed.) *Political Philosophy*, Oxford: Oxford University Press.

Berthoud, R. (1998) *Disability Benefits: A review of the issues and options for reform*, York: Joseph Rowntree Foundation.

Bevan, A. (1952) *In Place of Fear*, 1978 edition, London: Quartet.

Bevan, P. (2001) 'The dynamics of African in/security regimes and some implications for "global social policy"', paper presented at *Social Policy in Developing Contexts* workshop, University of Bath, 1–2 March.

Beveridge, W. (1942) *Social Insurance and Allied Services* (The Beveridge Report), Cmd.6404, London: HMSO.

Blackwell, J. (1994) 'Changing work patterns and their implications for social protection', in Baldwin, S. and Falkingham, J. (eds) *Social Security and Social Change*, Hemel Hempstead: Harvester Wheatsheaf.

Blair, T. (1996) 'Battle for Britain', *The Guardian*, 29 January.

Blair, T. (1998) *The Third Way*, London: Fabian Society.

Blair, T. (2000) *Values and the Power of Community*, speech to the Global Ethics Foundation, Tubigen, 30 June.

Blair, T. (2001) *Reform of Public Services*, speech at the Royal Free Hospital, London, 16 July.

Blake, C. (2000) 'Access to justice: The reform of legal service provision', in Dean, H., Sykes, R. and Woods, R. (eds) *Social Policy Review 12*, Newcastle: Social Policy Association.

Bloch, A. (1997) 'Ethnic inequality and social security policy', in Walker, A. and Walker, C. (eds) *Britain Divided: The growth of social exclusion in the 1980s and 1990s*, London: CPAG.

Bobbio, N. (1996) *The Age of Rights*, Cambridge: Polity.

Booth, C. (1889) *The Life and Labour of the People in London*, 1902 edition, London: Macmillan.

Bottomore, T. (1992) 'Citizenship and Social Class: Forty years on', in Marshall, T.H. and Bottomore, T. (1992) *Citizenship and Social Class*, London: Pluto Press.

Boyson, R. (1971) *Down With the Poor*, London: Churchill.

Bradshaw, J. (1972) 'The Concept of Social Need', *New Society*, 30 March.

Bradshaw, J. (1993) *Household Budgets and Living Standards*, York: Joseph Rowntree Foundation.

Bradshaw, J. and Holmes, H. (1989) *Living on the Edge: A study of living standards of families on benefit in Tyne and Wear*, Tyneside Child Poverty Action Group, London: CPAG.

Breugal, I. (1989) 'Sex and Race in the Labour Market', *Feminist Review*, no. 32.

Brook, L., Hall, J. and Preston, I. (1996) 'Public spending and taxation', in Jowell, R., Curtice, J., Park, A., Brook, L. and Thompson, K. (eds) *British Social Attitudes: The 13th report*, Aldershot: Dartmouth.

Bulmer, M. and Rees, A. (eds) (1996) *Citizenship Today*, London: UCL Press.

Burghes, L. (1993) *One-parent Families: Policy options for the 1990s*, York: Family Policy Studies Centre/Joseph Rowntree Foundation.

Burghes, L. and Stagles, R. (1983) *No Choice at 16: A study of education maintenance allowances*, London: CPAG.

Butler, J. (1993) 'A case study in the National Health Service: Working for patients', in Taylor-Gooby, P. and Lawson, R. (eds) *Markets and Managers: New issues in the delivery of welfare*, Buckingham: Open University Press.

Butler, J. and Calnan, M. (1999) 'Health and health policy', in Baldock, J., Manning, N., Miller, S. and Vickerstaff, S. (eds) *Social Policy*, Oxford: Oxford University Press.

Cabinet Office (1999) *Modernising Government*, Cm.4310, London: The Stationery Office.

Callinicos, A. (1989) *Against Postmodernism*, Cambridge: Polity.

Campbell, J. and Oliver, M. (1996) *Disability Politics*, London: Routledge.

Campbell, T. (1983) *The Left and Rights*, London: Routledge & Kegan Paul.

Campbell, T. (1988) *Justice*, Basingstoke: Macmillan.

Castles, F. (1982) *The Impact of Parties*, London: Sage.

Castles, F. and Mitchell, D. (1993) 'Worlds of welfare and families of nations', in Castles, F. (ed.) *Families of Nations: Patterns of public policy in Western democracies*, Aldershot: Dartmouth.

Cebulla, A. (1999) 'Government plans and individuals' intentions: The case of unemployment insurance', *Benefits*, Issue 26.

Central Statistical Office (CSO) (1992) *Social Trends No. 22*, London: HMSO.

Child Poverty Action Group (CPAG) (1994a) 'The Incapacity for Work Bill: Hitting the sick for six', *Welfare Rights Bulletin*, 119, April.

Child Poverty Action Group (CPAG) (1994b) 'JSA White Paper: Targeting the "workshy" and cutting benefit', *Welfare Rights Bulletin*, 123, December.

Citizen's Charter Complaints Task Force (1994) *If Things Go Wrong . . . A discussion Paper Series, No. 6, 'Redress'*, London: Cabinet Office.

Clapham, D., Kemp, P. and Smith, S. (1990) *Housing and Social Policy*, Basingstoke: Macmillan.

Clarke, J. and Newman, J. (1997) *The Managerial State*, London: Sage.

Clarke, P. Barry (1996) *Deep Citizenship*, London: Pluto.

Coleman, J. (1988) 'Social capital in the creation of human capital', *American Journal of Sociology*, vol. 94.

Coles, B. (1995) *Youth and Social Policy*, London: UCL Press.

Commission for Local Administration (1978) *Complaints Procedures*, London: CLA.

Commission for Local Administration (1992) *Devising a Complaints System*, London: CLA.

Commission of the European Communities (CEC) (1993) *European Social Policy: Options for the Union*, Luxembourg: Office for Official Publications of the European Communities.

Commission on Social Justice (CSJ) (1994) Social Justice: Strategies for National Renewal, The Report of the Commission on Social Justice, London: IPPR/Vintage.

Cook, J. and Watt, S. (1992) 'Racism, Women and Poverty', in Glendinning, C. and Millar, J. (eds) *Women and Poverty in Britain: The 1990s*, Hemel Hempstead: Harvester Wheatsheaf.

Cooper, J. (1994) *The Legal Rights Manual*, second edition, Aldershot: Ashgate.

Cooper, M. (1983) *Public Legal Services*, Sweet and Maxwell: London.

Coote, A. (1992) 'Introduction', in Coote, A. (ed.) *The Welfare of Citizens: Developing new social rights*, London: IPPR/Rivers Oram Press.

Cowan, D. (1999) *Housing Law and Policy*, Basingstoke: Macmillan.

Craig, G. (1992) 'Managing the poorest: The social fund in context', in *Social Work and Social Welfare Yearbook*, Buckingham: Open University Press.

Craig, G. (1999) ' "Race", social security and poverty', in Ditch, J. (ed.) *Introduction to Social Security: Policies, benefits and poverty*, London: Routledge.

Cranston, M. (1973) *What are Human Rights?* London: Bodley Head.

Cranston, M. (1976) 'Human Rights, Real and Supposed', in Timms, N. and Watson, D. (eds) *Talking about Welfare*, London: Routledge & Kegan Paul.

Cranston, R. (1985) *Legal Foundations of the Welfare State*, London: Weidenfeld and Nicholson.

Crosland, C.A.R. (1956) *The Future of Socialism*, London: Jonathan Cape.

Dahrendorf, R. (1996) 'Citizenship and Social Class', in Bulmer, M. and Rees, A. (eds) *Citizenship Today: The contemporary relevance of T.H. Marshall*, London: UCL.

Dale, J. and Foster, P. (1986) *Feminists and State Welfare*, London: Routledge & Kegan Paul.

Daniel, P and Ivatts, J. (1998) *Children and Social Policy*, Basingstoke: Macmillan.

Davis, A., Ellis, K. and Rummery, K. (1998) *Access to Assessment: Perspectives of practitioners, disabled people and carers*, Bristol: The Policy Press.

Davis, P. (2001) 'Calamity and coping in rural Bangladesh', paper presented at *Social Policy in Developing Contexts* workshop, University of Bath, 1–2 March.

Daycare Trust (2000) 'Achieving potential: How childcare tackles poverty amongst young children', *Childcare for All: The next steps*, No. 1, London: Daycare Trust.

de Schweinitz, K. (1961) *England's Road to Social Security*, University of Pennsylvania: Perpetua.

de Sousa Santos, B. (1979) 'Popular justice, dual power and socialist strategy,' in Fine, B., Kinsey, R., Lea, J., Picciotto, S. and Young, J. (eds) *Capitalism and the Rule of Law*, London: Hutchinson.

de Sousa Santos, B. (2001) 'Towards a multicultural conception of human rights', *World Social Forum*, Library of alternatives, www.worldsocialforum.org.

Deacon, B. (1993) 'Developments in East European social policy', in Jones, C. (ed.) *New Perspectives on the Welfare State in Europe*, London: Routledge.

Deacon, B. (2000) 'Globalisation: A threat to equitable social provision', in Dean, H., Sykes, R. and Woods, R. (eds) *Social Policy Review 12*, Newcastle: Social Policy Association.

Deacon, B. with Hulse, M. and Stubbs, P. (1997) *Global Social Policy*, London: Sage.

Deakin, N. (1994) *The Politics of Welfare*, Hemel Hempstead: Harvester Wheatsheaf.

Dean, H. (1988/9) 'Disciplinary partitioning and the privatisation of social security', *Critical Social Policy*, Issue 24.

Dean, H. (1991) *Social Security and Social Control*, London: Routledge.

Dean, H. (1992) 'Poverty discourse and the disempowerment of the poor', *Critical Social Policy*, Issue 35.

Dean, H. (1993) 'Social Security: the income maintenance business', in Taylor-Gooby, P. and Lawson, R. (eds) *Markets and Managers: New issues in the delivery of welfare*, Buckingham: Open University Press.

Dean, H. (1994) 'Social security: The cost of persistent poverty', in George, V. and Miller, S. (eds) *Social Policy Towards 2000*, London: Routledge.

Dean, H. (1996) 'Who's complaining? Redress and social policy', in May, M., Brunsdon, E. and Craig, G. (eds) *Social Policy Review 8*, London: Social Policy Association.

Dean, H. (1997) 'Underclassed or undermined? Young people and social citizenship', in MacDonald, R. (ed.) *Youth, the 'Underclass' and Social Exclusion*, London: Routledge.

Dean, H. (1999) 'Citizenship', in Powell, M. (ed.) *New Labour, New Welfare State?* Bristol: The Policy Press.

Dean, H. (2000) 'Managing risk by controlling behaviour: Social security administration and the erosion of welfare citizenship', in Taylor-Gooby, P. (ed.) *Risk, Trust and Welfare*, Basingstoke: Macmillan.

Dean, H. (2001) 'Green citizenship', *Social Policy and Administration*, vol. 35, no. 5.

Dean, H. (2002) 'Business *versus* families: Whose side is New Labour on?' *Social Policy and Society*, vol. 1, no. 1.

Dean, H. and Doheny, S. (2001) 'Human rights, social responsibility and the squeeze on welfare citizenship', paper to the annual conference of the Social Policy Association, *Reconstituting Social Policy: Global, national, local*, Queen's University, Belfast, 24–6 July.

Dean, H. and Khan, Z. (1997) 'Muslim perspectives on welfare', *Journal of Social Policy*, vol. 26, no. 2.

Dean, H. and Khan, Z. (1998) 'Islam: A challenge to welfare professionalism', *Journal of Interprofessional Care*, vol. 12, no. 4.

Dean, H. and Melrose, M. (1997) 'Manageable discord: Fraud and resistance in the social security system', *Social Policy and Administration*, vol. 31, no. 2.

Dean, H. and Shah, A. (2002) 'Insecure families and low-paying labour markets: Comments on the British experience', *Journal of Social Policy*, vol. 30, no. 1.

Dean, H. and Taylor-Gooby, P. (1990) 'Statutory sick pay and the control of sickness absence', *Journal of Social Policy*, vol. 19, no. 1.

Dean, H. and Taylor-Gooby, P. (1992) *Dependency Culture: the Explosion of a Myth*, Hemel Hempstead: Harvester Wheatsheaf.

Dean, H. with Melrose, M. (1999) *Poverty, Riches and Social Citizenship*, Basingstoke: Macmillan.

Dean, H., Gale, K. and Woods, R. (1996) ' "This isn't very typical, I'm afraid": Observing community care complaints procedures', *Health and Social Care in the Community*, vol. 4, no. 6.

Department for Education and Employment (DfEE) (1998) *The Learning Age: A renaissance for a new Britain – Higher Education: Meeting the challenge*, London: The Stationery Office.

Department for Education and Skills (DfES) (2001) *Schools: Achieving success*, London: DfES.

Department of Education and Science (DES) (1978) *Special Educational Needs* (The Warnock Report), London: HMSO.

Department of Education and Science (DES) (1991) *The Parent's Charter*, London: DES.

Department of Employment/Department of Social Security (DE/DSS) (1994) *Jobseeker's Allowance*, Cm.2687, London: HMSO.

Department of Health (DoH) (1992) *The Patient's Charter*, London: DoH.

Department of Health (DoH) (1997) *The New NHS – Modern and Dependable*, Cm.3807, London: The Stationery Office.

Department of Health (DoH) (1998) *Modernising Social Services*, London: The Stationery Office.

Department of Health (DoH) (2000a) *The NHS Plan: A plan for investment, a plan for reform*, Cm.4818–1, London: The Stationery Office.

Department of Health (DoH) (2000b) *Reforming the Mental Health Act*, London: DoH.

Department of Health and Social Security (DHSS) (1985) *The Reform of Social Security*, vol. 1, Cmnd.9517, London: HMSO.

Department of Health and Social Security (DHSS) (1989) *Caring for People: Community care in the next decade and beyond*, Cm.849, London: HMSO.

Department of Social Security (DSS) (1998a) *New Ambitions for our Country: A new contract for welfare*, Cm.3805, London: The Stationery Office.

Department of Social Security (DSS) (1998b) *A New Contract for Welfare: Partnership in pensions*, Cm.4179, London: The Stationery Office.

Department of Social Security (DSS) (1999a) *A New Contract for Welfare: Children's rights and parents' responsibilities*, Cm.4349, London: The Stationery Office.

Department of Social Security (DSS) (1999b) *Annual Report on the Social Fund 1998/99*, Cm.4351, London: The Stationery Office.

Department of Social Security (DSS) (1990) *Children Come First*, Cm.1264, HMSO, London.

Department of the Environment, Transport and the Regions (DETR) (1998) *English Housing Conditions Survey 1996*, London: The Stationery Office.

Department of the Environment, Transport and the Regions (DETR) (2000) *Quality and Choice: A decent home for all*, Cm.9021, London: The Stationery Office.

Department of Trade and Industry (DTI) (1998) *Fairness at Work*, Cm.3968, London: The Stationery Office.

Department of Trade and Industry (DTI) (2000) *Work and Parents: Competitiveness and choice*, Cm.5005, London: The Stationery Office.

Department of Work and Pensions (DWP) (2001) *Changes to Invalid Care Allowance: A consultation paper*, London: DWP.

Destremau, B. (2000) 'Poverty, exclusion and the changing role of the state in the Middle East', in Dean, H., Sykes, R. and Woods, R. (eds) *Social Policy Review 12*, Newcastle: Social Policy Association.

Dicey, A. (1885) *Introduction to the Law of the Constitution*, ninth edition (1939), edited by Wade, E., London: Macmillan.

Dilnot, A., Kay, J. and Morris, C. (1984) *The Reform of Social Security*, Oxford: Institute of Fiscal Studies/Clarendon.

Donnison, D. (1982) *The Politics of Poverty*, Oxford: Martin Robertson.

Doyal, L. (1979) *The Political Economy of Health*, London: Pluto.

Doyal, L. and Gough, I. (1984) 'A Theory of Human Needs', *Critical Social Policy*, Issue 10.

Doyal, L. and Gough, I. (1991) *A Theory of Human Need*, Basingstoke: Macmillan.

Driver, S. and Martell, L. (1997) 'New Labour's communitarianisms', *Critical Social Policy*, vol. 7, no. 3.

Drover, G. and Kerans, P. (eds) (1993) *New Approaches to Welfare Theory*, Aldershot: Edward Elgar.

Dryzek, J. (1997) *The Politics of the Earth*, Oxford: Oxford University Press.

Dworkin, R. (1977) *Taking Rights Seriously*, London: Duckworth.

Dwyer, P. (2000) *Welfare Rights and Responsibilities: Contesting social citizenship*, Bristol: The Policy Press.

Dyke, G. (1998) *The New NHS Charter – A different approach*, Wetherby: Department of Health.

Eardley, T. and Sainsbury, R. (1991) *Housing Benefit Reviews: An evaluation of the effectiveness of the review system in responding to claimants dissatisfied with housing benefit decisions*, Department of Social Security Research Report, Series No. 3, London: HMSO.

Economides, K. and Hansen, O. (1992) 'Critical Legal Practice: Beyond abstract radicalism', in Grigg-Spall, I. and Ireland, P. (eds) *The Critical Lawyers' Handbook*, London: Pluto Press.

Eide, A. (1997) 'Human rights and the elimination of poverty', in Kjonstad, A. and Veit-Wilson, J. (eds) *Law, Power and Poverty*, Bergen: CROP/ISSL.

Ellis, K. (1993) *Squaring the Circle: User and carer participation in needs assessment*, York: Joseph Rowntree Foundation/Community Care.

Esam, P., Good, R. and Middleton, R. (1985) *Who's to Benefit? A radical review of the social security system*, London: Verso.

Esping-Andersen, G. (1990) *The Three Worlds of Welfare Capitalism*, Cambridge: Polity Press.

Esping-Andersen, G. (1999) *Social Foundations of Post-Industrial Economies*, Oxford: Oxford University Press.

Esping-Andersen, G. (ed.) (1996) *Welfare States in Transition*, London: Sage.

Etzioni, A. (1995) *The Spirit of Community*, London: Fontana.

Evason, E. (1999) 'British pensions policies', in Ditch, J. (ed.) *Introduction to Social Security: Policies, benefits and poverty*, London: Routledge.

Exell, R. (2001) 'Employment and poverty', in Fimister, G. (ed.) *Tackling Child Poverty in the UK: An end in sight?* London: Child Poverty Action Group.

Fairclough, N. (2000) *New Labour, New Language*, London: Routledge.

Falk, R. (1994) 'The making of a global citizenship', in van Steenbergen, B. (ed.) *The Condition of Citizenship*, London: Sage.

Falkingham, J. and Rake, K. (1999) ' "Partnership in Pensions" – delivering a secure retirement for women?' *Benefits*, Issue 26.

Ferguson, C. (1999) *Global Social Policy: Human rights and social justice*, London: Department for International Development.

Ferris, J. (1991) 'Green politics and the future of welfare', in Manning, N. (ed.) *Social Policy Review 1990–91*, Harlow: Longman.

Field, F. (1995) *Making Welfare Work*, London: Institute of Community Studies.

Finch, J. (1989) *Family Obligations and Social Change*, Cambridge: Polity.

Finch, J. and Mason, J. (1993) *Negotiating Family Responsibilities*, London: Routledge.

Fine, B. (1984) *Democracy and the Rule of Law*, London: Pluto Press.

Finer, M. (1974) *Report of the Committee on One-Parent Families*, Cmnd.5629, London: HMSO.

Fitzpatrick, P. (1992) 'Law as Resistance', in Grigg-Spall, I. and Ireland, P. (eds) *The Critical Lawyers' Handbook*, London: Pluto Press.

Fitzpatrick, T. (1998) 'The implications of ecological thought for social welfare', *Critical Social Policy*, vol. 18, no. 1.

Ford, J., Hughes, M. and Ruebain, D. (1999) *Education Law and Practice*, London: Legal Action Group.

Forster, W. (1870) 'Speech introducing Elementary Education Bill, House of Commons', in Maclure, S. (ed.) (1996) *Education Documents*, London: Methuen.

Foucault, M (1977) *Discipline and Punish*, Harmondsworth: Penguin.

Foucault, M. (1979) *The History of Sexuality: An introduction*, Harmondsworth: Penguin.

Foucault, M. (1980) *Power/Knowledge*, edited by Gordon, C., Hemel Hempstead: Harvester Wheatsheaf.

Foweraker, J. and Landman, T. (1997) *Citizenship Rights and Social Movements: A comparative and statistical analysis*, Oxford: Oxford University Press.

Franks, O. (1957) *Report of the Committee on Administrative Tribunals and Enquiries*, Cmnd.218, London: HMSO.

Fraser, N. (1989) *Unruly Practices*, Cambridge: Polity.

Fraser, N. (1995) 'From redistribution to recognition: Dilemmas of social justice in a "post-socialist" age', *New Left Review*, vol. 212, pp. 68–93.

Friere, P. (1972) *Pedagogy of the Oppressed*, Harmondsworth: Penguin.

Gamble, A. (1988) *The Free Economy and the Strong State*, Basingstoke: Macmillan.

Ganz, G. (1974) *Administrative Procedures*, London: Sweet and Maxwell.

Gardiner, K. (1997) *Bridges from Benefit to Work*, York: Joseph Rowntree Foundation.

Garland, D. (1981) 'The birth of the welfare sanction', *British Journal of Law and Society*, vol. 8, no. 1.

Garnham, A. and Knights, E. (1994a) *Child Support Handbook*, second edition 1994/5, London: Child Poverty Action Group.

Garnham, A. and Knights, E. (1994b) *Putting the Treasury First*, London: Child Poverty Action Group.

Genn, H. (1995) 'Access to just settlements: The case of medical negligence', in Zuckerman, A. and Cranston, R. (eds) *Reform of Civil Procedure: Essays on 'Access to Justice'*, Oxford: Clarendon Press.

Genn, H. and Genn, Y. (1989) *The Effectiveness of Representation at Tribunals*, London: Lord Chancellor's Department.

George, V. (1973) *Social Security and Society*, London: Routledge.

George, V. (1988) *Wealth, Poverty and Starvation: An international perspective*, Hemel Hempstead: Harvester Wheatsheaf.

George, V. (1993) 'Poverty in Russia: from Lenin to Yeltsin,' in Page, R. and Baldock, J. (eds) *Social Policy Review 5*, Canterbury: Social Policy Association.

George, V. and Wilding, P. (1985) *Ideology and Social Welfare*, London: Routledge & Kegan Paul.

Gibb, K. (2001) 'Helping with housing costs? Unravelling the political economy of personal subsidy', in Cowan, D. and Marsh, A., *Two Steps Forward: Housing policy and the new millennium*, Bristol: Policy Press.

Giddens, A. (1990) *The Consequences of Modernity*, Cambridge: Polity.

Giddens, A. (1991) *Modernity and Self-Identity*, Cambridge: Polity.

Giddens, A. (1994) *Beyond Left and Right*, Cambridge: Polity.

Giddens, A. (1998) *The Third Way*, Cambridge: Polity.

Gilbert, B. (1966) *The Evolution of National Insurance in Great Britain*, London: Michael Joseph.

Glendinning, C. and Millar, J. (eds) (1992) *Women and Poverty in Britain: The 1990s*, Hemel Hempstead: Harvester Wheatsheaf.

Glennerster, H. (1998) 'Welfare with the lid on', in Glennerster, H. and Hills, J. (eds) *The State of Welfare*, second edition, Oxford: Oxford University Press.

Glennerster, H. and Hills, J. (eds) (1998) *The State of Welfare*, second edition, Oxford: Oxford University Press.

Gold, M. and Mayes, D. (1993) 'Rethinking a social policy for Europe', in Simpson, R. and Walker, R. (eds) *Europe: for richer or poorer?* London: Child Poverty Action Group.

Goode, J., Callender, C. and Lister, R. (1998) *Purse or Wallet? Gender inequality and income distribution within families*, London: Policy Studies Institute.

Goodin, R., Headey, B., Muffels, R. and Dirven, H. (1999) *The Real Worlds of Welfare Capitalism*, Cambridge: Cambridge University Press.

Goodman, A. and Webb, S. (1994) *For Richer, for Poorer: The changing distribution of income in the United Kingdom, 1961–91*, London: Institute of Fiscal Studies.

Goodman, R. and Peng, I. (1996) 'The East Asian welfare states: Peripatetic learning, adaptive change and nation-building', in Esping-Andersen, G. (ed.) *Welfare States in Transition*, London: Sage.

Goodwin, B. (1987) *Using Political Ideas*, second edition, Chichester: John Wiley.

Gordon, D. and Pantazis, C. (eds) (1997) *Breadline Britain in the 1990s*, Aldershot: Ashgate.

Gordon, D., Townsend, P., Levitas, R., Pantazis, C., Payne, S., Pastios, D., Middleton, S., Ashworth, K., Adelman, L., Bradshaw, J., Williams, J. and Bramley, G. (2000) *Poverty and Social Exclusion in Britain*, York: Joseph Rowntree Foundation.

Gordon, P. (1989) *Citizenship for Some? Race and government policy 1979–1989*, London: Runnymede Trust.

Gordon, R. (1993) 'Challenging community care assessments', *Legal Action*, August.

Gough, I. (1979) *The Political Economy of the Welfare State*, Basingstoke: Macmillan.

Gough, I. (1997) 'Social aspects of the European model and its economic consequences', in Beck, W., van der Maesen, L. and Walker, A. (eds) *The Social Quality of Europe*, Bristol: The Policy Press.

Gough, I. (2001) 'Globalisation and regional welfare regimes: The East Asian case', paper presented at *Social Policy in Developing Contexts* workshop, University of Bath, 1–2 March.

Gough, I., Bradshaw, J., Ditch, J., Eardley, T. and Whiteford, P. (1997) 'Social Assistance in OECD countries,' *Journal of European Social Policy*, vol. 7, no. 1.

Gramsci, A. (1971) *Prison Notebooks*, London: Lawrence & Wishart.

Gramsci, A. (1988) *A Gramsci Reader*, ed. Forgacs, G., London: Lawrence & Wishart.

Gray, A. and Jenkins, B. (1993) 'Markets, managers and the public service: the changing of a culture', in Taylor-Gooby, P. and Lawson, R. (eds) *Markets and Managers: New issues in the delivery of welfare*, Buckingham: Open University Press.

Griffiths, J. (1991) *The Politics of the Judiciary*, fourth edition, London: Fontana.

Groves, D. (1992) 'Occupational pension provision and women's poverty in old age', in Glendinning, C. and Millar, J. (eds) *Women and Poverty in Britain: The 1990s*, Hemel Hempstead: Harvester Wheatsheaf.

Habermas, J. (1976) *The Legitimation Crisis*, London: Heinemann.

Habermas, J. (1985) 'Modernity – an incomplete project', in Foster, H. (ed.) *Postmodern Culture*, London: Pluto Press.

Habermas, J. (1986) *Autonomy and Solidarity: Interviews with Jurgen Habermas*, ed. P. Dews, London: Verso.

Habermas, J. (1987a) *The Theory of Communicative Action: Vol. 2: Lifeworld and System*, Cambridge: Polity.

Habermas, J. (1987b) *The Philosophical Discourse of Modernity*, Cambridge: Polity.

Habermas, J. (1994) 'Citizenship and national identity', in van Steenbergen, B. (ed.) *The Condition of Citizenship*, London: Sage.

Hadley, R. and Hatch, S. (1981) *Social Welfare and the Failure of the State*, London: Allen and Unwin.

Hall, S. and Held, D. (1989) 'Citizens and citizenship', in Hall, S. and Jacques, M. (eds) *New Times: The changing face of politics in the 1990s*, London: Lawrence & Wishart.

Hall, S. and Jacques, M. (1990) 'The manifesto for New Times,' in Hall, S. and Jacques, M. (eds) *New Times: The changing face of politics in the 1990s*, London: Lawrence & Wishart.

Harden, I. and Lewis, N. (1986) *The Noble Lie: The Bitish Constitution and the rule of law*, London: Hutchinson.

Harlow, C. and Rawlings, R. (1984) *Law and Administration*, London: Weidenfeld & Nicolson.

Harlow, C. and Rawlings, R. (1992) *Pressure Through Law*, London: Routledge.

Hayek, F. (1944) *The Road to Serfdom*, London: Routledge & Kegan Paul.

Hayek, F. (1960) *The Constitution of Liberty*, London: Routledge & Kegan Paul.

Hayek, F. (1976) *Law, Legislation and Liberty: Vol. 2 – The Mirage of Social Justice*, London: Routledge & Kegan Paul.

Hegel, G. (1821) *Elements of the Philosophy of Rights*, 1991 edition, ed. Wood, A., Cambridge: Cambridge University Press.

Held, D. (1994) 'Inequalities of power, problems of democracy', in Miliband, D. (ed.) *Reinventing the Left*, Cambridge: Polity.

Held, D., McGrew, A., Goldblatt, D. and Perraton, J. (1999) *Global Transformations*, Cambridge: Polity.

Henwood, M. and Wicks, M. (1984) *The Forgotten Army: Family care and elderly people*, London: Family Policy Studies Centre.

Hewitt, M. (1993) 'Social movements and social need: Problems with post-modern political theory', *Critical Social Policy*, vol. 13, no. 1.

Hewitt, M. (1994) 'Social policy and the question of postmodernism', in Page, R. and Baldock, J. (eds) *Social Policy Review 6*, Canterbury: Social Policy Association.

Hindess, B. (1987) *Freedom, Equality and the Market*, London: Tavistock.

Hindess, B. (1996) 'Liberalism, socialism and democracy: Variations on a governmental theme', in Barry, A., Osborne, T. and Rose, N. (eds) *Foucault and Political Reason*, London: UCL Press.

Hirsch, F. (1977) *The Social Limits to Growth*, London: Routledge & Kegan Paul.

Hirst, P. (1980) 'Law, socialism and rights,' in Carlen, P. and Collison, M. (eds) *Radical Issues in Criminology*, Oxford: Martin Robertson.

Hirst, P. (1994) *Associative Democracy*, Cambridge: Polity.

Hobsbawm, E. (1962) *The Age of Revolution, 1789–1848*, New York: Mentor.

Holliday, I. (2000) 'Productivist welfare capitalism: Social policy in East Asia', *Political Studies*, vol. 48, no. 4.

Holloway, J. and Picciotto, S. (eds) (1978) *State and Capital: A Marxist debate*, London: Arnold.

Holman, R. (1978) *Poverty: Explanations of social deprivation*, Oxford: Martin Robertson.

Holmans, A. (1999) 'British housing in the twentieth century: An end-of-century review', in Wilcox, S., *Housing Finance Review 1999/2000*, York: Joseph Rowntree Foundation/Chartered Institute of Housing/Council of Mortgage Lenders.

Home Office (1998) *Supporting Families*, Cm.3991, London: The Stationery Office.

Hood, C. (1991) 'A public management for all seasons?' *Public Administration*, vol. 69, no. 1.

Horsman, M. and Marshall, A. (1994) *After the Nation State*, London: Harper Collins.

Huber, E. (1996) 'Options for social policy in Latin America; Neoliberal versus social democratic models', in Esping-Andersen, G. (ed.) *Welfare States in Transition*, London: Sage.

Hudson, B. (1999) 'Dismantling the Berlin Wall: Developments and the health–social care interface', in Dean, H. and Woods, R. (eds) *Social Policy Review 11*, Luton: Social Policy Association.

Hunt, A. (1978) *The Sociological Movement in Law*, Basingstoke: Macmillan.

Hunt, A. (1990) 'Rights and social movements: Counter-hegemonic strategies,' *Journal of Law and Society*, vol. 17, no. 3.

Hunter, I. (1996) 'Assembling the school', in Barry, A., Osborne, T. and Rose, N. (eds) *Foucault and Political Reason*, London: UCL Press.

Hurd, D. (1989) 'Freedom will flourish where citizens accept responsibilities', *The Independent*, 13 September.

Hutton, W. (1996) *The State We're In*, revised edition, London: Vintage.

Ignatieff, M. (1984) *The Needs of Strangers*, London: Chatto and Windus.

Illich, I., McKnight, J., Zola, I, Caplan, J. and Shaiken, H. (1977) *Disabling Professions*, London: Marion Boyars.

Inland Revenue (2001) *New Tax Credits: Supporting families, making work pay and tackling child poverty*, London: Inland Revenue.

Jackson, S. (1998) *Britain's Population: Demographic issues in contemporary society*, London: Routledge.

Jefferson, M. (2000) *Principles of Employment Law*, fourth edition, London: Cavendish.

Jenkins, S. (1994) *Winners and Losers*, Department of Economics, University of Swansea.

Johnson, N. (1987) *The Welfare State in Transition*, Brighton: Wheatsheaf.

Johnson, N. (1990) *Reconstructing the Welfare State*, Hemel Hempstead: Harvester Wheatsheaf.

Johnson, N. (1999) 'The personal social services and community care', in Powell, M. (ed.) *New Labour, New Welfare State?* Bristol: The Policy Press.

Jones Finer, C. (1999) 'Trends and developments in welfare states', in Classen, J. (ed.) *Comparative Social Policy: Concepts, theories and methods*, Oxford: Blackwell.

Jones, C. (1993) 'The Pacific challenge: Confucian welfare states', in Jones, C. (ed.) *New Perspectives on the Welfare State in Europe*, London: Routledge.

Jones, P. (1994) *Rights*, Basingstoke: Macmillan.

Jordan, B. (1973) *Paupers: The making of the claiming class*, London: Routledge & Kegan Paul.

Jordan, B. (1989) *The Common Good: Citizenship, morality and self-interest*, Oxford: Blackwell.

Jordan, B. (1993) 'Framing claims and the weapons of the weak', in Drover, G. and Kerans, P. (eds) *New Approaches to Welfare Theory*, Aldershot: Edward Elgar.

Jordan, B. (1996) *A Theory of Poverty and Social Exclusion*, Cambridge: Polity.

Jordan, B. (1998) *The New Politics of Welfare*, London: Sage.

Joseph, K. (1972) 'The cycle of deprivation', speech to Pre-school Playgroups Association, 29 June.

Joseph, K. and Sumption, J. (1979) *Equality*, London: John Murray.

Jowell, J. (1975) *Law and Bureaucracy: Administrative discretion and the limits of legal action*, New York: Dunellan.

Kahn-Freund, O. (1977) *Labour and the Law*, London: Stevens.

Kamenka, E. and Tay, A. (1975) 'Beyond bourgeois individualism: The contemporary crisis in law and legal ideology', in Kamenka, E. and Neale, R. (eds) *Feudalism, Capitalism and Beyond*, London: Edward Arnold.

Keane, J. (1988) *Democracy and Civil Society*, London: Verso.

Keithly, J. (1991) 'Social security in a single European market', in Room, G. (ed.) *Towards a European Welfare State?* Bristol: SAUS.

Kelly, A. (1994) *The National Curriculum: A critical review*, London: Paul Chapman.

Kemp, P. (1990) 'Foreword,' in Wall, D. (ed.) *Getting There: Steps to a green economy*, London: Green Print.

Kemp, P. (1999) 'Making the market work? New Labour and the housing question', in Dean, H. and Woods, R. (eds) *Social Policy Review 11*, Luton: Social Policy Association.

Kemp, P. (2000) 'Housing benefit and welfare retrenchment in Britain', *Journal of Social Policy*, vol. 29, no. 2.

Kemp, P. and Wall, D. (1990) *A Green Manifesto for the 1990s*, Harmondsworth: Penguin.

Kincaid, J. (1975) *Poverty and Equality in Britain*, Harmondsworth: Penguin.

Kingdom, J. (1999) *Government and Politics in Britain*, second edition, Cambridge: Polity.

Korpi, W. (1983) *The Democratic Class Struggle*, London: Routledge & Kegan Paul.

Labour Party (1996) *New Labour: New life for Britain*, London: Labour Party.

Labour Party (1997) *New Labour: Because Britain deserves better*, London: Labour Party.

Labour Party (2001) *Ambitions for Britain: Labour's manifesto*, London: Labour Party.

Laclau, E. and Mouffe, C. (1985) *Hegemony and Socialist Strategy*, London: Verso.

Land, H. (1975) 'The introduction of family allowances,' in Hall, R., Land, H., Parker, R. and Webb, A. (eds) *Change Choice and Conflict in Social Policy*, London: Heinemann.

Land, H. (1992) 'Whatever happened to the social wage?' in Glendinning, C. and Millar, J. (eds) *Women and Poverty in Britain: The 1990s*, Hemel Hempstead: Harvester Wheatsheaf.

Land, H. (1999) 'New Labour, new families?' in Dean, H. and Woods, R. (eds) *Social Policy Review 11*, Luton: Social Policy Association.

Langan, M. (1998) 'The personal social services', in Ellison, N. and Pierson, C. (eds) *Developments in British Social Policy*, Basingstoke: Macmillan.

Langan, M. and Ostner, I. (1991) 'Gender and welfare: towards a comparative framework', in Room, G. (ed.) *Towards a European Welfare State?* Bristol: SAUS.

Lawson, R. (1993) 'The new technology of management in the personal social services', in Taylor-Gooby, P. and Lawson, R. (eds) *Markets and Managers: New issues in the delivery of welfare*, Buckingham: Open University Press.

Leather, P. (2001) 'Housing Standards in the private sector', in Cowan, D. and Marsh, A. (eds) *Two Steps Forward: Housing policy and the new millennium*, Bristol: The Policy Press.

LeGrand, J. (1982) *The Strategy of Equality*, London: Allen & Unwin.

LeGrand, J. (1990) *Quasi-Markets and Social Policy*, Studies in Decentralisation and Quasi-Markets, No. 1, School for Advanced Urban Studies, University of Bristol.

Leibfried, S. (1993) 'Towards a European welfare state? On integrating poverty regimes into the European Community', in Jones, C. (ed.) *New Perspectives on the Welfare State in Europe*, London: Routledge.

Lenaghan, J. (1997) 'Citizens' rights to health care in the UK', in Lenaghan, J. (ed.) *Hard Choices in Health Care*, London: BMJ.

Leung, J. (1994) 'Dismantling the "iron rice bowl": Welfare reforms in the People's Republic of China', *Journal of Social Policy*, vol. 23, no. 3.

Levitas, R. (1996) 'The concept of social exclusion and the new Durkeimian hegemony', *Critical Social Policy*, vol. 16, no. 2.

Levitas, R. (1998) *The Inclusive Society?* Basingstoke: Macmillan.

Lewis, J. (1992) 'Gender and the development of welfare regimes', *Journal of European Social Policy*, vol. 2, no. 3.

Lewis, J. and Glennerster, H. (1996) *Implementing the New Community Care*, Buckingham: Open University Press.

Lewis, N. and Birkinshaw, P. (1993) *When Citizens Complain*, Buckingham: Open University Press.

Lilley, P. (1993) Speech to Conservative Party Annual Conference, 6 October.

Lipsky, M. (1976) 'Towards a theory of street-level bureaucracy', in Hawley, W. and Lipsky, M. (eds) *Theoretical Perspectives on Urban Politics*, Englewood Cliffs, NJ: Prentice Hall.

Lister, R. (1990) *The Exclusive Society: Citizenship and the poor*, London: Child Poverty Action Group.

Lister, R. (1997) *Citizenship: Feminist perspectives*, Basingstoke: Macmillan.

Locke, J. (1690) *Two Treatises on Civil Government*, 1960 edition, ed. Laslett, P., New York: Mentor.

Lord Chancellor's Department (LCD) (2000) Press Release, 3 April.

Luhmann, N. (1987) 'The self-regulation of law and its limits', in Teubner, G. (ed.) *Dilemmas of Law in the Welfare State*, Berlin: Walter de Gruyter.

Lund, B. (1999) ' "Ask not what your community can do for you"; Obligations, New Labour and welfare reform,' *Critical Social Policy*, vol. 19, no. 4.

Lund, B. (2000) 'Work and need', in Dean, H., Sykes, R. and Woods, R. (eds) *Social Policy Review 12*, Newcastle: Social Policy Association.

Lynes, T. (1975) 'Unemployment Assistance Tribunals in the 1930s', in Adler, M. and Bradley, A. (eds) *Justice, Discretion and Poverty*, Abingdon: Professional Books.

MacCormick, N. (1982) *Legal Right and Social Democracy*, Oxford: Clarendon.

Machin, S. (2000) 'How are the mighty fallen: What accounts for the dramatic decline of unions in Britain? *CentrePiece*, vol. 5, no. 2.

Mack, J. and Lansley, S. (1985) *Poor Britain*, London: Allen & Unwin.

Maguire, M., Maguire, S. and Vincent, J. (2001) *Implementation of the Education Maintenance Allowance Pilots: The first year*, London: DfES.

Mamdani, M. (1996) *Citizen and Subject: Contemporary Africa and the legacy of late colonialism*, Princeton, NJ: Princeton University Press.

Mann, J., Gostin, L., Gruskin, S., Brennan, T., Lazzarini, Z. and Fineberg, H. (1999) 'Health and human rights', in Mann, M., Gruskin, S., Grodin, M. and Annas, G. (eds) *Health and Human Rights*, Routledge: London.

Mann, K. (1992) *The Making of an English 'Underclass': The social division of welfare and labour*, Buckingham: Open University Press.

Mann, M. (1987) 'Ruling class strategies and citizenship', *Sociology*, vol. 21, no. 3.

Marshall, G. (1997) *Repositioning Class: Social inequality in industrial societies*, London: Sage.

Marshall, P. (1993) *Demanding the Impossible: A history of anarchism*, London: Fontana.

Marshall, T.H. (1950) 'Citizenship and social class', reprinted in Marshall, T.H. and Bottomore, T. (1992) *Citizenship and Social Class*, London: Pluto Press.

Marshall, T.H. (1981) *The Right to Welfare and Other Essays*, London: Heinemann.

Marx, K. (1847) *The Poverty of Philosophy* – extract reproduced in *Selected Writings in Sociology and Social Philosophy*, eds Bottomore, T. and Rubel, M. (1963) Harmondsworth: Penguin.

Marx, K. (1848) 'The Revolutions of 1848', in *Political Writings Vol. 2*, 1973 edition, Harmondsworth: Penguin.

Marx, K. (1859) 'Preface to a Contribution to the Critique of Political Economy', in *Marx and Engels Selected Works Vol. 1*, 1969 edition, Moscow: Progress.

Marx, K. (1887) *Capital*, Vol. 1, 1970 edition, London: Lawrence & Wishart.

Maslow, A. (1943) 'A theory of human motivation', *Psychological Review*, vol. 50.

Mathieson, T. (1980) *Law, Society and Political Action*, London: Academic Press.

McAteer, M. (2000) *The Community Legal Service: Access for all?* London: The Consumer's Association.

McCarthy, P., Simpson, B., Hill, M., Walker, J. and Corlyon, J. (1992) *Grievances, Complaints and Local Government: Towards the responsive local authority*, Aldershot: Avebury.

McKay, S. and Rowlingson, K. (1999) *Social Security in Britain*, Basingstoke: Macmillan.

McLaughlin, E. (1991) *Social Security and Community Care: The case of the invalid care allowance*, Department of Social Security Research Report No. 4, London: HMSO.

McLaughlin, E. (1999) 'Social security and poverty: Women's business', in Ditch, J. (ed.) *Introduction to Social Security: Policies, benefits and poverty*, London: Routledge.

McLaughlin, E., Millar, J. and Cooke, K. (1989) *Work and Welfare Benefits*, Aldershot: Avebury.

McMahon, W. and Marsh, T. (1999) *Filling the Gap: Free school meals, nutrition and poverty*, London: Child Poverty Action Group.

Mead, L. (1986) *Beyond Entitlement*, New York: Free Press.

Meadows, D., Meadows, M., Randers, J. and Behrens, W. (1972) *The Limits to Growth*, London: Pan Books.

Means, R. and Smith, R. (1998) *Community Care: Policy and practice*, second edition, Basingstoke: Macmillan.

Midgley, J. (1997) *Social Welfare in Global Context*, London: Sage.

Miles, R. and Phizacklea, A. (1984) *White Man's Country: Racism in British politics*, London: Pluto.

Millar, J. (2000) *Keeping Track of Welfare Reform: The New Deal programmes*, York: Joseph Rowntree Foundation.

Miller, S. and Peroni, F. (1992) 'Social politics and the Citizen's Charter', in Manning, N. and Page, R. (eds) *Social Policy Review 4*, Canterbury: Social Policy Association.

Mishra, R. (1984) *The Welfare State in Crisis*, Hemel Hempstead: Harvester Wheatsheaf.

Mishra, R. (1990) *The Welfare State in Capitalist Society*, Hemel Hempstead: Harvester Wheatsheaf.

Mishra, R. (1993) 'Social policy in the postmodern world: The welfare state in Europe by comparison with North America,' in Jones, C. (ed.) *New Perspectives on the Welfare State in Europe*, London: Routledge.

Moore, J. (1989) 'The end of the line for poverty', speech to Greater London Conservative Party Constituencies meeting, 11 May.

Morris, J. (1993) *Independent Lives? Community care and disabled people*, Basingstoke: Macmillan.

Moss, P. (2000) 'Uncertain start: A critical look at some of New Labour's "early years" policies', in Dean, H., Sykes, R. and Woods, R. (eds) *Social Policy Review 12*, Newcastle: Social Policy Association.

Moss, P. and Melhuish, E. (1991) *Current Issues in Day Care for Young Children*, London: HMSO.

Mulcahy, L. and Lloyd-Bostock, S. (1992) 'Complaining – What's the use?' in Dingwall, R. and Fenn, P. (eds) *Quality and Regulation in Health Care: International experiences*, London: Routledge.

Mullins, D. and Niner, P. (1998) 'A prize of citizenship? Changing access to social housing', in Marsh, A. and Mullins, D. (eds) *Housing and Public Policy: Citizenship, choice and control*, Buckingham: Open University Press.

Murray, C. (1984) *Losing Ground: American Social Policy 1950–1980*, New York: Basic Books.

Muschamp, Y., Jamieson, I. and Lauder, H. (1999) 'Education, education, education', in Powell, M. (ed.) *New Labour, New Welfare State?* Bristol: The Policy Press.

Naidoo, R. and Callender, C. (2000) 'Towards a more inclusive system: Contemporary policy reform in higher education', in Dean, H., Sykes, R. and Woods, R. (eds) *Social Policy Review 12*, Newcastle: Social Policy Association.

National Association of Citizens Advice Bureaux (NACAB) (1991) *Barriers to Benefit*, London: NACAB.

National Consumer Council (NCC) (1977) *The Fourth Right of Citizenship: A review of local advice services*, London: NCC.

Newman, B. and Thompson, R. (1989) 'Economic growth and social development: A longitudinal analysis of causal priority', *World Development*, vol. 17 no. 4.

Novak, T. (1988) *Poverty and the State*, Milton Keynes: Open University Press.

Nozick, R. (1974) *Anarchy, State and Utopia*, Oxford: Blackwell.

O'Connor, J. (1973) *Fiscal Crisis of the State*, New York: St. Martin's Press.

Offe, C. (1992) 'A non-productivist design for social policies', in von de Parijs P. (ed.) *Arguing for Basic Income*, London: Verso.

Offe, C. (1984) *Contradictions of the Welfare State*, Cambridge, Mass.: MIT Press.

Ogus, A. and Barendt, E. (1988) *The Law of Social Security*, third edition, London: Butterworths.

O'Higgins, N. (2001) *Youth Unemployment and Employment Policy*, Geneva: International Labour Office.

Oldfield, A. (1990) *Citizenship and Community, Civic Republicanism and the Modern World*, London: Routledge.

Oldfield, N. and Yu, A. (1993) *The Cost of a Child*, London: Child Poverty Action Group.

Oliver, M. (1990) *The Politics of Disablement: A sociological approach*, Basingstoke: Macmillan.

Oliver, M. and Barnes, M. (1998) *Disabled People and Social Policy*, Harlow: Longman.

Oppenheim, C. (1993) *Poverty: The facts*, London: Child Poverty Action Group.

Oppenheim, C. (ed.) (1998) *An Inclusive Society: Strategies for tackling poverty*, London: IPPR.

Oppenheim, C. and Harker, L. (1996) *Poverty: The facts*, third edition, London: Child Poverty Action Group.

Orshansky, M. (1969) 'How Poverty is Measured', *Monthly Labour Review*, vol. 92.

Osborne, T. (1996) 'Security and vitality: Drains, liberalism and power in the nineteenth century', in Barry, A., Osborne, T. and Rose, N. (eds) *Foucault and Political Reason*, London: UCL Press.

Pahl, J. (1989) *Money and Marriage*, Basingstoke: Macmillan.

Paine, T. (1791) *The Rights of Man*, 1984 edition, Harmondsworth: Penguin.

Pakulski, J. and Waters, M. (1996) *The Death of Class*, London: Sage.

Papadakis, E. and Taylor-Gooby, P. (1987) *The Private Provision of Public Welfare*, Brighton: Wheatsheaf.

Parker, G. (2000) 'The Royal Commission on Long Term Care for the Elderly: New vision or more of the same for social care policy', in Dean, H., Sykes, R. and Woods, R. (eds) *Social Policy Review 12*, Newcastle: Social Policy Association.

Parker, G. and Clarke, H. (1998) 'Paying for long-term care in the UK: Policy, theory and evidence', in Taylor-Gooby, P. (ed.) *Choice and Public Policy*, Basingstoke: Macmillan.

Parker, H. (1989) *Instead of the Dole*, London: Routledge.

Parker, H. (ed.) (1998) *Low Cost but Acceptable: A minimum income standard for the UK*, Bristol: The Policy Press.

Partington, M. (1997) 'The re-introduction of rent control?' *Journal of Housing Law*, vol. 1, no. 1.

Pascal, G. (1986) *Social Policy: A feminist analysis*, London: Tavistock.

Pascal, G. (1997) *Social Policy: A new feminist analysis*, London: Routledge.

Pashukanis, E. (1978) *General Theory of Law and Marxism*, London: Ink Links.

Paton, C. (1999) 'New Labour's health policy: The new healthcare state', in Powell, M. (ed.) *New Labour, New Welfare State?* Bristol: Policy Press.

Patterson, T. (2001) 'Welfare rights advice and the new managerialism', *Benefits*, Issue 30.

Peck, J. (2001) 'Job alert! Shifts, spins and statistics in welfare-to-work policy', *Benefits*, Issue 30.

Peden, G. (1991) *British Economic and Social Policy*, second edition, Hemel Hempstead: Philip Allan.

Pepinsky, H. (1975) 'Reliance on formal written law, and freedom and social control in the United States and The People's Republic of China', *The British Journal of Sociology*, vol. 26, pp. 330–42.

Performance and Innovation Unit (2000) *Adding it Up*, London: Cabinet Office.

Perry, R. (ed.) (1964) *Sources of Our Liberties*, New York: McGraw-Hill.

Pfeffer, N. and Coote, A. (1991) *Is Quality Good for You? A critical review of quality assurance in welfare services*, London: IPPR.

Piachaud, D. (1981) 'Peter Townsend and the Holy Grail, *New Society*, 10 September, reprinted in Townsend, P. (1993) *The International Analysis of Poverty*, Hemel Hempstead: Harvester Wheatsheaf.

Piachaud, D. (1999) 'Security for old age?' *Benefits*, Issue 26.

Piachaud, D. and Sutherland, H. (2001) 'Child poverty and the New Labour government', *Journal of Social Policy*, vol. 30, no. 1.

Pierson, C. (1998) *Beyond the Welfare State*, Cambridge: Polity.

Pirie, M. (1991) *The Citizens' Charter*, London: Adam Smith Institute.

Piven, F. and Cloward, R. (1974) *Regulating the Poor*, London: Tavistock.

Piven, F. and Cloward, R. (1977) *Poor People's Movements*, New York: Pantheon Books.

Plant, R. (1988) *Citizenship, Rights and Socialism*, Fabian Society Pamphlet No. 531, London: Fabian Society.

Plant, R. (1992) 'Citizenship, rights and welfare', in Coote, A. (ed.) *The Welfare of Citizens: Developing new social rights*, London: IPPR/Rivers Oram Press.

Plant, R. (1995) 'Market place for everyone,' *The Guardian*, 20 March.

Plant, R., Lesser, H. and Taylor-Gooby, P. (1980) *Political Philosophy and Social Welfare*, London: Routledge & Kegan Paul.

Polanyi, K. (1944) *The Great Transformation*, New York: Rinehart.

Portillo, M. (1993) Interview on *Westminster Live*, BBC television, 7 December.

Powell, E. (1972) *Still to Decide*, London: Elliot Right Way Books.

Powell, M. (ed.) (1999) *New Labour, New Welfare State?* Bristol: The Policy Press.

Prime Minister's Office (1991) *The Citizen's Charter: Raising the Standard*, Cm.1599, London: HMSO.

Prosser, T. (1983) *Test Cases for the Poor*, London: Child Poverty Action Group.

Putnam, R. (1993) *Making Democracy Work*, Princeton, NJ: Princeton University Press.

Rahman, M., Palmer, G., Kenway, P. and Howarth, C. (2000) *Monitoring Poverty and Social Exclusion 2000*, York: Joseph Rowntree Foundation.

Raphael, D. (1989) 'Enlightenment and revolution', in MacCormick, N. and Bankowski, Z. (eds) *Enlightenment, Rights and Revolution*, Aberdeen: Aberdeen University Press.

Rawls, J. (1972) *A Theory of Justice*, Oxford: Oxford University Press.

Redcliffe-Maud, Lord (1969) *The Report of the Royal Commission on Local Government in England*, Cmnd.4040, London: HMSO.

Reich, C. (1964) 'The new property', *Yale Law Journal*, vol. 73, no. 5.

Reidy, A. (1980) 'Legal rights and housing policy', *Social Policy and Administration*, vol. 14, no. 1.

Rentoul, J. (1989) *Me and Mine: The triumph of the new individualism?* London: Unwin Hyman.

Robson, P. (2001) 'Housing benefit', in Cowan, D. and Marsh, A. (eds) *Two Steps Forward: Housing policy and the new millennium*, Bristol: The Policy Press.

Roche, M. (1992) *Rethinking Citizenship*, Cambridge: Polity Press.

Rodger, J. (2000) *From a Welfare State to a Welfare Society*, Basingstoke: Macmillan.

Room, G. (ed.) (1995) *Beyond the Threshold: The measurement and analysis of social exclusion*, Bristol: The Policy Press.

Room, G., Lawson, R. and Laczko, F. (1989) 'New poverty in the European Community', *Policy and Politics*, vol. 17, no. 2.

Rose, H. (1981) 'Rereading Titmuss: The sexual division of welfare', *Journal of Social Policy*, vol. 10, no. 4.

Rose, H. (1982) 'Who can de-label the claimant?' in Adler, M. and Bradley, A. (eds) *Justice Discretion and Poverty*, Abingdon: Professional Books.

Rose, N. (1996) 'The death of the social?' *Economy and Society*, vol. 25.

Rose, R. (1988) *Ordinary People in Public Policy*, London: Sage.

Rose, R. (1993) 'Bringing Freedom back in: Rethinking priorities of the welfare state', in Jones, C. (ed.) *New Perspectives on the Welfare State in Europe*, London: Routledge.

Rowntree, B.S. (1901) *Poverty: A study of town life*, London: Macmillan.

Royal Commision on Legal Services (1979) *Report of the Royal Commission on Legal Services*, Cmnd.7648, London: HMSO.

Royal Commission on Long-term Care for the Elderly (1999) *With Respect to Old Age: Long-term care – rights and responsibilities*, Cm.4192, London: The Stationery Office.

Saville, J. (1958) 'The Welfare State: An historical approach', *New Reasoner*, vol. 1, no. 3.

Schiengold, S. (1974) *The Politics of Rights*, New Haven: Yale University Press.

Scott, A. (1990) *Ideology and New Social Movements*, London: Unwin Hyman.

Scott, J. (1985) *Weapons of the Weak: Everyday forms of peasant resistance*, New Haven: Yale University Press.

Scott, J. (1990) *Domination and the Arts of Resistance: Hidden transcripts*, New Haven: Yale University Press.

Scruton, R. (ed.) (1991) *Conservative Texts: An anthology*, Basingstoke: Macmillan.

Sen, A. (1984) *Resources Values and Development*, Oxford: Blackwell.

Sen, A. (1985) *Commodities and Capabilities*, Amsterdam: Elsevier.

Sevenhuijsen, S. (1998) *Citizenship and the Ethics of Care*, London: Routledge.

Sevenhuijsen, S. (2000) 'Caring in the third way: The relation between obligation, responsibility and care in "Third Way" discourse', *Critical Social Policy*, vol. 20, no. 1.

Short, J. (1982) *Housing in Britain: The post-war experience*, London: Methuen.

Simpson, R. (1993) 'Fortress Europe?' in Simpson, R. and Walker, R. (eds) *Europe: For richer or poorer?* London: Child Poverty Action Group.

Slapper, G. and Kelly, D. (1999) *The English Legal System*, third edition, London: Cavendish.

Smart, C. (1989) *Feminism and the Power of Law*, London: Routledge.

Smith, A. (1776) *An Inquiry into the Nature and Causes of the Wealth of Nations*, 1900 edition, London: George Routledge.

Smith, T. and Noble, M. (1995) *Education Divides: Poverty and schooling in the 1990s*, London: Child Poverty Action Group.

Social Exclusion Unit (SEU) (1997) *Social Exclusion Unit: Purpose, work priorities and working methods*, briefing document, London: Cabinet Office.

Solomos, J. (1989) *Race and Racism in Contemporary Britain*, Basingstoke: Macmillan.

Soper, K. (1993) 'The thick and thin of human needing', in Drover, G. and Kerans, P. (eds) *New Approaches to Welfare Theory*, Aldershot: Edward Elgar.

Soysal, Y. (1994) *Limits of Citizenship: Migrants and postnational membership in Europe*, Chicago: Chicago University Press.

Spicker, P. (1988) *Principles of Social Welfare*, London: Routledge.

Spicker, P. (1993) 'Needs as claims', *Social Policy and Administration*, vol. 27, no. 1.

Squires, P. (1990) *Anti-Social Policy: Welfare ideology and the disciplinary state*, Hemel Hempstead: Harvester Wheatsheaf.

Stacey, F. (1978) *Ombudsmen Compared*, Oxford: Oxford University Press.

Standing, G. (1996) 'Social protection in Central and Eastern Europe: A tale of slipping anchors and torn safety-nets', in Esping-Andersen, G. (ed.) *Welfare States in Transition*, London: Sage.

Stein, J. (2001) *The Future of Social Justice in Britain: A new mission for the Community Legal Service*, CASEpaper 48, London: London School of Economics.

Stephenson, S. (2000) 'Civil society and its agents in the post-communist world: The case of the Russian voluntary sector', in Dean, H., Sykes, R. and Woods, R. (eds) *Social Policy Review 12*, Newcastle: Social Policy Association.

Street, H. (1975) *Justice in the Welfare State*, London: Stevens & Sons.

Sullivan, H. and Potter, T. (1998) *Getting a Job is Not Always the Answer: Social exclusion and the hidden economy in urban areas*, University of Birmingham, School of Policy Studies Occasional Paper 2.

Tam, H. (1998) *Communitarianism: A new agenda for politics and citizenship*, Basingstoke: Macmillan.

Taylor-Gooby, P. (1990) 'Social welfare: The unkindest cuts', in Jowell, R., Witherspoon, S. and Brrok, L. (eds) *British Social Attitudes: The 7th report*, Aldershot: Gower.

Taylor-Gooby, P. (1991) *Social Change, Social Welfare and Social Science*, Hemel Hempstead: Harvester Wheatsheaf.

Taylor-Gooby, P. (1993) 'The new educational settlement: National Curriculum and local management', in Taylor-Gooby, P. and Lawson, R. (eds) *Markets and Managers: New issues in the delivery of welfare*, Buckingham: Open University Press.

Taylor-Gooby, P. (1994) 'Postmodernism and Social Policy: A great leap backwards?' *Journal of Social Policy*, vol. 23, no. 3.

Taylor-Gooby, P. (1995) 'Comfortable, marginal and excluded', in Jowell, R., Curtice, J., Park, A., Brook, L. and Ahrendt, D. (eds) *British Social Attitudes: The 12th report*, Aldershot: Dartmouth.

Teubner, G. (ed.) (1987) *Dilemmas of Law in the Welfare State*, Berlin: Walter de Gruyter.

Thompson, E.P. (1968) *The Making of the English Working Class*, Harmondsworth: Penguin.

Thompson, E.P. (1975) *Whigs and Hunters*, New York: Parthenon.

Thornton, P. (2000) ' "Work for those who can, security for those who cannot"? Welfare reform and disabled people', in Dean, H., Sykes, R. and Woods, R. (eds) *Social Policy Review 12*, Newcastle: Social Policy Association.

Titmuss, R. (1958) *Essays on the Welfare State*, London: Allen & Unwin.

Titmuss, R. (1968) *Commitment to Welfare*, London: Allen & Unwin.

Titmuss, R. (1971) 'Welfare rights, law and discretion', *Political Quarterly*, vol. 42, no. 2.

Townsend, P. (1979) *Poverty in the United Kingdom*, Harmondsworth: Penguin.

Townsend, P. (1991) 'The structured dependency of the elderly: A creation of social policy in the twentieth century', *Ageing and Society*, vol. 1, no. 1.

Townsend, P. (1992) *Hard Times: The prospects for European social policy*, Eleanor Rathbone Memorial Lecture, Liverpool: Liverpool University Press.

Townsend, P. (1993) *The International Analysis of Poverty*, Hemel Hempstead: Harvester Wheatsheaf.

Townsend, P. and Davidson, N. (eds) and Whitehead, M. (1988) *Inequalities in Health: 'The Black Report' and 'The Health Divide'*, Harmondsworth: Penguin.

Travers, M. (1994) 'The phemomenon of the radical lawyer', *Sociology*, vol. 28, no. 1.

Treasury, The (2001) *Pre-Budget Report 2001*, London: The Treasury.

Trickey, H. and Walker, R. (2001) 'Steps to compulsion within British labour markets', in Lodemel, I. and Trickey, H. (eds) *'An Offer You Can't Refuse': Workfare in international perspective*, Bristol: The Policy Press.

Turner, B. (1986) *Citizenship and Capitalism*, London: Allen & Unwin.

Turner, B. (1990) 'Outline of a theory of citizenship', *Sociology*, vol. 24, no. 2.

Turner, B. (1991) 'Prolegomena to a general theory of social order', position paper for ESRC workshop, *Citizenship, Civil Society and Social Cohesion*, London, 23 February.

Turner, B. (1993) 'Outline of a theory of human rights', *Sociology*, vol. 27, no. 3.

Turok, I. and Webster, D. (1998) 'The New Deal: Jeopardised by the geography of unemployment?' *Local Economy*, no. 13, pp.309–28.

Tweedie, J. and Hunt, A. (1994) 'The future of the welfare state and social rights: Reflections on Habermas, *Journal of Law and Society*, vol. 21, no. 3.

Twine, F. (1994) *Citizenship and Social Rights: The interdependence of self and society*, London: Sage.

Ungerson, C. (1994) 'Housing: need, equity, ownership and the economy', in George, V. and Miller, S. (eds) *Social Policy Towards 2000: Squaring the welfare circle*, London: Routledge.

United Nations (UN) (1948) 'Universal Declaration of Human Rights', reprinted in Centre for Human Rights, Geneva (1988) *Human Rights: A compilation of international instruments*, New York: UN.

United Nations Development Programme (UNDP) (1993) *Human Development Report 1993*, New York: Oxford University Press.

United Nations Development Programme (UNDP) (1996) *Human Development Report 1996*, New York: Oxford University Press.

United Nations Development Programme (UNDP) (2000) *Human Development Report 2000*, New York: Oxford University Press.

Vail, J. (1999) 'Insecure times: Conceptualising insecurity and security', in Vail, J., Wheelock, J. and Hill, M. (eds) *Insecure Times: Living with insecurity in contemporary society*, London: Routledge.

van-Praag, B., Hagenaars, A. and van Weeren, H. (1982) 'Poverty in Europe', *Review of Income and Wealth*, vol. 28.

Veit-Wilson, J. (1992) 'Muddle or mendacity? The Beveridge Committee and the poverty line', *Journal of Social Policy*, vol. 21, no. 3.

Veit-Wilson, J. (1994) *Dignity not Poverty: A minimum income standard for the UK*, The Commission on Social Justice, London: IPPR.

Veit-Wilson, J. (1999) 'Poverty and the adequacy of social security', in Ditch, J. (ed.) *Introduction to Social Security: Policies, benefits and poverty*, London: Routledge.

Vickerstaff, S. (1999) 'Education and training', in Baldock, J., Manning, N., Miller, S. and Vickerstaff, S. (eds) *Social Policy*, Oxford: Oxford University Press.

Wadham, J. and Mountfield, H. (1999) *Blackstone's Guide to the Human Rights Act 1998*, London: Blackstone.

Waine, B. (1999) 'The future is private', *Benefits*, Issue 26.

Walker, A. (1987) 'The social construction of dependency', in Loney, M., Bocock, R., Clarke, J., Cochrane, A., Graham, P. and Wilson, M. (eds) *The State or the Market?* London: Sage.

Walker, A. (1990) 'Community care', in McCarthy, M. (ed.) *The New Politics of Welfare: An agenda for the 1990s*, Basingstoke: Macmillan.

Walker, C. (1993) *Managing Poverty: The limits of social assistance*, London: Routledge.

Waltzer, M. (1983) *Spheres of Justice*, Oxford: Blackwell.

Ward, C. (1973) *Anarchy in Action*, London: Allen & Unwin.

Ward, S. (2000) 'New Labour's pension reforms', in Dean, H., Sykes, R. and Woods, R. (eds) *Social Policy Review 12*, Newcastle: Social Policy Association.

Warde, A. (1994) 'Consumers, consumption and post-Fordism', in Burrows, R. and Loader, B. (eds) *Towards a Post-Fordist Welfare State?* London: Routledge.

Watson, D. (1980) *Caring for Strangers*, London: Routledge & Kegan Paul.

Watson, T. (1995) *Sociology, Work and Industry*, third edition, London: Routledge.

Weale, A. (1983) *Political Theory and Social Policy*, New York: St. Martin's Press.

Webb, B. and Webb, S. (1935) *Soviet Communism: A new civilisation?* two volumes, London: Longman.

Webb, S. (1994) 'Social insurance and poverty alleviation', in Baldwin, S. and Falkingham, J. (eds) *Social Security and Social Change*, Harvester Wheatsheaf: Hemel Hempstead.

Webb, S. and Webb, B. (1909) *Break up the Poor Law*, London: Fabian Society.

Whiteley, P. and Winyard, S. (1983) 'Influencing social policy: The effectiveness of the poverty lobby in Britain', *Journal of Social Policy*, vol. 12, no. 1.

Wilcox, S. (1999) *Housing Finance Review 1999/2000*, York: Joseph Rowntree Foundation/Chartered Institute of Housing/Council of Mortgage Lenders.

Wilensky, H. (1975) *The Welfare State and Equality*, Berkeley: University of California Press.

Wilkinson, R. (1996) *Unhealthy Societies: The afflictions of inequality*, London: Routledge.

Williams, F. (1989) *Social Policy: A critical introduction*, Cambridge: Polity.

Williams, F. (1992) 'Somewhere over the rainbow: Universality and diversity in social policy', in Manning, N. and Page, R. (eds) *Social Policy Review 4*, Canterbury: Social Policy Association.

Williams, F. and Pillinger, J. (1996) *New Thinking on Social Policy Research into Inequality, Social Exclusion and Poverty*, Bath: Centre for the Analysis of Social Policy.

Wilson, A. (1994) *Being Heard: A report of a Review Committee on NHS complaints procedures*, Leeds: Department of Health.

Wistow, G., Knapp, M., Hardy, B. and Allen, C. (1994) *Social Care in a Mixed Economy*, Buckingham: Open University Press.

Wood, E.M. (1986) *The Retreat from Class*, London: Verso.

Wood, G. (2001) 'Governance and the common man: Embedding social policy in the search for security', paper presented at *Social Policy in Developing Contexts* workshop, University of Bath, 1–2 March.

World Bank (2001) *World Development Report 2000/2001: Attacking poverty*, New York: Oxford University Press.

Wraith, R. and Hutchinson, P. (1973) *Administrative Tribunals*, London: Allen & Unwin.

Yeates, N. (2001) *Globalization and Social Policy*, London: Sage.

Zander, M. (1978) *Legal Services for the Community*, London: Temple-Smith.

Index

Note: Page references in *italics* refer to tables.